Nurses' Guide to Children's Eyes

Andrea Kovalesky, R.N., M.S.N.

Pediatric Clinical Nurse Specialist
Department of Nursing
Childrens Hospital of Los Angeles
Los Angeles, California

G&S

Grune & Stratton, Inc.
(Harcourt Brace Jovanovich, Publishers)
Orlando   San Diego   New York
London   Toronto   Montreal   Sydney   Tokyo

Library of Congress Cataloging in Publication Data

Kovalesky, Andrea.
Nurses' guide to children's eyes.

Includes index.
1. Pediatric ophthalmology. 2. Ophthalmic nursing.
I. Title. [DNLM: 1. Eye Diseases—in infancy & child-
hood—nurses' instruction. 2. Eye Diseases—nursing.
WY 158 K88n]
RE48.2.C5K68   1984   618.92'0977   84-19280
ISBN 0-8089-1689-0

Grune & Stratton, Inc.
Orlando, Florida 32887

Distributed in the United Kingdom by
Grune & Stratton, Ltd.
24/28 Oval Road, London NW 1

Library of Congress Catalog Number   84-19280
International Standard Book Number   0-8089-1689-0

Printed in the United States of America
85 86 87 10 9 8 7 6 5 4 3 2 1

Contents

Preface

A lthough a number of books that deal with children's eye problems are currently available, none address the specific concerns of nurses or consider the unique background and experiences of our profession. Nursing is one of the few health disciplines that has the opportunity to promote optimal visual health in a wide variety of settings. Nurses outnumber other groups of health professionals by a large margin, and we frequently have the opportunity to spend more time with patients than do other health professionals. In addition, the broad scope of nursing allows us the flexibility and versatility to adapt to our patients' needs.

This book is intended not only to enhance the nurse's knowledge of the more common eye problems seen in childhood and adolescence, but also to promote the expansion of related services, which are becoming increasingly important in view of current economic trends. This book is not meant to replace standard nursing references, such as a detailed pharmacology text or general pediatric nursing book.

The reader should keep in mind that many of the approaches discussed in this book are those used at the Childrens Hospital of Los Angeles, and that other institutions and agencies may have different but equally acceptable procedures and practices.

Acknowledgments

A lthough writing is basically a singular experience, this book would never have been possible without the assistance of many people. First thanks goes to Gerald T. Bowns, M.D., Assistant Clinical Professor of Ophthalmology at the University of Southern California School of Medicine, and Attending Ophthalmologist at Childrens Hospital of Los Angeles. Without his input and support I would have given up long ago. Much gratitude must also be extended to Elaine Angone, R.N.; Paula Edelman, C.O.; Robert Lingua, M.D.; A. Linn Murphree, M.D.; Bernard Szirth, Ophthalmic Photographer; all of whom are on staff at Childrens Hospital of Los Angeles; and to Patrick J. Caroline, C.O.T., formerly of the Estelle Doheny Eye Foundation of the University of Southern California. In addition, unending thanks must be given to my sister, Denise Mary Pope, also a writer; to my parents and other family members for their encouragement and understanding; to my nieces and nephews, who patiently posed for many illustrations; to Andy Gauthier, a child with retinoblastoma, to whom this book is dedicated; and of course, to God, who somehow got me through this whole thing.

Chapter One

Guidelines for Visual Acuity Screening

M any health professionals consider visual acuity screening routine and assign it to clerks or aides. Hence, it is no wonder that nurses find themselves ambivalent toward the process. But if you have special knowledge and a positive attitude, visual acuity screening can be both challenging and rewarding. For example, it takes keen perception and skill to detect amblyopia in a wiggling, 6-month-old infant and even more ability with a severely disabled or frightened child. Yet how nice it is to see that infant return after treatment with equal vision in both eyes or that disabled child gain an entirely new perspective of the world with glasses.

Over the years the vision screening of children has changed dramatically. For example, the late Dr. Mary Sheridan, a pioneer in visual screening and the developer of the STYCAR (Screening Test for Young Children and Retardates) Vision Test, once remarked, "I became interested in the vision-testing of young children many years ago. . . . In those days school medical officers were not required to test the vision of 5-year-old school entrants because the testing was considered to be too time-consuming and the results unreliable."[1] Yet statistics currently used by the National Society to Prevent Blindness (NSPB) show that up to 5 percent of preschool children have an eye problem that may need professional care; an even higher incidence exists among school-aged children.[2] Unfortunately, the rate is considerably higher for children with physical or developmental disabilities. For example, in one study children with cerebral palsy had a 50 percent incidence of ocular problems.[3] In another, 72 percent of children with IQs lower than 60 had abnormal vision![4]

When a child successfully passes a distance visual acuity screening, you can be fairly confident in making the following assumptions. First, the cornea and lens are sufficiently clear to allow the child to fixate on an object of regard. Hence, if any corneal scars or cataracts are present, they do not interfere with the transmission of the image along the visual axis (Fig. 1-1). Second, the images transferred along the visual axis are not significantly distorted by such refractive

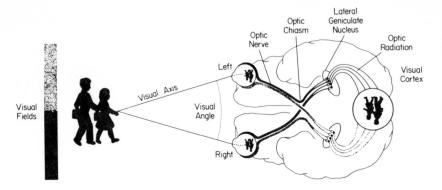

Fig. 1-1. The visual pathway. Note that images are relayed upside down through the visual cortex (see Chapter 7). From Kuffler SW and Nicholls JG: From Neuron to Brain: A Cellular Approach to the Function of the Nervous System. Sunderland, Mass., Sinauer Associates, 1976. Adapted with permission.

errors as myopia or astigmatism. Third, the area on the retina specifically designed for sharp vision, the fovea centralis, is functioning well. This section of the retina serves as a computer network, sending images of the object along the visual pathway to the brain. Therefore, you can also assume that no significant defects are present along this pathway, which consists of the optic (second) cranial nerve, optic chiasm, optic radiation or tract, and the visual cortex. Finally, if the child passes the screening equally with each eye, the diagnosis of amblyopia can usually be excluded.

The NSPB endorses central distance visual acuity screening as the most important single test of visual ability.[5] The findings of Köhler and Stigmar (1973) support this conclusion. In examinations of more than 2000 children in Swedish nursery schools, they discovered that 97 percent of all significant eye problems were found through visual acuity screening alone.[6] Although the success rates from other studies have been lower (especially among children with other disabilities) the value of visual acuity screening is indisputable.

DEFINITIONS

The term *visual acuity* refers to sharpness of vision, or the ability to distinguish fine detail. It is technically a measurement of the ability to resolve the visual angle that separates two parts of a test object. Formal determination of visual acuity is largely performed by ophthalmologists, optometrists, and orthoptists. Professionals from other specialties and disciplines usually screen for visual acuity. Observations from their screenings serve to refer the child to the proper practitioner.

An *ophthalmologist* (or *oculist*) is a physician who specializes in the diagnosis and treatment of the eye, including surgical procedures and medications. Only ophthalmologists can provide complete eye care. On the other hand, an *optometrist* (O.D.) is a licensed nonphysician who has completed extensive graduate training in refractive problems of the eye. Optometrists may use prisms and glasses or contact lenses as methods of treatment, but they may not perform surgery, and in most states, they may not prescribe medications. Optometrists often dispense lenses, as well.

Opticians are persons who have completed intensive short-term courses in the grinding and fitting of lenses and frames, which they make according to prescriptions written by ophthalmologists and optometrists. An *ocularist* is a person who specializes in making prosthetic devices for the eye. An *orthoptist* (C.O.) has completed a graduate-level training course and is certified to diagnose and treat *ocular motility* (muscle) problems with special equipment and techniques.

Other practitioners include the certified allied health personnel in ophthalmology. An *ophthalmic assistant* (C.O.A.) has completed a short-term course and 1 year of guided work experience. An *ophthalmic technician* (C.O.T.) has completed 2 years of work experience and higher-level courses in ophthalmic techniques and procedures. Finally, the *ophthalmic technologist* (C.O.M.T.) has completed a 4-year post–secondary school program or has been a certified ophthalmic technician, has completed extensive course work, and has passed written and performance examinations.

NURSING GOALS, OUTCOME STANDARDS AND DIAGNOSES

The primary nursing goal in Chapters 1 and 2 is that *each child should have maximal visual acuity for his or her particular age and health status.* A child's visual acuity must be at its maximum for the child's best development and school performance. Ideally, professional eye examiners should determine a child's visual acuity at regular intervals, but current geographical, financial, and other parameters often preclude this level of care. Hence, nurses in a variety of roles and settings continue to provide this valuable service for children of all ages.

Outcome Standard 1

All children have valid documentation of their visual acuity every 2–3 years (R/O vision *sensory deficit*).

Suggested interventions:

- Nurses document a child's visual acuity by identifying and correctly using an age-appropriate method of visual acuity screening for each child and recording the results appropriately or by requesting such information from the child's primary care provider or professional eye examiner, or from the child's medical or school records.

- Nurses who conduct screenings identify and alter factors that affect a child's *anxiety* regarding the screening process (and hence, may affect the child's performance). Such steps include properly preparing the child for the screening or assisting others in doing so; arranging for proper lighting during the screening; setting up and maintaining a nonthreatening screening environment, free from distraction; and arranging for a gamelike, unhurried, and private screening atmosphere. In addition, nurses recognize and are sensitive to a possible *fear of failure* by some children before or during the screening.
- Nurses who conduct screenings request input from family members, teachers, and caretakers about the child's vision, history, and behaviors that may be visually related.
- Nurses who conduct screenings share the results with the child and his or her parents and teachers, whether the child has passed or failed. This intervention counteracts the parents' or educators' *knowledge deficit* about the screening.
- In addition, nurses working with pediatric patients participate in educating parents, teachers, and the public about the warning signs of possible eye problems in children. They stress the importance of frequent visual acuity checks (or preferably vision examinations) for children of all ages.
- Nurses assist volunteers who perform visual acuity screenings with in-service training, consultation, and supervision.

Outcome Standard 2

Children who do not have maximal visual acuity for their ages are cared for by professional eye examiners.

Suggested interventions:
- Nurses refer children who do not pass their visual acuity screening to an appropriate eye care specialist.
- Nurses follow all children who do not pass their visual acuity screening to ensure that each child is examined by a professional eye examiner and receives the examiner's recommended treatment. (This procedure counteracts *noncompliance* about follow-up or treatment.)
- Nurses assist in decreasing any financial, psychosocial, or other problems that might otherwise inhibit a child in receiving the recommended treatment. (Assistance can counteract *anxiety*, *noncompliance*, *knowledge deficit* and/or *ineffective coping*.)

Outcome Standard 3

Children with decreased visual acuity can identify factors that maximize or minimize their vision (for example, lighting or glasses).

Suggested interventions:
- See individual chapters for interventions that correspond to a child's particular problem.

Outcome Standard 4

Older children and the families and significant others of all children with decreased vision can verbalize (1) the benefits of treatment (such as increased school performance, increased sports participation, and decreased complaints of pain or related behaviors); (2) the *potential for injury* if a child does not receive or use the recommended follow-up care and treatment; and (3) any new sources of stress that the identification or treatment of a decreased visual acuity has caused (such as *disturbances in body image* or *ineffective individual* or *family coping* resulting from financial or time constraints, peer problems, and so on).

Suggested interventions:

- Nurses provide the patient and family individual opportunities to discuss these issues, on several different occasions if possible.
- Nurses make referrals as necessary to community or other professional resources that can assist in any related matters. (See individual chapters for additional information about a child's specific eye problem.)

VOLUNTEERS

Although these chapters are directed to nurses as visual acuity screeners, you may also supervise or consult volunteers, teachers, or other laypersons who perform screenings. The NSPB recognizes the importance of these screeners; in fact, it initially developed its screening program using nonprofessionals in 1951. Since then, volunteers have performed a large part of the visual acuity screenings in this country, especially in areas that do not have access to professional eye examiners or allied health professionals; in day-care centers, American Indian reservations, and migrant worker facilities, for example.

To assist the efforts and training of volunteers, the NSPB has produced two inexpensive publications. *The Home Eye Test Program Guide* for Preschoolers ($2.00) assists volunteers and groups in distributing the Home Eye Test for Pre-schoolers in their local communities and helps them promote the test to the public. *The Children's Eye Health Guide* ($3.00) (a must for volunteer groups) is a 32-page source of the who, what, where, when and how of screenings and referrals. It also briefly reviews anatomy, eye safety, and common eye disorders in children.

Volunteers can also assist with publicity programs (the NSPB's "Lazy Eye Alert") that relay the importance of preschool vision checks. For example, at the Milwaukee Zoo, volunteers and staff staged a weekend of vision screening that received television and newspaper coverage.

A key factor for the success of volunteers as screeners is to give them ample opportunity to become comfortable with the screening process before they begin formal screening. They should participate in a number of actual practice sessions.

To assist them, LADOCA Publishing Foundation has two films (and videotapes) about the Denver Eye Screening Test that can be purchased or rented. (The Denver test includes the E Test, the Allen picture cards, the Fixation Test, a cover test, and the pupillary light reflex test for strabismus.) The first is a training film, and the second emphasizes developing proficiency in administration of the test.

GUIDELINES FOR VISUAL ACUITY SCREENING

Who Needs Screening?

Although school and health personnel may determine their own criteria for who should be screened, the NSPB recommends screening children 3–4 years old; those in kindergarten, grades 2, 5, 8, 10, or 11; all new students; all teacher referrals; children with behavioral changes or learning disabilities; all children who are currently under the care of an eye specialist; and those who have medical problems such as diabetes that can increase their risk for visual disorders. Of course, the Society recommends a professional eye examination whenever possible. In addition, newborns and 6-month-old infants should receive a professional eye examination whenever possible.

Occasionally, some eye care specialists prefer that children currently under their care not be screened simultaneously at school or in your office. In such cases, request that records be sent to you at regular intervals so that you can assess the need for any special considerations in the school and home environments. In addition, such ongoing communication with the eye specialist can assure you that the child is continuing to receive regular care.

Because of the time parents and teachers spend with their children, their observations are a vital component in determining who should be screened. To assist them, various organizations have compiled lists delineating signs of possible eye trouble. These are summarized in Table 1-1.

These observations can become quite useful when a child's visual acuity screening does not produce clear-cut results. For example, Jamie, a child with special developmental needs, may not be able to comply with the screening process satisfactorily. However, his teachers may notice that he can pick up various small objects, look at airplanes in the sky, or see his mother enter the opposite side of the room. Therefore, we can assume that Jamie has functional vision, even though we cannot quantify it.

On the other hand, 8-year-old Michele may successfully pass her visual acuity screening. Yet her teachers, knowing the signs of possible eye trouble in children, notice that Michele squints when reading and has begun daydreaming in class in the past few months. Because of these observations, they refer Michele for a more complete eye evaluation, which results in a prescription for glasses to

Table 1-1
Signs of Possible Eye Trouble in Children

Rubs eyes frequently	Is unable to see distant things, such as the chalkboard, clearly
Blinks more than usual	
Shuts or covers one eye	Prefers to view objects at a distance rather than close by
Has crossed or wandering eye	
	Avoids close work
Has red-rimmed, encrusted, or swollen eyelids	Doesn't like to read or has difficulty reading
Has inflamed, bloodshot, or watery eyes	Holds books or other objects unusually close to eyes
Has recurring styes	
Has abnormal sensitivity to light	Complains that eyes itch, burn, hurt, or feel scratchy or dusty
Has pupils that are unequal in size or shape	Complains of not being able to see well
Frowns, squints, or makes other facial distortions	Complains of dizziness, headaches, or nausea after doing close work
Tilts head to the side or thrusts head forward	Complains of blurred or double vision
Is tense or irritable when doing close work	Has unusual pencil grasp
Has usually short attention span or reputation as "daydreamer"	Turns paper often during work
	Loses place frequently

Data from National Association for Visually Handicapped: *About Children's Eyes* (available in English and Spanish); National Society to Prevent Blindness: *Signs of Eye Trouble in Children* (also in Spanish); American Optometric Association: *A Teacher's Guide to Vision Problems;* American Academy of Ophthalmology: *Eye Cues for Eye Care for Children.*

treat her astigmatism. Michele's squinting ceases and she becomes more interested in her school work.

As with observations by parents or teachers, a significant history should always temper the findings of a visual acuity screening, even when the screening is within normal limits. Children who have a history of prematurity, a positive family history for such significant eye problems as retinoblastoma, or whose mothers had a TORCH infection during the child's pregnancy should be referred immediately to an ophthalmologist for a complete eye examination unless this has already been done.

Matching the Test to the Child

Some methods of visual acuity screening are more reliable than others. In addition, all vary in the skills that they require of the child. Thus, you must select the most reliable and appropriate method based on each child's age and development.

Table 1-2

Appropriate Visual Acuity Screening Methods for Various Groups of Children

	Newborns (0–1 month)	Infants (1–12 months)	Severely Delayed	Toddlers (12–30 months)	Preschool (30–60 months)	Aphasic	Non-English-Speaking	Illiterate	Moderately Delayed	Kindergarten (5–6 years)	School-aged (7 years +)
Reflexes	X	X	X								
Optokinetic Nystagmus	X	X	X	Y							
Preferential Looking	X	X	X	X	Y						
Fixation Test	X	X	X	X	Y						
STYCAR Graded-balls		X	X	X							
STYCAR Miniature Toys			X	Y							
Improvised Methods			Y								
Allen Picture Cards				Y	X	Y	Y	X	X		
H:O:T:V Matching				Y	X	X	X	X	X	X	

	School-aged (7 years +)	Kindergarten (5–6 years)	Moderately Delayed	Illiterate	Non-English-Speaking	Aphasic	Preschool (30–60 months)	Toddlers (12–30 months)	Severely Delayed	Infants (1–12 months)	Newborns (0–1 month)
STYCAR Matching		X	X	X	X	X	X	Y			
Blackbird Vision Screening		Y	X	X	X	X	X				
Sjögren's Hand		Y	X	X	X	X	X				
E Game		X	X	X	X	X	X				
Landolt Rings	X	Y		X	X	X					
Letter Charts	X	Y									
Machines	X	X	Y	Y		X	Y				
Near Vision	X	X	X	X	X	X	X				
Hyperopia	X	Y	Y	Y	Y	Y					

X = Strongly age appropriate
Y = May be age appropriate

Table 1-2 summarizes methods of visual acuity screening that are appropriate for various groups of children. Although you may not have access to all of these methods, try to have several available and to become comfortable and proficient in their use.

In brief, the Snellen and Sloan letters and the Landolt rings are the most complex and reliable methods, since they measure retinal resolution. As a result, they are often administered only to school-aged children. Therefore, when these methods are inappropriate, use the matching methods such as the H:O:T:V (British STYCAR) or the directional "E" method. These are still quite reliable, and can be used with children who are aphasic, illiterate, non-English-speaking, as well as preschool children or those with mild developmental special needs. If these are still not suitable, try the other directional methods such as the Sjögren's Hand, the Blackbird, or the Allen picture cards. Finally, use the Fixation Test for all infants and any children who cannot participate in any of the other methods.

Methods such as the wall charts allow you to show an entire line at once or one symbol on the line at a time. If this is possible with the tool that you are using, use the linear method for children over 4 years of age to help rule out the crowding phenomenon often seen in amblyopia (Chapter 4). However, younger children tend to become confused when they have an entire line presented to them at one time; therefore, present one character at a time. Between the linear and singular methods is a "pointed" approach, whereby you show a line at a time but point out each letter individually. This may be useful for the more mature 3-year-old and may provide you with more accurate results than the singular method.

Preparing the Child

Make sure that the child understands the screening procedure before the actual testing. For younger children, preparation can occur in small groups in the classroom or day care center, or in the home. For example, the NSPB publishes a pamphlet on the home eye testing of preschool children that prepares them for more formal screening at school or in the office or allows parents to screen their children themselves. Other preparatory materials are listed in Tables 1-3 and 1-4. Through such booklets the children become familiar with the screening procedure in a comfortable environment, and as a result, the number of children who can successfully participate in the screening procedure increases. In addition, the children realize that the screening procedure is nonthreatening and will not cause them any pain or discomfort.

Students in the elementary and high school grades can also benefit from a brief presentation on the hows and whys of visual acuity screening. Comments such as "What's this 20/20 business?" and "Why do I need to go to an eye doctor; I can see fine!" are not uncommon among school children, so try to arrange for a brief in-service session before the actual screening occurs.

Table 1-3
Suggested Equipment for Infant Vision Screening

Equipment	Source	Cost*
Junior size eye patches	Opticlude (3M)	$4.00/box of 25
	Coverlet (Beiersdorf)	$4.00/box of 25
Penlight		
One or two small black-and-white or colored objects to attract the infant's attention	Toy or department stores (consider finger puppets, keys, spinning toys, balls)	
Teaching pamphlets for parents		
"Parent's Guide to Infant Stimulation"	Infant Stimulation Education Association	$1.00 each
"Charlie Brown, Detective"	National Society to Prevent Blindness	$5.00/100
"Your Baby's Eyes"	American Optometric Association	$12.00/100
Optokinetic nystagmus drum**	Da-Laur or WCO	$80.00–135.00
Optokinetic nystagmus tape**	Keeler or Richmond	$80.00
Train or stuffed animal that can be activated**		
STYCAR Graded-balls**	National Foundation for Education Research	$20.00

*Prices approximate (1984) and do not include postage or handling fees; inclusion of product in table does not necessarily indicate endorsement.
**Optional

Table 1-4

Suggested Equipment for Screening Preschool and School-Aged Children

Equipment	Source
Pinhole occluder	Da-Laur, Richmond, or WCO ($20.00 each) or make your own
Regular occluders	Regular size eye patches (3M or Beiersdorf) ($5.00/box of 20) or
	Disposable spectacles by Blackbird Vision ($5.00/25), or clip-ons for children with glasses by Keeler or Richmond ($15.00–20.00) or
	Plastic nondisposable occluders; set of six from Good-Lite ($9.00) or single one from LADOCA ($3.00), or make your own
Selection of teaching and preparatory materials "Home Eye Test for Pre-schoolers"	National Society to Prevent Blindness ($6.00/100); available in English, Spanish, German, Chinese, Japanese, and Arabic
"Signs of Eye Trouble in Children"	National Society to Prevent Blindness ($1.00 each)
"About Children's Eyes"	National Society to Prevent Blindness ($3.00/100); available in Spanish
"A Teacher's Guide to Vision Problems"	National Association for Visually Handicapped ($4.00/100); available in Spanish
"A Visit to the Eye Doctor"	American Optometric Association ($12.00/100)
	Wisconsin Optometric Association, 16-page storybook, ($1.00 each, plus postage and handling)
	National Foundation for Educational Research ($20.00 with manual and forms)
STYCAR miniature toys**	Allen cards from Ophthalmix, Da-Laur, Richmond, or WCO ($17.00–25.00 for plastic set)
Picture card method	Denver Eye Screening Test by LADOCA ($4.00 for cards made from cardboard; $10.00 for entire test)
	Schering (Faye) wall chart by Lighthouse or Good-Lite ($10.00 each)
	Efron visual acuity wall chart ($10.00) or cards ($35.00) from WCO

Equipment	Source
Matching method	H:O:T:V from Good-Lite or WCO ($18.00/complete set or $9.00/wall chart)
	Sheridan-Gardiner Test from Keeler ($25.00/set)
	Complete STYCAR from National Foundation for Educational Research ($115.00)
One or more directional methods	Wall chart with E from NSPB ($2.00/chart); made on coated paper
	Cover and window cards for charts from NSPB ($1.25/set)
	E or hand chart from Good-Lite, WCO, or Richmond [$4.00 each (cardboard) or $10.00 (plastic)]
	Blackbird Vision Screening Kit (includes 25 screening spectacles) from Blackbird Vision ($48.00/kit, $9.00/wall chart, or $8.00/home eye test)
	Denver Eye Screening Test by LADOCA ($10.00)
	E flash cards from Ophthalmix, Richmond, or WCO ($17.00–20.00)
	E cube from Ophthalmix, WCO, or Keeler ($22.00–32.00)
	E cut-out for demonstration from Richmond ($10.00)
	Pad of training Es from WCO or Richmond ($5.00–7.00)
Letter chart	Wall chart with Es on reverse side from NSPB ($2.00)
	Wall charts, regular or with reversed letters for use with mirrors from Good-Lite, Richmond, or WCO [$4.00 (plastic) or $10.00 (cardboard)]
Mirror**	Hanging type or with adjustable stand from Good-Lite ($40.00–85.00)
Vision screening machines**	Bausch and Lomb, Good-Lite, Keystone, or Titmus; $100.00–200.00 for the self-illuminating types; $550.00–1100.00 for the multifeature type
Forms**	National Society to Prevent Blindness ($1.00–$5.00)

*Prices approximate (1984) and do not include any postage or handling fees; inclusion of product names does not necessarily indicate endorsement.
**Optional

Lighting

Arrange even, diffuse lighting, without glare, that does not shine directly into the child's eyes. If a light meter is available (they can often be borrowed from power companies), it should measure between 10 and 30 foot-candles (f-c) of daylight. Most fluorescent ceiling lights, and 75-watt (W) goose-neck lamps set 4–5 ft to the side of the screening tool, provide appropriate lighting. Of course, self-illuminating screening devices such as the Good-Lite Company portable model provide ideal illumination. Avoid using a screening tool in front of a window, however, unless all light can be blocked out to prevent glare or shadow.

The Environment

Children must feel relaxed to promote their best performance. Yet many health care settings are threatening to them, despite one's best efforts to provide an unhurried and comfortable atmosphere. Therefore, cover scales and other examining equipment when possible to help a child focus on the tasks at hand. In addition, place the screening tool against a light wall, free from bright colors and excess clutter, at the child's eye level; these precautions also help eliminate distractions. Pieces of cardboard or plastic with a slit cut out to expose only the letter or line you are testing can be held in front of the chart to further decrease distraction. Screen individual children privately. Finally, although a fair amount of speed is desirable, try to appear relaxed and unhurried yourself. Use a cheerful, gamelike approach. For children who continue to find the health care setting uncomfortable, encourage the parents or teachers to use a home eye screening test and forward the results to you.

Distance

The desired distance for most visual acuity screenings is 6 meters (20 feet). At this range, rays of light from the object to the eye are almost parallel, and therefore the lens of a normal eye can focus with a minimal amount of accommodation.

For any distance, measure from the back of the child's chair to the screening device; if the child is standing, measure from the heels. Younger children frequently find that footprints taped to the floor help them remember where to stand.

Remember that different charts are made for different distances. If you use a mirror because of limited space availability, select a chart with reversed symbols. Place the mirror and screening device so that your desired total distance equals the distance from the child's chair or heels to the mirror plus the distance from the mirror to the screening device. For example, if you are using a 20-foot chart in a 12-foot room, place the child 8 feet from the mirror and the chart on the back wall. The child should stand 4 feet in front of the chart, slightly to one side of it, so there will be adequate visualization from the child's eyes to the mirror and back to the chart.

It is also helpful to premeasure the distance between selected objects in the screening area and the location of the child. For instance, the front of one's desk may be 6 feet from the child, the back of the desk 8 feet, and the baby scale 11 feet. These measurements are helpful for methods that require the examiner to move about, such as the E cube or Allen cards.

Finally, as discussed in the section on recording your findings, the distance at which the child successfully passes the screening becomes the numerator of the child's visual acuity score.

Test One Eye at a Time

Unless a child has nystagmus (involuntary rhythmic movements of an eye [See Chapter 8]) always test each eye separately. When both eyes are tested together, the visual acuity almost always equals that of the better eye; therefore, the decreased visual acuity of the weaker eye may go unnoticed. In addition, testing both eyes defeats the purpose of visual acuity screening: to identify and refer children who need a more complete eye examination. Children who pass their screenings using both eyes should be referred if they fail their screening with either eye. However, children with nystagmus must have both eyes tested together because covering one eye often accentuates the nystagmoid movements of the uncovered eye and therefore decreases its visual acuity.

Children with a loss of vision in one eye will often attempt to peek when their better eye is covered. To assure that only one eye is being tested, use those visual acuity screening methods that allow observation of the child during the entire procedure. If you observe frowning, squinting, tilting or moving the head, blinking excessively, tearing, or peeking, record your observations and gently request the children (if they are old enough) to refrain from them. These behaviors often assist children in seeing better. For instance, squinting is similar to the pinhole test because both techniques channel light to enhance vision. However, children may not be aware of what they are doing, so they may not be able to stop.

Finally, another method for assuring that one eye only is being tested is to use a good, age-appropriate occlusion method (Figure 1-2). When selecting such a method, consider quantity, cost, disposability, safety, and acceptability to the child. For example, the Coverlet (Beisdorf) and Opticlude (3M) eye patches are relatively inexpensive, provide good occlusion, and are disposable. They are also soft and pliable so that they cannot accidentally injure the external eye area. However, they may make young children apprehensive. Disposable construction paper shapes (fishes or other objects) may be more acceptable to the child. However, their sharp edges may cause accidental injury to the cornea or lids, and the child may inadvertently peek around them. In addition, when one is screening a large

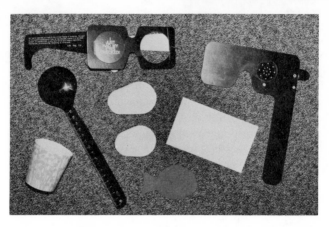

Fig. 1-2. Various types of occluders. Clockwise, from top: Blackbird vision screening specs, commercial pinhole occluder, 3-inch x 5-inch index card, home-made construction paper fish, commercial Gulden occluders, paper cup. Center: commercial patches in regular and junior sizes.

number of children, constructing these more appealing types of occlusion devices may be too time-consuming. Other adequate types of occlusion sometimes used are paper cups, 3 by 5 inch cards, and the commercially produced, nondisposable occluders. Whichever method is selected, the examiner should be sure that both eyes are kept open throughout the screening, both for greater comfort and to avoid any pressure on the occluded eye.

Recording Your Findings

$$V_{\bar{s}c} \qquad \begin{matrix} 20/40 \\ 20/60^{-1} \end{matrix} \qquad \text{single E's} \qquad \text{PH} \qquad \begin{matrix} 20/30 \\ \text{NI} \end{matrix} \quad N \quad \begin{matrix} J2 \\ J5 \end{matrix}$$

To those unfamiliar with interpreting and recording visual acuity results, these symbols may look very foreign. However, they are really not as difficult as they appear.

The large V (sometimes V_A) on any eye care note refers to visual acuity. The $\bar{s}c$ and its opposite cc indicate "without correction or corrective lenses" and "with correction," respectively.

If children are wearing glasses to correct myopia or astigmatism, screen them first with their glasses on; otherwise, they may become frustrated or embarrassed by their poor performance. In contrast, children with hyperopia may do better on a distant visual acuity screening without their glasses.

It is common practice to record the visual acuity from the right eye first, above the visual acuity of the left eye. This practice also encourages the examiner to screen the right eye first, thus establishing a consistent pattern and decreasing possible confusion. The numerator refers to the distance at which the visual acuity screening was performed; in most cases, it is 20 feet (6 meters). The denominator refers to the distance at which a person with normal eyes can satisfactorily read the chart. For example, we know that a child who has 20/40 vision was tested at a 20-foot distance (numerator) and could see what a child with normal vision would be able to see from 40 ft (denominator). Similarly, we know that a child with 12/30 vision was tested at 12 feet and could see from that distance what a child with normal eyesight could see 30 feet away. We obtain the number in the denominator from the specific screening method itself.

Many people have difficulty in comprehending how "good" or "bad" a child's vision is unless the number 20 is in the numerator. They probably understand better because $20/x$ is a common referral point: 20/20 for normal vision, 20/70 for the baseline of the visually impaired, and 20/200 for the definition of legal blindness. Therefore, to convert other visual acuity results to a $20/x$ format, divide the numerator into 20 and multiply the denominator by the result. For example, to find the $20/x$ equivalent for 10/30, first divide 10 into 20, which equals 2. Then multiply the denominator (in this case, 30) by 2, for a product of 60 or 20/60.

Remember that visual acuity is actually a measurement of the visual angle that separates two parts of a test object. Therefore, 20/40 represents double the visual angle of 20/20, for example.

The numbers that are preceded by a plus or minus sign and immediately follow the denominator in a visual acuity result indicate small changes in a person's vision; these changes are important in such problems as amblyopia. A plus sign indicates that the child has successfully read that amount of symbols on the next line of the visual acuity screening tool. A minus sign indicates that a specific number of symbols was missed on that same line recorded as the visual acuity for that eye.

To promote continuity and communication between examiners, it is helpful to record the type of visual acuity method used, such as Snellen, Es, or Allen cards. In addition, examiners often differentiate between a linear method and a singular, or letter, procedure in their notes because children with amblyopia may experience the crowding phenomenon when viewing a line of symbols. Hence, they may fail a line that they would pass if they viewed each symbol individually. Data collected from any pinhole (PH) or near vision (N) testing should also be recorded. These procedures are discussed in later sections in this chapter and in Chapter 2. Some examiners also let older children record their own results to reinforce the results and their meaning.

Regardless of the notation system that you use, record your findings systematically, so others will have quick access to your observations and findings. If your school or agency does not use specific forms for such recording, consider using those produced by the NSPB.

When a Child Fails a Screening

Whenever possible, a child should be given another opportunity to pass a screening before the examiner recommends referral. A child may be sick, tired, or upset during a first screening or may misunderstand the screening procedure. Preferably the retesting should occur within 10 days of the first. Some organizations prefer that a nurse retest all children if volunteers or lay persons have performed the initial screening.

Each method of visual acuity screening has criteria for passing or failing. For example, the Good-Lite Company specifies that a child who passes more than half a line receives credit for that line. For other sources, two mistakes or more may indicate failure for that line.

In addition, the visual acuity level considered appropriate for the different ages varies. The NSPB and certain state educational systems refer 3-year-olds when their vision is less than or equal to 20/50. Children 4 to 6 years old and those in kindergarten through grade three whose vision is less than or equal to 20/40 are referred, whereas fourth grade and older children are referred when their vision is less than or equal to 20/30. Furthermore, children who have a difference greater than one line between the visual acuity of both eyes are likewise referred. Some authorities use even higher screening criteria; for example, they refer a 5- or 6-year-old with vision less than or equal to 20/30. Therefore, it is important that you become familiar with the referral criteria in your area or organization.

When a child fails a visual acuity screening, there are several techniques of gathering information to supplement your referral. One simple yet informative method is the pinhole test *(PH)*. To determine whether the loss of vision is due to an uncorrected refractive error instead of amblyopia or an organic problem, repeat the screening, placing a pinhole occluder in front of the child's eyes. These occluders can be purchased, or made from a sheet of cardboard with a number of holes poked into it with a pencil. The occluder is placed in front of the eye being screened (remember to keep the other eye totally occluded), and the child is asked to select one hole to look through. If the child has better results when the screening is repeated, an uncorrected refractive error is likely. This finding is noted as *PH 20/x* after the original notation; for example, *V (OD) 20/40 PH 20/25* indicates that the visual acuity in the right eye was initially 20/40 but increased to 20/25 with the pinhole test. Pinhole testing never results in 20/20 vision, however.

If there is no improvement *(NI),* the child may have amblyopia or an organic cause of his decreased vision. Children who have improved results on the pinhole test can be referred to either an optometrist or an ophthalmologist, but children who show no improvement should be referred to an ophthalmologist for a complete eye evaluation to rule out organic problems. Since finances are often a consideration in your referrals, this technique will assist you in deciding the most appropriate referrals, and it will improve your assessment skills.

Another technique is appropriate for children who cannot see the top line on a chart. In such cases, ask them to walk toward the chart (or move the chart toward them) until they can see it. If the top line on your chart represents 20/100 vision, and the child walks up to 10 feet in order to see this line, you can either record ''20/100 seen at 10 feet'' or place the 10 in the numerator and keep the old denominator, for 10/100 (20/200).

Additional methods of assessing the vision of a child who fails the initial screening use fingers, hand motion and light. Children who require these measures have failed their screening by a significant margin and are legally blind. However, each method can assist the nurse, the family, and educators in determining a child's specific visual capabilities. (As discussed in Chapter 13, these children are also referred to low-vision centers when appropriate for equipment and techniques that can maximize their visual capabilities.)

To use these techniques, first hold several fingers close to the child's face and ask how many fingers the child sees. If the child can see some, write CF (counts fingers) beside the distance at which the child can perform the test successfully *(CF at 6 inches)*. If the child is not successful, move your hand before the child's face in the different quadrants and ask if and where she or he can see your hand. If successful, write *HM* (''hand movements''). If that test produces no better result, shine a pocket light or flashlight before the child's face, again in the various quadrants, and ask whether the child can see and possibly localize the light. *PLL* describes children who can both perceive and localize the light source; *LP* stands for ''light perception,'' which, some examiners use for children who can perceive light but are unable to localize it. Children who have no light perception *(NLP)* are considered totally blind in that eye.

Once you have finished the screening, you need to discuss your findings with the child's parents (in person or by letter or phone). Figure 1-3 is the parent notification form regarding a visual problem used by the Arizona state school system. As seen in this example, the signs of eye trouble noted by school personnel are also listed; these signs assist the eye care specialist in understanding the specific reason for the referral.

You should develop a list of referrals before beginning visual acuity screening. Parents often have no idea where to receive follow-up care, and it is useless to refer a child when services for treatment are unknown or unavailable.

Include in your list the names of ophthalmologists, optometrists, and opticians. Remember, though, that children with the following problems should be referred to an ophthalmologist: sudden loss of vision or acute onset of other symptoms;

SCHOOL DISTRICT NAME AND ADDRESS
PARENT NOTIFICATION REGARDING VISION PROBLEM

Date _____

Student's Name _____

Address _____

Grade _____ Teacher _____

To Parent or Guardian:

A recent vision screening shows that your child may have some vision difficulty for the reason or reasons indicated below. A complete eye examination is recommended. Please take this form to the eye doctor. When completed, form should be returned to the school nurse. If you will have any financial difficulty in paying for eye examination, glasses or treatment, please contact school nurse or principal.

| | SIGNS OF EYE TROUBLE NOTED |
| FOR THE EXAMINER: | BY SCHOOL PERSONNEL: |

Visual Acuity ☐ _____

Far Sightedness ☐ _____

Binocular Vision–Far ☐ _____

Binocular Vision–Near ☐ _____

Depth Perception ☐ _____

_____
SCHOOL NURSE

•••

EXAMINER'S REPORT

Student's Name _____ Address _____

Diagnosis _____

_____

_____

When should glasses be worn? _____

When should student be reexamined? _____

Recommendation for school health program _____

Date of examination _____

_____
EXAMINER'S SIGNATURE AND TITLE

_____
ADDRESS

EXAMINER: Please return this form to the school nurse or administrator in order that vision referral records may be completed.

Fig. 1-3. One recommended form for reproduction and use by schools. Reprinted with permission from the Arizona Vision Screening Guidelines, Arizona Department of Health Services.

known eye or systemic diseases (such as diabetes, sickle cell anemia, or hypertension); high myopia (greater than 6 diopters [D]) or high hyperopia (greater than 4-1/2 [D]) because of the increased risk of retinal detachment and glaucoma, respectively; and injury to the eye area, and children with ocular problems who are under the age of 3 years because of the increased risk of such eye pathology as tumors.

Follow-up

Once you have made a referral, you can act as the liaison between the eye care specialist and the family and school or daycare staff. Using a form similar to that in Fig. 1-3 encourages communication and feedback. The specialist can then contact you about any questions regarding the referral or for additional information, such as observations of the child in the school setting.

As with any referral, never consider it complete until you know that appropriate care and treatment have been given. For this reason, many nurses establish a follow-up system, such as noting in their calendars when they should contact a parent if they receive no feedback. But allow 1 to 2 months before such follow-up, as finances and a filled appointment schedule of an examiner may interfere with any earlier care.

It is also suggested that you keep track of your referrals by comparing your findings with those of the eye care specialists. An approximate 15–25 percent overreferral rate is standard among visual acuity screeners. This rate indicates that for every 100 children referred, 15-25 will not have any problem noted by an eye care specialist. If you find that your overreferral rate is much higher, you should seek assistance or re-evaluate your techniques and criteria for referrals, since excessive overreferrals may undermine your judgments. On the other hand, if your rate is considerably lower, for instance in the 5 percent range, you should also re-evaluate your techniques and criteria, since you are probably letting children with eye problems slip through the screening process.

REFERENCES

1. Sheridan MD: Diagnosis of visual defect in early childhood. Brit Orthop J 20:31, 1963
2. National Society to Prevent Blindness: Children's eye health guide. New York, 1982, p 3
3. Oberman JW: Vision needs of America's children. Sight Sav Rev 36:217, 1966
4. Lawson LJ, Schoofs G: A technique for visual appraisal of mentally retarded children. Am J Ophthalmol 72:623, 1971
5. National Society to Prevent Blindness: Children's eye health guide. New York, 1982, p 3
6. Köhler L, Stigmar G: Vision screening of four-year-old children. Acta Paediatr Scand 62:25, 1973

Chapter Two

Methods of Visual Acuity Screening

SCREENING OF INFANTS AND TODDLERS

Most methods of visual acuity screening require a subjective response by the child; that is, the examiner relies upon the child's speech or gestures to help determine how well the child sees. But since infants cannot tell us what they see, we must base our estimations on such objective measures as their behaviors and reflexes. In the past, these estimations have varied greatly. For example, one ophthalmologist in 1950 estimated that a baby's visual acuity in Snellen equivalents was approximately 20/2000 at age 4 months, with improvement to 20/150 by 1 year of age.[1] Nowadays, however, more sophisticated equipment and techniques have allowed us to refine these views considerably.

Preferential Looking

One exciting innovation has been assessment of *preferential looking*. In this method, an infant is placed facing one side of a partition. The examiner, who observes the infant through a peephole, is seated on the other side. Two panels then simultaneously appear on the partition at the sides of the infant's visual field. Both panels have the same brightness, but one has black and white stripes, and the other has a gray hue. As long as an infant can see the contrast of the black and white stripes, he will usually attend to them.

However, if the infant cannot see any contrast he will gaze randomly. Therefore, by presenting different widths of stripes to the infant, each width corresponding to a specific visual acuity, researchers have been able to determine visual capabilities by noting which panels an infant prefers. As a result, some researchers now believe that an infant can see 20/1000 by the age of 4 weeks. By 17 weeks of age, vision is estimated to be 20/200, and by 1 year 20/50 or better.[2] Such findings differ considerably from earlier ones. Unfortunately, preferential looking is still in the experimental stages and is not available in most areas as a routine method of visual acuity determination. In addition, it requires equipment that is not yet commercially available, and it is inappropriate for infants who may have impaired head turning abilities. Therefore, preferential looking is currently not a useful screening tool.

Fixation Test (Fix and Follow Test)

The most common method of screening an infant's vision involves the use of the *Fix and Follow (f & f)* or *Fixation Test*. This method is based upon an infant's ability to fixate, or visually focus on an item of interest, and then to follow the item as it moves in various directions. It has long been used by professionals in assessing infants' vision and development, since the two are closely interrelated.

Many of you are already familiar with the Neonatal Behavioral Assessment Scale, developed by T. Berry Brazelton to assess a baby's interactive behavior. Using this tool, you can often demonstrate to parents how babies less than 30 days old can focus on an item of interest. Of course, the babies must be in the right mood, neither hungry nor sleepy. In addition, some babies need to be correctly positioned to help them attend. By placing a newborn in your lap at a 45 degree angle, with the infant's face and body facing yours, you can often increase the baby's attention. Then, by using your face or a brightly colored object, you can observe the newborn's ability to fixate. Once the baby has fixated, move the stimulus first horizontally, then vertically, and see whether the baby follows it, either by moving the eyes or turning the head. Also note whether these movements of the eye or head are smooth or jerky. Although no specific determinations about a baby's vision can be made from Brazelton's tool, you and the parents will develop a ''feel'' for the infant's visual capabilities.

In Gesell's Developmental Screening Examination, a dangling ring made from a 4-inch red embroidery hoop is used to assess the baby's adaptive behavioral skills. At 4 weeks, the ''average'' baby in a supine position can fixate on the ring when it is dangled on a 10-inch string and presented 1 foot above his level of vision from a pedal approach. By 8 weeks, the baby can follow the ring to midline; by 12 weeks, he can follow it 180 degrees.

In the Bayley Scales of Infant Development, a red light (pen light with red filter) is used in addition to the red ring and the face of the examiner or parent. The Denver Developmental Screening Test also makes use of these stimuli, and the Denver Eye Screening Test provides a spinning toy and flashlight for your assessments. These and other infant developmental tests also note a baby's ability to search with the eyes for sounds (bell, rattle) at approximately 2 months of age, and by turning the head at 4 months; eye-hand coordination with a block or ring, also at approximately 4 months; and ability to follow dropped objects (a beginning of depth perception skills) around the age of 6 months. Sturner and co-workers have likewise demonstrated that visual acuity screening of preschool children allows the investigator to note both the child's developmental status and visual capabilities.[3]

Usually, however, the Fixation Test is performed outside the setting of formal developmental examinations. It has proved most helpful for children whose mental ages are under 2 years, until they are old enough to participate in more formal visual acuity screening methods. For infants who were premature, age is based upon conception instead of birth.

To perform the Fixation Test, first make sure that the child is content, preferably sitting on the parent's lap or being held by the parent. If possible, arrange for the screening to occur between naps and feeding time. Then occlude one eye with your thumb, your hand, or an eye patch. To use your thumb, rest the fingers of one hand on the child's head, hold a stimulus in place with your other hand, and then quickly lower your thumb over one pupil, being careful not to touch the lashes (Fig. 2-1). Continue this process until you can determine whether the child can adequately fix and follow with the unoccluded eye.

If you use your hand, don't hold it too close, since it may be threatening to

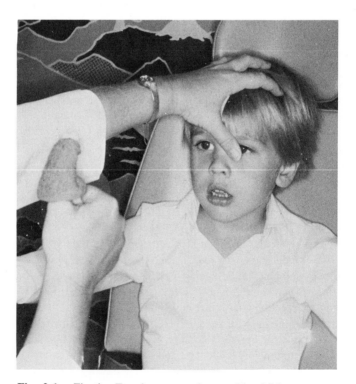

Fig. 2-1.   Fixation Test demonstrated on an older child.

some children. The use of your thumb or hand as an occluder is preferred for those children who automatically fuss at the application of an eye patch; otherwise, it may be difficult for you to determine whether their behavior is influenced by the patch or by an inability to see.

The success of the Fixation Test can be influenced by your choice of stimulus; the more interesting it is, the more attention it may elicit from the baby. "Wiggle" pictures, finger puppets, flashlights, keys, and interesting sounds are best for testing at a near range (14 inches). Some examiners test infants with a stimulus in the distance (such as a train that can be activated or a stuffed animal that can be animated). However, since many infants live in a "near world," they may not be interested in distant stimuli and hence may not respond well. Finally, be as quick as accuracy allows, since many infants tire or lose interest rapidly.

Infants "pass" the Fixation Test when they centrally fixate and follow a stimulus—in the directions of gaze appropriate for their ages—*with each eye separately*. As the developmental tests indicate, babies from birth to 4 weeks will at least focus briefly on a stimulus and perhaps follow it horizontally to midline. From 4 to 12 weeks of age, they should be able to follow the stimulus in a complete 180-degree horizontal arc, and probably vertically as well (in infants, the horizontal sense develops before the vertical). By the age of 4 months and after, they should follow the object 180 degrees in all directions, including diagonally.

Infants who have amblyopia, organic disease, or an asymmetrical refractive problem fuss and cry when their better eye is occluded, since they are being forced to see with their weaker eye. Hence, the child's response to having one eye occluded during the Fixation Test is quite important. Refer any child who fusses when one eye is covered but allows the other eye to be occluded.

Keep in mind, however, that until the age of 3 months, the two eyes often work separately. Therefore, if you occlude the eye of a 2-month-old and note that one of the eyes moves or shifts, although the infant appears to see well, advise the parents to have the test repeated at the age of 3 months. If the shifting continues at 3 months, refer the child to an ophthalmologist at once. If the eye is always misaligned, refer the child, whatever the age.

The STYCAR Graded-balls and Miniature Toys Tests

The STYCAR Test (see also Table 1-3) has several components that may be particularly helpful for those nurses who screen children with developmental special needs. Introduced by Dr. Mary Sheridan in the 1960s, it is designed for children whose mental age ranges from 6 months to 2-1/2 years.

The Graded-balls Test is an adaptation of Worth's Ivory Ball Test developed in 1903. Dr. Sheridan uses 10 white balls of various diameters (1/8–2-1/2 inches) that are rolled horizontally at various speeds across the floor on a dark, soundproof carpet or mounted on a black stick and presented from behind a dark screen.

In the first method, it is recommended that one examiner attract the child's attention and roll each ball at 10 feet from the child, while another notes the child's fix and following responses. A trial at 5 feet may be helpful for some children. Older children may wish to pursue or point at the balls.

To perform the mounted method, attach a dark cloth over a cardboard box of about 24 × 28 inches and insert a 3 × 1/4-inch peephole 6 inches from the top. Then present the balls at random locations from behind the box, holding them in place for 2 to 3 seconds and noting the child's reaction. Alternate the balls from one side to the other, being careful to vary your style of presentation; otherwise, a child who appears to be seeing the smaller balls may actually be responding to a pattern of delivery.

In both methods, a child is credited with seeing a particular ball if the child regards it successfully three times. Remember, however, to test each eye separately. Children from 6 to 8 months of age are able to see the 1/4-inch rolling ball at 10 feet and the 1/2-inch mounted ball from the same distance. The 8- to 12-month-olds, as well as older children, can see all of the balls. However, children from 12 to 24 months may be difficult to test, since they have shorter attention spans. Children older than 2 years seem to enjoy retrieving the balls as part of a game.

Dr. Sheridan has clearly stated that the Graded-balls Test is an assessment tool of everyday vision, not a precision measurement of visual acuity. At one point, her colleagues encouraged her to develop Snellen equivalents. She complied but re-emphasized that the test basically provides information about a child's ability to fix and follow small moving objects or to fixate small stable objects. Such information does not tell us what characteristics a child sees about an object, only that a child knows that the object is there. (This is the difference between discriminatory and observable distance vision.)

Also in the STYCAR is a set of miniature toys: a doll; chair; car; plate; and doll's knife, fork, and spoon. Children 21 months or older are asked to name the toys or to match them with a duplicate set. This test is first done at near and then at 10 feet on a dark carpet. If a child can recognize the larger toys, vision is estimated to be about 20/30. If a child can see the small toys (the cutlery items), the estimate is 20/20. Because the value of the Snellen equivalents has been questioned, Dr. Sheridan stresses that the test should mainly be used to identify myopia or to notice a difference between the vision of both eyes. Other criticisms about the Miniature Toys Test include the language-motor skill requirements and the problem that some children want to keep the toys and become upset when they cannot!

Optokinetic Nystagmus

Before the development of the preferential looking method, G. V. Catford, an ophthalmologist, developed an apparatus using optokinetic nystagmus to establish a quantitative measure of infant visual acuity.[4]

Nystagmus is a periodic involuntary movement of the eyes from side to side, or less frequently, up and down. *Optokinetic nystagmus (OKN)* is a physiologic response that can be elicited by viewing repetitive objects in motion. A positive response, written as + *OKN,* occurs when the eyes fix on one of the moving items, slowly follow it to the periphery until it disappears from sight, and then quickly return to the center (hence, nystagmus) to repeat the process. These eye movements are similar to those of someone viewing telephone poles from a car window.

Catford's tool consists of two interchangeable cylinders with various premeasured sizes of black dots on the sides of each cylinder. Only one dot is visible at any time through a small viewing square.

To perform the test, the motor is activated; the selected dot begins to move slowly toward the other end of the viewing square and then quickly returns to the original side. If an infant is capable of seeing the dot, similar patterns of movement are mirrored in the baby's eyes. By correlating the sizes of the dots with specific visual acuities, Catford concluded that when a dot was too small for an individual baby to see, no *(–OKN)* would be elicited for that dot. However, researchers have since questioned the correlations and recommend the Catford apparatus as a qualitative screening, but not as a quantitative one.[5]

At Childrens Hospital of Los Angeles, we have used OKN qualitatively to help rule out cortical blindness in selected infants, such as those who are post meningitis or post intraventricular hemorrhage. If the results are positive, the infants probably have some vision; however, if the results are negative, they may or may not.

OKN is also used in adult neurologic examinations. For these purposes, the nystagmus drum and tape are the two common methods of testing for OKN (Fig. 2-2). The drum is made of a 6- or 12-inch cylinder with either alternating vertical black-and white lines or pictures of animals. It is held 20 inches from the baby and slowly rotated at about 6–8 frames/sec to elicit a horizontal OKN. The tape is approximately 1 inch wide and 40 inches long and has alternating 1/2-inch segments of black and white. It is used more frequently with adults.

Nystagmus is also used to help determine the presence of vision by holding infants under their arms and spinning them (and yourself) around in a complete circle. This method is especially helpful for infants with impaired motor abilities. Once you stop, note how long the nystagmus continues. Babies with some vision will be able to suppress the nystagmus within a few seconds by fixating their surroundings. However, an infant who is blind will have the nystagmus for 20 to 30 seconds.

Reflex Tests

The blink reflex is tested in young babies by the confrontation method and is only used when the presence of any vision is being questioned. One mother of a blind baby explained that she had used this technique in her home, hoping to

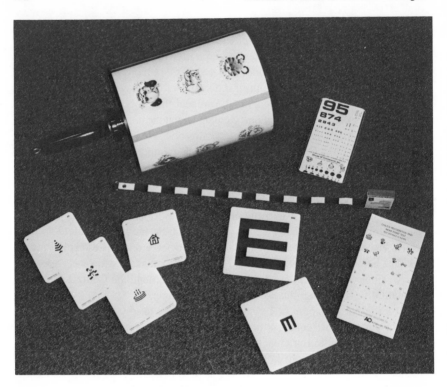

Fig. 2-2. Tools used in visual acuity screening. From top left, clockwise: optokinetic nystagmus drum, Rosenbaum near vision card, nystagmus tape, Child's Near Point Test, *E* cards, Allen cards.

elicit some response. A negative response, however, does not always imply blindness.

To elicit the blink reflex, quickly move your fist toward the baby's eyes, obviously being careful not to hit the infant or to cause a tactile stimulant (such as wind) that might also make the baby blink. If parents or uninformed bystanders are present, explain the test first, since it naturally appears quite inappropriate. Another method for testing the blink reflex—lightly touching the cornea with a piece of cotton—is inaccurate for assessing an infant's vision, since the cotton is a tactile stimulant.

Improvised Methods for Children with Multiple Needs

If you do not have access to the tools described previously (some of which can be quite expensive), you can estimate the vision of a child with severe developmental needs by observing the child's ability to pick up small objects. Several authors have devised practical methods for this procedure that allow you to make approximate visual acuity estimations.[6,7] As stated previously, the primary goal of assessing vision in a child with severe developmental special needs is to ensure that the child has functional vision. For example, does the child smile at a parent across a room or point to a plane in the air? Even though one cannot quantify such vision, such behavioral observations indicate whether the child has adequate vision for functioning or whether there has been some deterioration. Because nurses, educators, and parents can provide information about the visual functioning of a child with severe developmental needs that the examiner cannot observe in an office examination, they should record their observations of each child who is referred for the professional eye examiner's information.

Interventions

A number of interventions can be quite helpful in developing and maximizing a child's sight. Special interventions for the infant who has low vision are discussed in Chapter 13, but may also be useful for children who have normal vision.

In general, any interventions that correspond to the baby's developmental skills are helpful. To assist parents, the American Optometric Association prints the pamphlet *Your Baby's Eyes,* which lists such interventions for children from birth to 3 years of age. Furthermore, the Infant Stimulation Education Association serves as a clearinghouse for references on infant stimulation studies. It produces the booklet *Parent's Guide to Infant Stimulation,* which compiles the findings of many of these sources.

For example, it is now known that black-and-white patterned cards and mobiles and black-and-white bed linens provide excellent visual stimuli for premature infants in intensive care settings.[8] The patterns include stripes, checkerboards (2-inch squares), circles, dots or triangles (each 3 inches), or faces. These stimuli should be placed near and facing the infant. Furthermore, they should be changed at frequent intervals, especially if the infant loses interest in them. Several times a day the stimuli that a particular infant enjoys (each infant has preferences) should be presented at midline and moved around the infant's visual field for 1–2 minutes. Encourage parents to do this, and teach them to observe how the infant is developing fixating and following skills. Also, infants should be held near a mobile (or vice versa, if they cannot be easily moved) for 1 or 2 minutes several times a day.

For older infants at home, a total of 10 min/day of increased visual stimulation is adequate.[9] They also enjoy colored mobiles and objects (medium yellows, greens, and pinks seem to be best) and items with a light and dark contrast. Place mobiles near the feet in the early months, so that infants can learn to kick the mobile and further refine their motor and visual skills at the same time. In addition, suggest changing the baby's position (including moving the bed around at frequent intervals) often to provide new visual stimuli and place interesting pictures on the ceiling above the crib. As the baby grows, keep small yet safe objects in the near vision range (about 10 inches) to help develop eye-hand coordination and grasping abilities.

SCREENING OF PRESCHOOL AND SCHOOL-AGED CHILDREN

Allen Picture Cards

The Allen cards are the most widely used method of picture card screening in the United States. They were designed by H. F. Allen in 1957 to assist examiners in determining the presence of amblyopia or refractive errors in preschool children until the children were old enough to participate in the *E* method. Therefore, Allen cards find their greatest use among children 2½–3 years of age and older children and those with developmental special needs who cannot understand the *E* method. Another popular picture method, the Schering or Faye chart, uses a wall chart with pictures of apples, houses, and umbrellas. The new Efron picture method employs pictures of a shoe, a cup, and a circle (see Table 1-4).

To use the Allen card method you need a set of Allen cards, some type of occlusion, and a premeasured room 20 feet in length. The Allen cards contain seven pictures on four cards (Fig. 2-2). The pictures (horse, house, telephone, cake, bear, tree, and car) were selected by Allen both for their optical qualities and because they remind children of pleasurable things.

Preferably, the child should be introduced to the Allen card pictures in the home or school. In these environments children feel comfortable with the process, and you will obtain better results. To determine how the child will name each picture, show all of them before you start the screening. This is important because many children will say "Mickey Mouse" upon seeing the bear or "Happy Birthday" when they see the cake. As long as the child is consistent in naming each picture, it does not matter what name is used.

Delete any picture that the child hesitates to name, since that hesitation may indicate limited familiarization or language skills. Let a child who is shy or aphasic point to the answer on a piece of paper containing all seven pictures. Finally, if you work with a large non-English-speaking population, you may wish to learn the Allen card pictures in another language. The Spanish equivalents are *mono, monito, oso,* or *osito* ("bear"); *carro, carrito,* or *cameon* ("car"); *pastel* ("cake"); *arbol* or *piño* ("tree"); *teléfono* or *allo* ("telephone"); *caballo* ("horse"); *casa* or *casita* ("house").

Once you are sure that the child understands the screening process, occlude one eye and start the screening. The current preferred method is to ask children to name the pictures as you slowly move away from them. When two or three pictures have been named correctly at each distance, step back another foot or two.

This rapidity helps the child maintain attention as the pictures become more difficult to see.

In the original design of the Allen cards, however, the examiner immediately moved to the 15- or 20-foot locations, to see whether the child could correctly name four or more pictures from that distance. But such immediate relocation away from the child can occasionally decrease attention or full participation, making the child untestable.

Children 2 and 3 years old pass the Allen cards when they successfully see four or more pictures at a distance of 12 feet or more. Children 3 to 4 years old pass the screening when they can name the pictures at a distance of 15 feet or greater. Children 4 years or older pass at 20 feet. Record these findings as 12/30, 15/30, or 20/30, respectively, and repeat the process with the other eye. To prevent a child from memorizing the pictures, remember to vary their sequence.

However, if the child begins to name some of the pictures incorrectly, be careful not to indicate in any way that a mistake has been made. Instead, move forward again a foot or so to see whether four pictures (a statistically significant response) can be correctly named at this nearer distance. With that assurance, enter the distance in feet as the numerator of the visual acuity result. Remember that with Allen cards the numerator always corresponds to the best distance in feet at which the child correctly names four or more pictures; the denominator is always 30, a preset figure determined by the optics of the pictures.

An example of Allen card use follows. With the left eye patched, a 3-year-old can correctly name the Allen card pictures up to a distance of 12 feet. At that point, the child calls the car a boat, and the house a horse. When the examiner moves back to 10 feet, the child can correctly name four of the pictures. Therefore, vision for the right eye is recorded as 10/30, written as *V OD 10/30 Allens*.

In addition, the difference between the two eyes should be less than 3 feet. For example, a 2-1/2-year-old child with 12/30 vision in one eye and 15/30 vision in the other should be retested. If the difference continues, refer the child to an eye examiner, since the result may indicate amblyopia in the weaker eye.

As with all visual acuity screenings, the use of Allen cards can be a source of frustration for the parents who are so concerned that their child see well. Frustrated parents frequently scold a child who misses a picture or yell "No!" or "Look again." Other parents unconsciously say the beginning of the picture names or give hints such as "What do you eat on your birthday?" Therefore, it is most important to explain how the screening works before it actually occurs, to assist the parents in their own behavioral and verbal responses.

Finally, children who quickly respond to the Allen card method should be given information on the *E* game to take home, so that on a subsequent visit, they can be tested with a more optically mature screening. Preschool children who cannot participate in the Allen card method because they are unable to comprehend the screening procedure should have their fixation and following responses examined and be retested on a monthly basis when possible until more reliable results can be obtained.

Because the Allen cards have been used for over 20 years, they have received more study than some other methods have. Thus, they have been criticized for being potentially experientially and culturally biased and for using recognition—not resolution—as the optical principle behind the visual acuity determination. These criticisms, however, can be debated. First, through preparation materials young children can become familiar with the Allen card pictures, as well as with the process of screening, before the actual screening occurs. Second, Allen himself has suggested that picture card screening be used only when more mature methods cannot be understood by the child. For these reasons, the Allen cards have been incorporated into the Denver Eye Screening Test as a reliable method of testing the young (2–4 years) preschool child.

H:O:T:V and Other Matching Methods

The H:O:T:V, STYCAR, Sheridan-Gardiner, and Snellen letters as matching symbols are related visual acuity screening methods. That is, they are based upon the principle of matching, rather than the identification of pictures (as with the Allen cards) or directional responses (as in the *E* game). This concept of matching is fairly new, developed by Mary Sheridan in the early 1960s in Britain. Designed for young preschool children, matching methods can also be used for children with dyslexia, aphasia, developmental special needs, and those who speak a foreign language (see Table 1-4).

The STYCAR Test employs the letters, *H, O, T, V, X, U, A, C,* and *L.* Notice that most of these letters are reversible and therefore do not have a mirror image to confuse a child. In the Sheridan-Gardiner version, the four letters *H, O, T,* and *V* are used with 2-year-olds; the *X* is added for children 3–5 years, and the *U* and *A* are added for children 4–7 years old. Since the development of these other versions, however, Dr. Otto Lippmann has shown that the use of the first four symbols, *H, O, T,* and *V,* is sufficient for adequate screening with all children.[10]

Whatever method is used, the choice of the letters corresponds with developmental principles. For example, a vertical and horizontal line can be identified and copied by most children 2 years old. Circles can be copied by 3 years, crosses by 4 years, and squares and triangles by 5 years. In addition, children learn to respond manually before they can respond verbally, and the matching tests make full use of this principle.

To perform the H:O:T:V version you will need four training cards, each containing one symbol; a so-called response panel that has all four symbols easily visible on one side; and a 9 × 14-inch chart to be used at the 10-foot distance. Prepare children by using the four training cards and the response panel, asking them to place a hand on a similar symbol as you show one of the training cards. Unlike the original STYCAR test, Lippmann's method does not encourage the child to respond verbally, unless the child chooses to do so. Lippmann also suggests that you use names such as *donut* for the *O* instead of referring to the symbols by their letter names. Some children will prefer to recopy the letter in midair, rather than pointing it out on the response panel.

Once the child understands the procedure, you can start the screening by placing the child 10 feet from the chart. After occluding one eye, show one letter at a time to the younger children, and one line at a time for those 4 years old and older. Children pass each line when they can correctly match four of the six symbols for that line.

These matching tests, particularly H:O:T:V, have been widely received among visual acuity screeners. Their main advantage has been their high reliability, which is most likely due to their developmental base. In addition, they are quick to administer, requiring only a few minutes for children ages 3–4 years who have been previously prepared. Furthermore, the symbols do not presuppose previous familiarity, as pictures do.

The main disadvantage of matching methods is that a child needs to understand the concept of likeness in order to comply. In addition, some people are concerned that the use of only four symbols on the H:O:T:V allows a child to guess the appropriate answer correctly one out of four times, which is the same guess rate as for the *E* game. However, reliability studies have shown that such guessing is insignificant. Finally, when more than four symbols are used, some authorities feel that greater attention span is necessary than in picture card techniques.

The *E* and Other Directional Methods

The *E* game is one of the many directional methods of visual acuity screening now in use. Other popular ones include the Sjögren's Hand Test, the Michigan Preschool Test, the Blackbird System, and the Landolt Rings. All of these are based upon the concept of which direction the particular symbol—*E*, hand, bird, or ring—is facing (Fig. 2-3 and Table 1-4).

In the 1860s a Dutch ophthalmologist, Dr. Hermann Snellen, developed the first directional method of visual acuity screening (now known as the *E game*). Snellen based his test on *optotypes*, or symbols of graded optically measured sizes. To this day, the *E* game continues to be widely used, since it is a highly reliable method. It has proved most beneficial in screening children ages 42 months to 6 years, as well as those who are non-English-speaking, developmentally disabled, or asphasic. The NSPB continues to endorse the *E* method as the preferred method of visual acuity screening among preschoolers. The Denver Eye Screening Test and the Michigan Preschool Test also use the *E* method.

In 1909 in France E. Landolt developed the most valid method of visual acuity screening available today. Based totally on resolution power, the Landolt

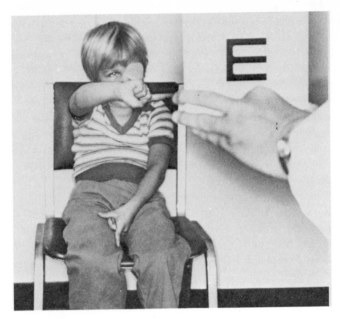

Fig. 2-3. *E* game. Note use of both hands, a common behavior in 4-year-olds.

rings or broken circles do not offer any false clues to assist the subject in answering. Because of this, they require increased maturity and are therefore not appropriate for preschoolers and some older children. However, the NSPB has recently produced a home eye test for adults, using the Landolt rings as its basis for distance vision screening.

In 1939 Sjögren modified the Snellen *E* into the shape of a hand to assist younger children in understanding the concept of direction. As a result, children as young as 36 months can often participate in a directional method with the use of the Sjögren's hand. However, the modifications have provided additional false clues available to the child. Therefore, this method is not as reliable as the *E* game or Landolt ring, although its use with younger children can prepare them for these more reliable methods.

Similarly, in the early 1970s Kiyo Sato-Viacrucis, a public health nurse in California, modified the standard *E* into the shape of a bird and developed the Blackbird Vision Screening System. The uniqueness of this system centers around the story of an adventurous blackbird, who flies in all different directions. The story background often enables a child who cannot participate in other directional methods to be screened successfully with this test. Included in the system are unique spectacles used for occlusion; reading "I just had my eyes checked," they are given to the child after the screening. However, as with the Sjögren's Hand, the modifications from the standard *E* into the shape of a bird increase the number of false clues, thus somewhat decreasing the reliability of this test.

Since any screening will be unreliable unless the child understands the process, try to allow adequate time for preparation. When a group of children, such as a daycare class, is to be tested, ask the teacher to prepare the children on several occasions prior to the actual screening. The teacher can use a plastic or paper model *E,* such as the one that accompanies the NSPB Home Eye Test for Preschoolers, to create a game. For those of you who work in an office setting, suggest that parents use these resources to prepare their child at home or have them perform the actual screening themselves.

With the directional methods, children can respond either verbally or with gestures. Sometimes two examiners are necessary in testing a child who uses gestures: one to note whether the child is responding correctly and the other to handle the chart. Often parents can assist with the first role, or you can use flash card methods so that you are constantly facing the child. Also encourage children who gesture to use a full hand or arm motion, to prevent confusion during the actual screening process when they become doubtful about the direction of a symbol being shown.

Children who respond verbally often have no difficulty in stating whether a symbol faces up or down but may become confused with the lateral directions and therefore use gestures for those responses. The Michigan Preschool Test was developed to assist with this problem; four pictures are placed next to the four directions of the *E,* and the child is asked, "To which picture is the 'E' pointing?" For persons using the wall chart, this technique has been modified by placing pictures of, for example, a boy to the left side, and a girl to the right. Then, a child who becomes confused in a lateral response simply replies "to the girl" or "to the boy" to indicate the direction of the *E* in question. Some examiners refer to the *E* as an object with which the child is already familiar (a hand, table, or bird), even though they are not specifically using these other methods. Once the child is prepared, you are ready to occlude an eye and begin the screening.

The directional methods are available in flash cards, cubes, and wall charts. If you select the wall chart, use a 15-foot distance whenever possible for children who are 3 years old, and a 20-foot distance for those 4 years old and above unless your instructions state otherwise. If you select the flash cards, you can go immediately to the prescribed distance, or you can present a larger symbol in various directions while continuing to back away quickly from the child at 1- to 2-foot intervals. This second approach may be beneficial for younger children who have difficulty when you remove yourself too quickly by going immediately to the 15- or 20-foot distance.

An alternative to the flash card is a cube that has six different-sized *E* figures on its various sides, usually measuring from 20/20 to 20/200. With both the cube and the flash card, start with a larger symbol, rotating it in three or four directions. If the child responds correctly to all of these, proceed to a smaller size until you determine the child's visual acuity for that eye.

Unless the instructions for the method you use state otherwise, a 3-year-old who cannot successfully respond to three of the five directions of the 20/50 card or line should be referred. A child 4–6 years old who cannot correctly respond to three of six responses of the 20/40 line should also be referred.

One advantage of the directional method is its reliability, although that varies among the methods used. The children appear to enjoy the gamelike atmosphere, and these methods are also quick to administer. In addition, you can sometimes pick up possible signs of dyslexia or other visual perceptual problems by using a directional method in older children.

The main disadvantage to directional screening is that many younger children have difficulty with the concept of direction. This is especially true of the lateral sense, since it is a learned response. Usually, 2-year-olds cannot be tested at all with these methods, and children with dyslexia may find them frustrating. In addition, some examiners state that a child has a one-in-four chance of correctly guessing the appropriate response, although reliability studies have continued to negate the significance of such guessing. Finally, some children find directional screening monotonous.

Letter Charts

The Snellen and Sloan letters continue to be two of the most highly reliable and valid methods of visual acuity screening, since they are based primarily on the principle of retinal resolution instead of recognition. Preferably, these screenings should be done at a 6-meter (20-feet) range and should follow the standard guidelines for lighting, occlusion, and preparation. To prevent memorization of the letters, you may ask the child to read one line from the beginning and the next line in reverse. Most examiners start the screening at around the 20/50 line, working up or down as needed. Criteria for passing vary; some examiners pass a child for each line if the child makes no mistakes or has only one error, but others give credit for the line if at least half of it is correctly identified.

Case history: Nine-year-old Barbara misses two letters on the 20/30 line of the letter chart with her right eye. This result is recorded as V_{OD} *20/30^{-2} letters*. Her results on the rescreening one week later are similar. In view of Barbara's age, her good school performance, lack of complaints, and borderline results, she is not referred to an eye examiner. Instead she is placed on a follow-up list to be rescreened in 6 months. Her teacher and parents are informed of these results and asked to notify the nurse if any changes in behavior or performance occur.

Machines

Nurses who perform a high number of visual acuity screenings may be interested in obtaining an automated machine to assist them in their work. Not only do these machines allow you to screen for distance visual acuity for the various age levels, but with appropriate parts you can also screen for hyperopia, color vision, muscle imbalance, stereopsis, and fusion. Newer models are now portable, and they can save you time and space (a 5-foot × 5-foot area is generally needed).

Some agencies (NSPB and various state educational systems) do not recommend such machines for younger children, however, because the machines can frighten the child.

Therefore, when determining whether a machine would help or hinder your work, consider the number and type of children that you screen, which screenings you are performing, and the finances available to you.

NEAR VISION SCREENING

Near vision is a person's visual acuity for objects held at a comfortable reading or working distance, usually 33–40 centimeters (cm) (13–16 inches) away. Since most authorities feel that a child's near vision mirrors the child's best corrected distance vision, this measurement is frequently not taken during routine screenings. However, as will be seen shortly, in selected cases it can provide important information to the examiner.

The tools for near vision screening are simple: a pocket-sized card and some type of occlusion. Near vision cards for children can be obtained free of charge from several pharmaceutical companies (Table 2-1). Others are available commercially in various designs, such as Allen pictures; the Snellen format; vocational-based (for example, Engineers' Drawing, telephone directory); recreational-based (playing cards, musical notations); and several foreign languages. Although the professional eye examiner needs a wide selection, you will need only one or two cards for an adequate screening.

Screening for near vision is essentially the same as distance visual acuity screening, except that the card is held about 13–16 inches away; other factors, such as preparation of the child, observations, occlusion, lighting, and so forth, remain the same. When performing near vision screening, most examiners learn to approximate the near distance, using perhaps the distance between their fingers and elbow as a guide.

The notation of near vision can be confusing to those unfamiliar with it, since numerous methods are currently in use. Table 2-2 compares many of these methods. Keep in mind, however, that such comparisons are for clinical use and are therefore not exact.

Near vision can be performed by inpatient or community health nurses who

Table 2-1
Near Vision and Hyperopic Screening Equipment

Near Tests*

Burroughs Wellcome provides a free reprint of a card based on Allen card pictures.

CooperVision Pharmaceuticals reproduces the Rosenbaum pocket vision screener (free); this chart uses numbers, Es, Xs and Os.

Good-Lite manufactures reading cards incorporating Snellen letters with first-grade words or Sloan letters at approximately $5.00/set of 12.

Keeler produces professional reading cards and near tests, including the vocation type, a four-page reading type, and a child's reading test using Peter Rabbit; these professional, high-quality cards vary from $20.00 to $30.00.

Lighthouse Industries sells the Schering-Faye picture cards and a card with numbers ($1.00 each); also Sloan near cards.

Richmond Products sells a wide variety of near cards, including some in Spanish; prices start at $2.00.
WCO also sells a wide assortment of near vision cards, including the Efron picture card; prices start at $2.00.

Hyperopic Glasses

Good-Lite Company and Richmond Products produce various plus-strength lenses for hyperopic screening at an approximate cost of $35.00/set.

*Occlusion is necessary in near testing but not in hyperopic screening.

do not have easy access to distance visual acuity screening equipment; they find the pocket-sized near vision cards a satisfactory way of estimating a child's vision. Similarly, the school nurse can use near vision screening cards to help determine a child's visual acuity after trauma (see Chapter 12) or to determine the functional visual ability of a child with low vision. For children with low vision, the nurse ignores the standard 33-cm distance from eye to test card and allows the child to view the card from whatever distance is most comfortable; at a closer distance, the child can often see at a much higher level. (Although, of course, the child has failed the vision screening.) This technique helps the staff determine what visual capabilities a child has, if selected environmental factors such as distance are altered.

On infrequent occasions, near vision cards or hyperopic screening may be used for a child in the lower grades who is a poor reader but has passed the distance visual acuity screening. If the child fails one of these additional screenings referral to a professional eye examiner is in order.

Finally, nurses who are around 40 years old (or older) may be acquainted with near vision cards from personal experience. Around this age the lens loses its

Table 2-2
Comparative Chart of Various Near Vision Notation Systems

Snellen Feet	Snellen Meters	AMA[a]	Jaeger[b]	Point[c]	Decimal Notation[d]	Pergentage[e]	Visual Angle[f]	Usual Text Type Size
20/20	6/6	14/14	1	3	1.00	100	5	Mail order catalogue
20/25	6/7.5	14/17	1-	4	0.80	100	6.25	
20/30	6/9	14/21	2	5	0.66	95	7.5	Want ads
20/40	6/12	14/28	4	6	0.50	90	10	Telephone directory
20/50	6/15	14/35	6	8	0.40	50	12.5	Newspaper text
20/60	6/18	14/42	8	9	0.33	40	15	Adult textbooks
20/70	6/21	14/49	9	10	0.29	30	17.5	
20/80	6/24	14/56	10	12	0.25	20	20	Children's books, 9–12 yr
20/100	6/30	14/70	11	14	0.20	15	25	Children's books, 8–9 yr
20/120	6/36	14/84	12	18	0.17	10	30	
20/200	6/60	14/140	17	24	0.10	2	50	Large type text
20/320	6/96	14/224	19			1.5		
20/400	6/120	14/280				1	100	

[a]American Medical Association system, developed in 1940; numerator indicates 14 inches; [b]System developed by Jaeger in the 1800s; now varies minimally from one source to the next; during recording, it is usually preceded by a *J* ; [c]Also known as *Times Roman*, the print typeface used; may be preceded by an *N* in the notation (*N9*); [d]Snellen equivalent converted to the decimal system (20/40 = 1/2 = 0.50); [e]Percentage of central visual efficiency for near; approved by Section on Ophthalmology, American Medical Association, 1955; [f]Technical measurement between two pieces of a visual acuity test symbol, in arc min.

ability to accommodate, and a person finds that she or he has increasing difficulty in seeing things at close range. This condition is called *presbyopia,* and its presence is often determined with near vision cards. If a person must hold the card at a distance in order to read it, presbyopia is often the cause, and reading glasses (or bifocals for those who have a refractive error) are prescribed. Fortunately, children rarely develop presbyopia.

SCREENING FOR HYPEROPIA

Depending upon your role, you may also wish to incorporate screening for *hyperopia* (farsightedness) into your visual assessment. Many authorities consider hyperopic screening to be more reliable than near vision screening in determining the accommodative ability of the lenses. As a result, screening for hyperopia is included in the widely used Massachusetts Battery of Vision Tests, along with tests for distance visual acuity, suppression, and muscle imbalance. However, other authorities feel that screening for hyperopia is not necessary when a child's vision is good and no strabismus is present.

As with all screening, organizations differ about some of the criteria used in hyperopic screening. For example, the Good-Lite Company, which manufactures hyperopic screening glasses, recommends that children in grades three through high school be tested for hyperopia every other year. In contrast, the Arizona Department of Health Services recommends that children in kindergarten or grade one and special education students participate in this screening. Although the NSPB suggests techniques for screening children from grades one through high school, they do not make any specific recommendations regarding hyperopic screening.

To perform hyperopic screening you need a set of glasses with certain plus lenses, and a distance visual acuity chart, preferably at the 20-foot range. The NSPB recommends + -2.25-D-strength lenses for grades one through three, and + -1.75-D-strength lenses for grades four and above. Other organizations may suggest lenses with slightly different specifications. In contrast to regular screening for visual acuity, however, no occlusion is needed, since both eyes are tested together.

A good time to screen for hyperopia is immediately after you finish the screening for distance visual acuity. Let the children wear the special glasses (if they already wear glasses, place these over the others) and wait about 1 minute before continuing. You must allow this time because the child's own lenses will tend to accommodate to the special glasses, and the child may see better (and thus *fail*) if this additional time is allowed for such accommodation.

To perform the screening, simply ask the child to read the 20/20 line (some agencies use the 20/30 or 20/40 lines). A child who *cannot* has *passed* the screening. However, a child who *can* read the line has *failed* the screening for hyperopia and must be referred. Some examiners refer children who fail the screening only if they are performing poorly in school or if they have complaints or appearances of excessive straining.

REFERENCES

1. Guibor G: Nonparalytic strabismus: Problems in treating infants and children with crossed eyes. Med Clin North Am 34:284, 1950
2. Jacobson SG, Mohindra I, Held, R: Visual acuity of infants with ocular diseases. Am J Ophthalmol 93:200, 1982
3. Sturner RA, Green JA, Funk SG, et al: A developmental approach to preschool vision screening. J Pediatr Ophthalmol Strabismus 18:61–67, 1981
4. Catford GV, Oliver A: Development of visual acuity. Arch Dis Child 48:47–50, 1973
5. Khan SG, Chen KF, Frenkel M: Subjective and objective visual acuity testing techniques. Arch Ophthalmol 94:2086–2091, 1976
6. Holland SH: 20/20 vision screening. Pediatr Nurs 8:81–87, March–April 1982
7. Frenkel M, Evans LS: The nonpareil test of visual acuity in the young and retarded. Ann Ophthalmol 13:811, 1980
8. Chaze BA, Ludington-Hoe SM: Sensory stimulation in the NICU. Am J Nurs 84:68–71, 1984
9. Ludington-Hoe SM: What can newborns really see? Am J Nurs 83:1286–1289, 1983
10. Lippmann O: Vision screening of young children. Amer J Public Health 61:1586–1601, 1971

SELECTED BIBLIOGRAPHY FOR CHAPTERS 1 AND 2

Allen HF: Testing of visual acuity in preschool children. Pediatrics 19:1093–1100, 1957
Barker J, Goldstein A, Frankenburg WK: Denver Eye Screening Test. Denver, LADOCA Publishing Foundation, 1972
Barker ER, Seeger PF: In the hands of volunteers. Sight Sav Rev 45:75–82, 1975
Bayley N: Manual for the Bayley Scales of Infant Development. New York, Psychological Corporation, 1969
Brazelton TB: Neonatal Behavioral Assessment Scale. Philadelphia, Lippincott, 1973
Knobloch H, Pasamanick B (Eds): Gesell and Amatruda's Developmental Diagnosis (ed 3). New York, Harper & Row, 1974
Larsen GL: Optokinetic nystagmus. Am J Nurs 73:1897–1898, 1973
Sheridan MD: The STYCAR graded-balls vision test. Develop Med Child Neurol 15:423–432, 1973

Chapter Three

Errors of Refraction

The term *refraction* refers to the bending of light rays as they pass from one medium to another, as when light travels from the atmosphere into our eyes. For us to see clearly, these light rays must be focused precisely on the retina, where they will be relayed by nerve endings to higher visual centers. When we speak of *errors of refraction,* we are referring to those variations within an eye that prevent perfect focusing of light rays upon the retina. Specifically, in children these errors are myopia, hyperopia, astigmatism, anisometropia, and aphakia.

Although a decrease in visual acuity may cause an adult to seek ophthalmic attention, young children may not realize that they are not seeing well. Many of you are familiar with the 6- or 7-year-old who, upon receiving a first pair of glasses, remarks, "I didn't know the world looked like this!" Yet refractive errors are responsible for at least 50 percent of all referrals of children to eye examiners.[1] In addition, it is estimated that 9 percent of all 6-year-olds and 15 percent of all 15-year-olds require treatment with corrective lenses for their refractive errors.[2]

NURSING GOALS, OUTCOME STANDARDS, AND DIAGNOSES

This chapter's goal is that *the visual acuity of every child with a refractive error improves as much as possible with the proper use of prescriptive lenses.* Successful treatment of refractive errors is the simplest and most easily available treatment of all chronic eye disorders. Its potential for improving a person's vision can be awesome: a child with 20/400 vision secondary to a refractive error, who had no other eye disorder, would be legally blind if prescriptive lenses did not exist. With lenses the child can usually attain a visual acuity of 20/20! Such a difference in vision no doubt has a tremendous impact on the child's development and daily functioning. Yet before a child can benefit from prescriptive lenses, that child must first be identified and examined and then obtain and use the recommended lenses. Nurses are frequently able to work with children in all aspects of this process, from the simple and quick screenings in schools and community settings, through assisting with the retinoscopy process in the office or clinic, to follow-up back in the local environment.

Outcome Standard 1

Each child has a valid documentation of visual acuity every 2–3 years.

Suggested Interventions:

* Because many children with refractive errors, particularly those with myopia, fail their visual acuity screenings at distance, a number of suggested interventions are the same as those listed for Outcome Standard 1, Chapter 1. In addition, place children with a positive family history of refractive errors at a high priority for screenings, since many refractive errors tend to be inherited. Furthermore, use the pinhole technique described in Chapter 1 as a simple and fairly reliable method of determining which children fail their visual acuity screening secondary to a refractive error and which fail because of an organic eye disorder.
* Nurses with adequate time and materials should incorporate screening for hyperopia into their visual acuity assessments (see Chapter 2).

Outcome Standard 2

Each child with a suspected or documented refractive error is seen by a professional eye examiner at recommended intervals.

Outcome Standard 3

Each child with a suspected or documented refractive error receives an accurate retinoscopy examination.

Suggested Interventions:

* The nurse refers children who do not pass their visual acuity screening to an appropriate eye care specialist. The nurse maintains a list of local ophthalmologists and optometrists who enjoy working with children and provides such information to families as necessary. Children whose vision improves with the pinhole technique can be referred to either an ophthalmologist or an optometrist. However, children who fail the pinhole test or children too young to participate in it must be referred to an ophthalmologist, since the possibility is greater that these children have organic causes for their decreased vision.
* The nurse follows all children who do not pass their visual acuity screening to ensure that each one has had an examination by a professional eye examiner.
* The nurse follows all children with prescriptive lenses to ensure that they return as necessary to their professional eye examiner for follow-up appointments and possible changes in the prescription.
* The nurse assists the patient and family in correctly carrying out any home instructions needed for the professional eye examination, such as the safe and proper administration of atropine or homatropine. (See Table 3-1, a nursing care plan for atropine eyedrop administration, and Table 3-2, the procedure for administering eyedrops to children.)
* The nurse assists the child and family in increasing their knowledge of the retinoscopy process and in decreasing their fears and anxieties through such

preparatory interventions as the use of dolls or other play equipment, story books, pictures, and preexamination visualization of the actual equipment.

• The nurse makes every possible effort to decrease the discomfort associated with the administration or aftereffects of eyedrops or ophthalmic instruments and equipment. For example, the nurse instructs children receiving eyedrops with mydriatic properties to protect their eyes from bright lights, or those receiving topical ophthalmic anesthetics to refrain from rubbing their eyes.

The nursing diagnoses associated with Outcome Standards 2 and 3 include *noncompliance, potential for physical injury, knowledge deficit, anxiety* or *fears* regarding procedures and equipment, *alterations in comfort,* and *sensory deficit* (visual).

Outcome Standard 4

Each child with a refractive error possesses a pair of glasses or contact lenses with the appropriate correction.

Outcome Standard 5

Each child with a refractive error uses the glasses or contact lenses at all recommended times.

Suggested Interventions:

• The nurse assists the child and family in identifying and removing any barriers to obtaining and using glasses or contact lenses (potential *noncompliance*). For example, financial problems may interfere with a family's ability to purchase prescriptive lenses *(impaired home maintenance management).* Or the child or family may not understand the purpose of the prescriptive lenses and may have such misconceptions *(knowledge deficit)* as thinking that using the glasses will "weaken the child's eyes."

Even when the lenses are purchased, numerous problems may interfere with their use. The sections on glasses and contact lenses describe these problems in detail. Briefly, the use of prescriptive lenses may *alter* a child's *body-image* or may cause additional *sensory perceptual alterations* if they are dirty or old, or if a period of adjustment is necessary. In addition, if they are poorly fitted or used at inappropriate times (for example, overuse by contact lens users), *alteration in comfort* may result. Furthermore, *social isolation* can result if peers or family members make fun of the child with glasses.

Children with moderate to severe refractive errors who do not wear their glasses or contact lenses will have an increased *potential for physical injury* and *impaired physical mobility* because of the associated decrease in their vision. Finally, *ineffective coping* by the child or parents may result in the child's not wearing the lenses. For example, parents of a 1-year-old with bilateral aphakia who are frustrated in their attempts to persuade the child to wear the glasses may simply stop trying. The nurse may use such techniques as counseling, education, role playing, behavior modification, or play therapy, to help these families.

Table 3-1

Nursing Care Plan for Atropine Eyedrop Administration

Nursing Diagnosis	Nursing Interventions	Rationale
Potential for poisoning to patient; Knowledge deficit	Instruct the parent to administer the medication only if the appointment will be kept	If the appointment is not kept, the child will receive atropine needlessly. If the appointment is changed, additional atropine may be required for the desired effects.
	Instruct the parent about the expected side effects of atropine (see other nursing diagnoses).	If parents are aware of the normal side effects, they will be able to identify abnormal effects. Signs of atropine allergy include itching, redness, and edema of the eye area.
	Give the parent a phone number to call in case other reactions occur.	
	When possible, use atropine ophthalmic drops instead of atropine ointment.	Signs of atropine toxicity include high fevers, tachycardia, visual hallucinations, delirium, tremors, weakness, irritability, enlarged bladder leading to a distended abdomen, cough, difficulty in swallowing, and rash on the face or trunk. A fatal dose for children is approximately 10 mg. Atropine toxicity is treated in children with 1 mg/m^2 of body surface of physostigmine, given IM,* IV,** or SC.† 0.25 mg every 15 min may be repeated until the child recovers. Atropine ointment yields unknown doses because of its random absorption. Premature babies and children with Down syndrome or CNS damage have a higher incidence of atropine toxicity.
	Ask the family to inform other health care providers that the child is receiving atropine, particularly if the child receives care in an emergency room setting secondary to trauma, because dilated pupils may also indicate brain damage.	
	Provide the parents with clear, written instructions, preferably in their native language, about the prescribed dose and frequency of atropine eyedrops.	Written instructions provide an additional safeguard against administration of incorrect dosage.

(continued)

Table 3-1 *(continued)*

Nursing Diagnosis	Nursing Interventions	Rationale
	Emphasize to the parent that one drop means one drop only and that unless the medication misses the child's eye entirely, it should not be repeated until the next prescribed time.	One drop of 1 percent contains 0.5 mg of the drug, the usual preoperative dose!
	Review the method of eyedrop administration listed in Table 3–2 and emphasize the mechanism of occluding the tear duct.	Obstruction of the tear duct is thought to help decrease systemic absorption by the nasal mucosa. It also decreases the complaint some children make of a funny taste from atropine going through the tear duct into the nose and throat. Atropine oil suspensions are not absorbed from the nasal mucosa.
	(Although few children have glaucoma, remember that atropine may increase intraocular pressure in persons having that condition.)	
Potential for poisoning to all family members	Counsel the parent to keep atropine out of reach of all children.	As stated, a little atropine goes a long way and can be life-threatening in large doses.
	When treatment is completed, instruct the parent to discard any remaining medicine down the toilet or sink, before discarding the container.	
	Encourage the use of 1.0 ml ampules for dispensing atropine, to limit availability of excess medication.	
	Counsel the parent not to use the atropine for any other purpose or person.	
Alteration in comfort: flushed skin with possible increased body temperature secondary to vasodilation.	Review or instruct the parent on reading a thermometer and taking a child's temperature.	Many parents stop the medication because the child feels warm, although the child may not have a fever; in addition, many parents hesitate to admit that they have difficulty reading a thermometer.
	Instruct the parent to take and record the temperature if the child feels warm; if the child has a fever, the parent should follow the physician's directions.	

Alteration in comfort: dry mouth and skin secondary to the effect of atropine on sweat gland production	Parent should offer fluids frequently; teething rings for infants and lollipops for older children may provide palliative relief.	One source states that a "70 percent inhibition of salivation has already occured at a dosage that reduces accommodation by only 10 percent."[3]
Alteration in comfort: photophobia secondary to enlarged pupils	Instruct the parents to cover the child's eyes with a hat or sunglasses in the sun and brightly lit areas as long as the pupils remain dilated.	Dilated pupils cannot restrict the amount of light entering the eye. Hence, discomfort can result from excess light rays hitting against the retina.
	Instruct the parents in identifying a dilated pupil and the normal pupillary response to light.	
Sensory deficit: blurred near vision secondary to enlarged pupils and loss of accommodation	Inform the parent (and the child, depending on age) that vision at near will be blurred for up to 14 days.	Because of the duration of its effect on vision, atropine is often used only for infants or young children with excessive accommodation.
	Explain that attendance at school is permissible if teachers are notified and near work is avoided.	
	Infants and children may initially be frustrated by the change in vision but usually adjust well within a few days. However, because such frustration may be confused with behavioral changes secondary to atropine toxicity, tell the parent to call about any concerns.	

*IM = intramuscular, **IV = intravenous, †SC = subcutaneous.

Table 3-2
Procedure for Administering Eyedrops to Children

1. Assemble the eyedrops and tissues or cotton balls; check that you have the correct medication by reading the label before each use.
2. Wash your hands.
3. Prepare the child by describing what you are going to do and demonstrating on a doll (using water for medication); simultaneously describe the sensations (cold, "funny," or stinging) as the eyedrops fall into the doll's eyes. Allow the child to administer drops to the doll if he desires.
4. Tell the child to sit or lie down. Depending on the age and coopertiveness, you may need assistance in holding the child's head or body. For safe administration, a squirming child requires a minimum of two people. In the home, a child can be held by another adult or mummified with a blanket. You may want to hold the child's arms above the head as the child lies on the table to limit both head and arm motion simultaneously.
5. If the child is cooperative, ask him to look up toward his forehead to help decrease the blinking reflex that occurs as a foreign body (the eyedrops, in this case) approaches the eye.
6. Pull the lower lid down gently to form a small pocket with the conjunctival sac.
7. Hold the eyedrops in a perpendicular position to the eye (hold ointments parallel) and be careful not to touch the eye (contaminated bottles must be discarded or cleaned); if you hold the bottle too far away, the drops will land uncomfortably on the eye.
8. Develop a system of always instilling the medication onto the right eye first. In this way, no confusion will result if the process is interrupted.
9. Instill the prescribed amount into the pocket and release the lower lid. If you are using an ointment, squeeze only a 1/2-inch ribbon onto the eye, unless otherwise instructed.
10. Let the child keep the eyes closed for about 15 seconds and, if possible, roll them around to help distribute the medication.
11. At the same time hold a clean tissue for about 30–60 seconds over the tear duct to help decrease systemic absorption (the benefit of this procedure is currently under debate); or turn the head toward the eye that received the medication, so that the excess can run down the side of the face. Clean away excess medication from around the eye with a clean tissue or cotton ball.
12. Wash your hands to remove any remaining medication.
13. If the child desires, let him re-enact the eyedrop administration procedure, using a doll or stuffed animal.

OPTICS

The term *optics* refers to the physical characteristics of light. The following discussion explains some of the optical characteristics of errors of refraction.

By convention, light rays are assumed to go from left to right. The direction and power of light rays is called *vergence,* and the unit of measurement of vergence is the *diopter (D).* When light rays (other than laser beams) leave a source of light, they fan out in all directions and hence are called *divergent rays* (Fig. 3-1). On the other hand, light rays that come together at a specific point are called *convergent* rays. Light rays that neither travel from a source nor toward a focus are said to be *parallel.*

Divergence and convergence are the principles upon which prescriptive lenses are based. For example, in myopia the light rays naturally fall short of the retina. By changing the refraction of these light rays through divergence, we can lengthen their point of focus to the retina. Divergence is achieved by using concave (or minus) lenses, which are thin in the center and thick at the edge. Hyperopia, however, involves the opposite problem. The light rays fall naturally behind the retina and require convex (or plus) lenses to shorten them through convergence.

These basic principles of optics can assist you in correcting some long-held myths regarding prescriptive lenses. For example, many parents believe that glasses either weaken a child's refractive problem or, conversely, stop its progression. In reality, however, corrective lenses simply neutralize the problem by refocusing light rays; the lenses themselves have no relation to the original cause of the refractive problem.

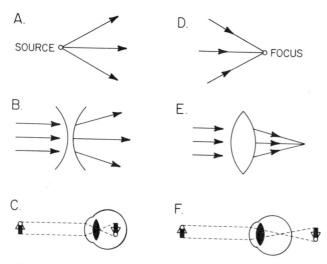

Fig. 3-1. Some optical principles regarding errors of refraction. A: Divergent light rays. B: A concave (minus) lens, which causes light rays to diverge or lengthen. C: A myopic eye. Note how the natural lens cannot focus the image on the retina, so the image falls before it. A concave lens would correct this error. D: Convergent light rays. E: A convex (plus) lens, which causes the light rays to converge or shorten. F: A hyperopic eye: the image falls beyond the retina and can be corrected with a convex lens.

ANATOMY

The eye's major anatomic components related to refractive errors involve the cornea, diameter of the eye, lens, and ciliary body (Fig. 3-2). In addition, the eyelids and lacrimal system play a significant role in the wearing of contact lenses.

The *cornea* is a clear five-layered cover protecting the iris and pupil. Its first and most anterior layer is the *epithelium,* which is also the most regenerative.

In order for light rays to be transmitted precisely through the lens onto the retina, the cornea must be well-curved and smooth. An unequal curvature will cause unequal focusing *(astigmatism).* Too flat a cornea will cause the rays to fall beyond the retina, resulting in *hyperopia.* Too much curvature will cause *myopia,* because the rays will fall before the retina.

Keratometry is the measurement of corneal curvature. Besides assisting in identifying children with refractive problems secondary to abnormal corneal curvatures, keratometry is also used in fitting contact lenses and for patients with keratoconus.

Because the cornea is avascular, it relies on the atmosphere and tears for assistance in its metabolism. When a contact lens is present, the cornea's meta-

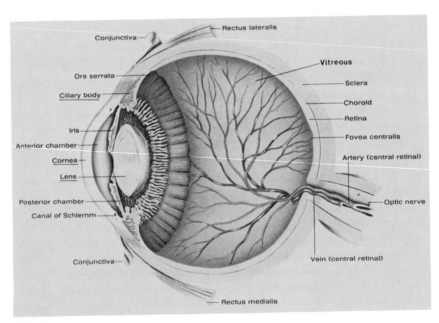

Fig. 3-2. A cross-secional view of the eye. The ciliary body, cornea, and lens play important roles in refractive errors, as does the diameter of the globe (eyeball). (Illustration reproduced with permission of Burroughs Wellcome Company)

bolic rate increases in order to continue the exchange of oxygen and other gases through the barrier of the lens. In contrast, the cornea's metabolic rate decreases during sleep.

The length or diameter of the *globe* (eyeball) is another primary variable that may cause errors of refraction. Averaging 16 millimeters (mm) in diameter at birth, the globe grows rapidly during the first year of life; it approaches its adult size of approximately 24 mm in diameter during a child's early school years. The approximate length of one's globe is influenced by heredity. When it is too long for the refractive power of the eye, images are focused in front of the retina, causing myopia. On the other hand, persons with hyperopia may have eyeballs that are too short, causing the rays of light to extend too far.

The *lens* also plays an important role in refraction. Like a camera lens, its purpose is to focus light, in this case, on the retina. The lens remains transparent because it lacks vascular and nerve supplies. Instead, aqueous solutions surrounding it provide metabolites, and the ciliary muscles control its size. When a cataract develops (that is, the lens loses its transparency), this ability to focus light is impaired and the person cannot see clearly.

In persons below the age of 40, the lens provides approximately 20 D, or one-third of the focusing power of the eye. (The cornea provides the other two-thirds.) The power of the lens can be varied to provide *accommodation,* whereby the lens becomes thicker and its surface more curved so that a person can focus nearby objects. Otherwise, when the eye is looking at objects in the distance, the lens is thin and has a flat surface; its ability to refract light rays is at a minimum. In the early years, the lens responds well to the movements of the ciliary muscles around it and is quite elastic, so that it can accommodate easily. In fact, the power of the lens in newborns and infants is higher than in older people because so much of infants' visual functioning is at close range. As a result, they require even greater accommodative powers. This elasticity, however, decreases with time. In the middle years we develop presbyopia. The elasticity of the lens decreases to such a point that it can no longer accommodate or change its shape from distant to near vision.

The *ciliary body,* located in a circle behind the iris, has two main functions. When its muscular component contracts, the fibers connecting it with the lens are relaxed, allowing the lens to accommodate; when the ciliary muscles relax, on the other hand, the tension on the zonular fibers increases and accommodation ceases. As will be seen in Chapter 9, the secretory component of the ciliary body assists in the fluid circulation within the eye, a phenomenon important to understanding glaucoma.

Finally, the *eyelids* and *lacrimal system* are important for persons who wear contact lenses. Normally a person blinks once every 4 seconds. At this frequency, enough tear fluid is transported to maintain the corneal metabolic equilibrium. In addition, blinking and tearing keep the contact lens clean and free of dust particles and hold the contact lens in place.

RETINOSCOPY

Retinoscopy is a simple, objective method for determining a refractive error. It is performed by professional eye examiners or their specially trained assistants. Eyes that are not in perfect focus during retinoscopy have a refractive error and are said to be *ametropic*. Those in perfect focus are called *emmetropic*.

Infants and toddlers are often frightened by the retinoscopy procedure, crying frequently and closing their eyes. To decrease these fears, examiners may ask children to sit on a parent's lap and view cartoons on a screen in the distance. If this does not work, however, it may be necessary to place the child in a blanket or special restraint and to insert a wire speculum in the eye to keep the lids separated (Fig. 3-3). In rare cases, the examiners may have to perform the refraction in the operating room under general anesthesia. Be aware that the restraints and wire speculums may appear barbaric to some parents, and that they may require additional support and clarification, despite the eye examiner's explanations.

During retinoscopy, all accommodation by the patient must be removed, so it does not interfere with the focusing process. To remove accommodation in adults, the examiner asks the patient to look at an object about 20 feet away. However, because accommodation is so strong in children, eyedrops must usually be administered to paralyze the ciliary muscles, which ultimately control accommodation temporarily; this process of paralysis is called *cycloplegia*. Errors in the prescription of a child's lenses can result when some accommodation remains during the retinoscopy; this is especially true for children with hyperopia.

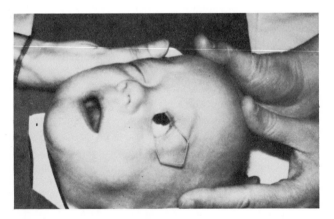

Fig. 3-3.   Some parents may become upset by the strange appearance of a speculum in their child's eye.

After the objective measurement of the refractive error has been completed through the use of the retinoscope, it is desirable to obtain a *manifest refraction,* or subjective opinion, from the patient regarding the selected lenses. Older children and adults sit in a chair and compare various lenses in the phoroptor. For younger children who are able to give a subjective response but have received eyedrops, the examiner will use a trial lens set and frame at a later visit. The *trial set* is a frame without lenses into which the examiner places selected lenses. Through trial and error, the examiner asks the child which lenses help the child to see best. For very young children or those with developmental special needs, the trial frame may be somewhat frightening; hence, the examiner may prefer to hold loose lenses before the child's eyes to help determine which are preferable.

LENS PRESCRIPTIONS

You can determine whether a child has astigmatism, myopia, or hyperopia by noting the numbers in a horizontal row on the ophthalmic report. The first number refers to the degree of hyperopia or myopia present. When it is preceded by a plus sign, it indicates hyperopia; when it is preceded by a minus sign, it refers to myopia. When no other numbers are present or the letters *sph* (for "sphere") are included, the child does not have astigmatism. For example, *+3.50* and *+3.50 sph* both indicate that the child has hyperopia and requires a correction of 3.50 D.

When a prescription for glasses contains additional numbers, the second number refers to the degree of astigmatism, and the third number refers to its location. If the eye is considered as a 360-degree circle, with 180 degrees being horizontal, then the location of the astigmatism is 90 degrees from what is written on the prescription. Depending upon the notation system, the astigmatism may be preceded by a plus or minus sign. An example of a notation indicating astigmatism is

$$+3.50 \qquad +1.00 \times 180°$$

These figures indicate that the child needs 3.50 D of correction for hyperopia, with an additional plus 1.00 D of correction in the vertical (90-degree) axis. Lenses used to correct myopia or hyperopia are called *spherical lenses; cylindrical lenses* are used to correct astigmatism. A child who loses a prescription can take the lenses to an eye examiner or optician, who can readily identify the exact prescription with a lensometer.

When you read a child's prescription for contact lenses, you will notice other measurements. The *base curve* of a contact lens is derived from the measurement of the corneal curvature. As its name implies, the base, or posterior, of the contact lens is made to match the corneal curvature of the child's eye. It usually ranges from 8 to 10 mm; the higher the number, the flatter the curve. The power of the lens (in the front of the contact lens) is usually written the same way it is for glasses. The diameter of the lens however, is also noted. For soft lenses, the diameter is written in millimeters, usually ranging from 13.5 to 16.0 mm. Since the average cornea is 12 mm in diameter, the soft lens extends slightly beyond the cornea.

CYCLOPLEGIC EYEDROPS

The word *cycloplegia,* from the Greek words meaning "circle" and "paralysis," refers to the chemical inhibition of the ciliary muscles. As a result of the process, accommodation is likewise inhibited. Although cycloplegia is preferred when refracting most children, it is mandatory in refracting those who have crossed eyes or hyperopia.

Cycloplegia is often confused with *mydriasis.* However, this latter process refers to the dilation of the pupil and accompanies cycloplegia. The use of mydriatic drugs is quite helpful when examining the retina, as described in Chapter 7.

The most common cycloplegia drugs are atropine sulfate, homatropine hydrobromide, isopto-hyoseine (Scopolamine; Elkins-Sinn); cyclopentolate (Cyclogyl; Alcon Laboratories); and tropicamide (Mydriacyl; Alcon Laboratories). Children with dark irides often require increased amounts of these drugs. Dark irides have higher amounts of melanin than lighter irides. Since melanin binds to many drugs, additional time and medication are necessary for creating the desired effect, and more time is required for the effect to disappear. In contrast, noticeably fair-skinned children require lower amounts of medication.

Atropine and Its Derivatives

Atropine, the oldest cycloplegic drug, is a natural alkaloid made from the deadly nightshade plant, belladonna. Used in 0.5 and 1.0 percent ophthalmic strengths, it acts on the smooth muscles and secretory glands. Although ophthalmologists vary in their selection, it is common to use the 0.5 percent or weaker strengths for infants less than 12–18 months. The usual regimen is one drop of atropine in each eye, given two or three times a day for 3 days preceding an appointment; in addition, one drop is usually placed into each eye on the morning of the appointment. Such a routine yields both cycloplegic and mydriatic effects, the former lasting up to 14 days. Because of this lengthy duration and resulting interference with near vision, atropine is rarely given to school-aged children.

Table 3-1 is a nursing care plan for children receiving atropine, which elaborates on the numerous side and toxic effects for which atropine is well known.

Because of these effects, some ophthalmologists prefer to use atropine on rare occasions only, since it is administered in the home and they cannot monitor its effects. However, other ophthalmologists consider atropine the drug of choice when refracting children with strabismus or excessive hyperopia. With proper instruction and preparation, the risks from its administration can be markedly decreased. Besides its use in refraction, atropine is employed in treating iridocyclitis, in providing occlusion in certain types of amblyopia, and during some ophthalmic surgeries.

Homatropine hydrobromide is a weaker relative of atropine. It is mainly used during cycloplegic refractions of preschool children, who may find the lengthy blurred vision from atropine inconvenient; the cycloplegic and mydriatic effects of homatropine last for several days only. At Childrens Hospital of Los Angeles, 5 percent homatropine is administered in the home eight times, at 15-minute intervals, starting about 2-1/2 hours before the child's appointment. Other examiners may use weaker strengths, 2 percent or 4 percent, and may administer the homatropine in their offices. Side effects, such as blurred vision, photophobia, fever, and flushing, are similar to those seen in the administration of atropine.

Isopto-hyoseine (Scopolamine; Elkins-Sinn) 0.2 percent is an older cycloplegic drug, which is now usually used only if a child is hypersensitive to atropine. It has a significant incidence of disorientation, hallucination, and other central nervous system (CNS) involvement, as well as an increased incidence of urinary incontinence. Its cycloplegic and mydriatic effects usually last from 3 to 8 days.

Synthetic Cycloplegics

Cyclopentolate (Cyclogyl; Alcon Laboratories) is administered in the office setting, since it requires only 30–60 minutes waiting time after the administration of one or two drops. Cycloplegia and mydriasis last about 24 hours; in some children the mydriasis has been known to last even longer.

Cyclopentolate is available in 0.5 percent, 1 percent, and 2 percent concentrations, although the 2 percent is used cautiously in children because of increased CNS disturbances. Even the 1 percent concentration (which is the most commonly used) can cause hallucinations and altered cerebellar functioning in children. Administration of cyclopentolate in children who have a history of brain damage should therefore be carefully considered. For example, a 4-year-old, blond-haired boy who had intraventricular hemorrhage at birth was seen in the office. About 40 minutes after the administration of 1 percent cyclopentolate the boy's face became flushed, and he began to act strangely. A few minutes later, he was hallucinating, quite fearful, and clinging tightly to his mother. Nursing interventions included notifying the physician, dimming the lights in the room to decrease visual stimuli, sitting with the parent and child while providing reassurance, and monitoring the child's vital signs. His behavior returned to normal about 90 minutes later.

In young infants, the 0.5 percent strength is more commonly used, since delayed gastric emptying has been reported with more potent strengths.

Cyclopentolate is also used for children who have an allergy to atropine. However, repeated use of cyclopentolate also can create allergic sensitivity. Although this reaction is rare and usually does not happen during the office visit, patients may report that they experienced redness and an eye discharge for a day or two following the administration of cyclopentolate.

Two other drugs frequently used in combination with cyclopentolate are tropicamide, 0.5 percent and 1 percent (Mydriacyl; Alcon Laboratories) and phenylephrine, 2.5 percent and 10 percent (Neo-Synephrine; Winthrop). Tropicamide provides both mydriasis and cycloplegia, although its cycloplegic effect is not so strong that it can be used alone. Its mydriatic effect lasts 4–6 hours, and it is generally considered a safe drug for children. Phenylephrine provides a short-acting mydriasis (3 hours) with no cycloplegia. The 2.5 percent strength has no reported systemic effects, even in infants. The 10 percent strength, however, can cause vasoconstriction with a resultant hypertension and reflex bradycardia. In addition, arrhythmias occur in rare instances, and a temporary topical blanching of the skin has been noted in a number of infants. Since phenylephrine is a pure mydriatic, children receiving only this drug will not have any disturbance in their vision; however, they may complain of photophobia and, as with all mydriatic drugs, should be advised to protect their eyes from the sun or bright lights with sunglasses or a hat.

Topical Anesthetics

Patients often report that cyclopentolate and tropicamide eyedrops sting their eyes. As a result, many eye examiners first administer a topical anesthetic. Proparacaine 0.5 percent (Ophthaine; Squibb; Alcaine; Alcon Laboratories; or Ophthetic; Allergan) is one such anesthetic commonly used in the United States, and 0.5 percent tetracaine (Pontocaine; Breon) is frequently used in the United Kingdom. Although proparacaine drops may also sting initially, they cause a numbing sensation, which develops 20 seconds after their administration and lasts approximately 10–15 minutes. Hence, eyedrops administered after proparacaine usually feel cold but do not sting. Proparacaine is usually helpful when the child will receive more than one dosage of cyclopentolate or tropicamide. To help them endure the initial stinging, suggest that your young patients sing a stanza of their favorite song or count to 10. By the time they finish, the stinging sensation from the proparacaine will have ceased. Also warn them to blot their eyes with their lids closed, rather than rubbing or wiping them; otherwise, they made abrade the cornea without realizing it because of the numbness from the anesthetic.

Proparacaine is also used during glaucoma testing *(tonometry),* and conjunctival scrapings, and removal of foreign bodies or sutures from the cornea. However, it should not be used on a regular basis, for instance, for corneal abrasion, since it tends to inhibit corneal healing. Instillation of one or two drops of proparacaine causes minimal side effects, but the solution should be clear when used.

Cocaine in concentrations of up to 4 percent has also been used as an ophthalmic anesthetic. However, it has an increased incidence of toxicity to the cornea, and federal narcotics laws make its use more difficult.

Preparation of the Child

To many children, the administration of eyedrops is a threatening procedure. Even with the use of a topical anesthetic they may not understand that the other drops will not hurt. Therefore, to minimize the negative effects, incorporate some play activities into the procedure. For example, keep a small doll that has blinking eyes and simple clothes nearby. In addition, fill an old ophthalmic drop bottle with water and label it carefully to show that it has nonsterile contents. Before administering drops to young children, show them the routine, using the doll as the patient. Be brief in your explanation but be sure to mention what the doll feels as you put in the drops. Then let the children place eyedrops into the doll's eyes (Fig. 3-4). Finally, administer the eyedrops to the children (Table 3-2). Although many children still scream or cry while receiving their eyedrops, they tend to have quicker recoveries; many will sit up and proceed to give the doll more drops, sometimes with much more intensity than before. A few children have been known to poke out the doll's eye! This play therapy works well even with children as young as 18 months; some use the eyedrop bottle to feed the doll, and others busy themselves dressing and undressing the doll.

A number of children feel threatened when they lie down, especially on an examining table. For this reason, some examiners use couches or let the child lie on the parent's lap during the administration of the eyedrops. Other children are quite influenced by modeling, and seeing a self-made slide or tape presentation using puppets or cartoon characters as patients may help decrease their own anxieties toward the eyedrop procedure. Whatever preparation techniques you choose to use, remember that the administration of eyedrops is a threatening procedure, and children should not be faulted for whatever coping behaviors they use during this process.

MYOPIA

Myopia (nearsightedness) can be divided into two types based on the clinical course. *Simple myopia* accounts for more than 99 percent of all myopic cases. It frequently progresses during the preteen and teenage years then stabilizes. Simple myopia results from a mismatch of corneal curvature and eye length that causes images to focus in front of the retina. *Pathologic myopia,* however, is a progres-

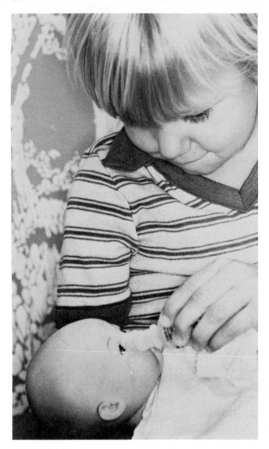

Fig. 3-4. This child is re-enacting the administration of eyedrops as part of the preparation program before and after this procedure.

sive myopia that can lead to a retinal degenerative process and can ultimately cause scarring and retinal detachment with possible permanent loss of vision. Pathologic myopia is sometimes seen in children with retrolental fibroplasia, Marfan's syndrome, or Down syndrome.

Over the years, two main theories have been used to explain the etiology of myopia. The current and most widely accepted theory, based on genetics, states that most cases of simple myopia are inherited through a recessive gene. For this reason, ask about a family history of myopia in any child who has suspicious symptoms. The older use–abuse theory has been disregarded until recently; however, some scientists have lately begun studying it again as a possible cause in certain cases of myopia. Proponents of the use–abuse theory state that close work over a long period of time causes excess tension on the ciliary muscles, which are already providing greater refractive strength for the close work. Finally, some studies are investigating whether certain vitamin deficiencies and other environmental factors can cause myopia; so far no correlations have been documented.

Infrequently, an infant may be diagnosed with *congenital myopia*. Most children with myopia, however, are of the "school variety" type: around the puberty years, the eyeball experiences growth at a faster rate than the rest of the body, causing myopia. By the age of 20 years, most persons with myopia will have reached a stable refraction and experience little change for the following 20 years or so. Then, around the 40-year mark, signs and symptoms of presbyopia develop.

Children with significant myopia often exhibit several classic symptoms. They rarely complain of headaches or fatigue. Instead, they prefer to sit close to the television or chalkboard because of their blurred distance vision. They likewise have a decreased interest in outside activities that require distance vision, such as ball games. In addition, they often squint or have a "closed-eye" appearance. The squinting, which is unconscious, allows them to see better by changing the refraction of the light rays; it is similar to the pinhole effect used during visual acuity screening.

Treatment for myopia employs prescription lenses, whether they are in glasses or contact lenses. Normally, myopia of less than 0.50 D is not treated. Children who have a refractive error between –0.5 and –1.5 D are considered to have mild myopia and may or may not need glasses for distance vision. Children with myopic changes of greater than –1.5 D, however, should be encouraged to use their glasses at all times. If their myopia is greater than –6.0 D, they are considered to have high myopia and may be advised to refrain from contact sports to help prevent retinal detachment, a complication associated with high myopia.

For children receiving their first prescription lenses, it is important to allow adequate time for adjustment to the lenses. This is especially true if a child is receiving a strong prescription, since objects in the environment may appear smaller and the child may see reflections from the edges of the glasses. Remind both parents and children that the lenses do not cure the eye problem but merely alter the light rays, causing them to focus back onto the retina for clear vision.

Once the myopia stabilizes in the late teens or early twenties, a person may prefer to have contact lenses. This preference may not be for the sake of cosmesis only, but also because contact lenses do not change the size of images the way regular lenses do, and because they cause no added reflection. The use of extended wear contact lenses for myopia is increasing; patients must remove them only every month or two for cleaning. Furthermore, an entire branch of optometry, *orthokeratology,* is pursuing the possibility of decreasing the lens curvature of myopes by using contact lenses (see the section on contact lenses).

In recent years a surgical procedure for the correction of myopia, known as *radial keratotomy,* has been studied. Developed in Russia and used in the United States since 1978, this painless 15-minute procedure is performed with local anesthesia. It attempts to decrease the curvature of the eye via small radial microincisions around the outside of the cornea. However, radial keratotomy is still considered experimental and the National Advisory Eye Council, in cooperation with the National Eye Institute, has established a multicenter study of adults to evaluate its short- and long-term effects.

Refractive keratoplasty is another surgical modification of the cornea that is being pursued for the treatment of myopia. In general, all or part of the cornea is removed, altered, and replaced. The results have been variable, with the development of lens opacities as one complication.

Visual training, or eye exercises, do not improve myopia, since myopia is a result of structural changes within the eye.

Finally, remind children with myopia to see their eye examiner at 6- to 12-month intervals until they reach the age of 16 or so. After this age, the myopia starts to stabilize, and fewer changes will be needed in the lens prescription.

HYPEROPIA (HYPERMETROPIA)

In hyperopia, either the diameter of the globe is too short *(axial hyperopia),* or less commonly, the cornea is too flat *(curvature hyperopia).* Either problem causes light rays to focus behind the retina (Fig. 3-1). In order to shorten the focal point of these rays naturally, the lenses of the eye accommodate, or become thicker in the center. A child who needs extensive accommodation may complain of frontal headaches, fatigue, nausea, burning, or blurring of vision. In addition, the child may refrain from close work, hold books farther away, or become irritable from increased tension.

Most young children are naturally hyperopic, with their refraction increasing to approximately + 3.00 D at about 7 years of age and decreasing subsequently. Hence, although hyperopia is technically defined as a refractive error of + 1.50 D or more, it is often not treated in the younger years until the + 4.00 D range or until the child develops some of the symptoms listed previously. Children not in these categories will often use their accommodative powers to correct the hyperopia themselves.

During an examination, a child with hyperopia or excessive accommodation requires cycloplegic drops. When the child returns for a second visit, the examiner can determine how much accommodation the child uses to compensate for the hyperopia naturally. From these results a prescription can be determined. Some examiners prefer to undercorrect or overcorrect a child's hyperopia, depending on the child's age and whether strabismus is present.

If the hyperopia is mild, the child may wear glasses only for reading or for close work. If strong hyperopia is present, however, or if accommodative esotropia occurs, the child will need glasses at all times. Bifocals are often prescribed for children with accommodative esotropia or a high accommodative convergence–

accommodation ratio. The top portion of the lens is used for distance vision and the bottom portion for close work.

As with myopia, contact lenses may also be used for the correction of hyperopia, but vision therapy is not applicable. Be aware that sometimes children with hyperopia may do slightly better on a distance vision acuity screening without their glasses than with them.

ASTIGMATISM

Astigmatism is related to irregularly shaped corneas. Although in reality no one has a perfectly rounded cornea, everyone does not have astigmatism. The unequalness in the curvature must be significant enough to cause an unequal refraction among the various meridians *(axes)*. Therefore, *significant astigmatism* is defined as a difference of 1.00 D or more between two opposite axes of the same eye. At this value, some light rays will be clearly focused onto the retina, and others will not. For example, a child may have no refractive error along the 180-degree axis but have a +2.00 D error along the 90-degree axis. The child will not be able to focus images clearly because of the astigmatism.

A child may have astigmatism with myopia, with hyperopia, or simply by itself. As in the cases of myopia and hyperopia, it is felt that astigmatism is usually inherited. In addition, we know that astigmatism can be induced by contact lenses, trauma to the cornea, masses that push on the eye, and eye surgery.

Although 3- and 4-year-old children may have a small degree of astigmatism, they may not become symptomatic for years. In late childhood, however, students may complain of decreased vision, headaches, burning eyes, and blurred or distorted vision. In addition, they may squint and prefer not to do prolonged close work. During a visual acuity screening, they may miss some, but not all, of the symbols on the lower lines of the eye chart.

As with myopia and hyperopia, the treatment for astigmatism is with spectacle or contact lenses. Children who receive glasses to correct their astigmatism may initially have blurred vision until they adapt to their lenses; you may have to encourage these children to give the glasses an adequate trial.

Finally, see that these children receive yearly eye examinations, as astigmatism changes with age. This is especially true for individuals in the preschool years, in junior high, and in old age.

ANISOMETROPIA

Anisometropia refers to a difference of 1.00 D or more between the refractive strength of the two eyes. It is believed that 2 percent of the population has significant anisometropia. In children, it is occasionally present at birth but more likely develops during the first 4 years of life.

As discussed in Chapter 4, anisometropia can lead to amblyopia, as the young child with anisometropia cannot focus both eyes simultaneously. Hence, the child unconsciously prefers to use the better eye. This preference allows the weaker eye to have a constant, blurred image and eventually to become amblyopic.

In addition, anisometropia can lead to *asthenopia,* which is visual fatigue manifested by headaches, dizziness, burning, and blurring of vision secondary to weak ocular muscles. This problem can occur because the ciliary muscles of the two eyes are working unevenly.

As with all the other refractive errors, anisometropia is treated with prescriptive lenses. However, in anisometropia contact lenses are often preferred; in this way each eye can be corrected individually. Otherwise, glasses can cause *aniseikonia,* or the difference in the size of the ocular image in each eye. Because glasses can magnify or reduce the real world by significant percentages, different powers will be used for each eye to correct the anisometropia and the amount of magnification or reduction before each eye will be different. Children with anisometropia need to wear their prescriptive lenses at all times. This is especially true if they are less than 9 years old because they have an increased risk for developing amblyopia.

APHAKIA

Aphakia (''without lens'') describes the resulting refractive error when a lens is removed because of cataracts or trauma. High plus lenses are prescribed, in the form of a contact lens if the aphakia is unilateral or in glasses or contact lenses if it is bilateral. Aphakia is discussed in greater detail in Chapter 10.

GLASSES

In 1972 a federal law requiring all lenses to resist a specific impact was passed; therefore, lenses are now made of either tempered glass or plastic. Plastic lenses are more commonly used by children, athletes, persons with seizures, and those with good vision in one eye only because they are unbreakable. In addition, they weigh only half as much as glass lenses and so are preferred for persons requiring high-power correction. Unfortunately, plastic lenses scratch more easily and are more difficult to clean than glass lenses.

Teach children with plastic lenses to blow dust away from the lenses before cleaning and never to wipe the lenses while they are dry, as this can promote scratching. With either glass or plastic lenses, instruct children to clean them with water at least once a day and to dry them with a soft, clean cloth. They can use a mild soap and warm water for the lenses and frames once or twice a week and occasionally use a toothbrush for around the nose pads and hinges. Children should also refrain from placing their glasses with the lens side down; instead they should place them with the ear-pieces on the bottom. Finally, they should avoid sprays when they are wearing their glasses, to prevent damage to the lenses, and they should be aware of when the nose bridge or hinges need adjustment.

Reading glasses can infrequently be used by children for near work. Such children must have the same refractive error in each eye and have an average pupillary distance, as these glasses normally come in one frame size only. Four states—Massachusetts, Minnesota, New York, and Rhode Island—do not allow reading glasses to be sold over the counter. Remind children with this type of glasses not to use them for any distant vision, such as watching television, driving, or looking at the blackboard.

Prescription glasses can be obtained from an optometrist, optician, or ophthalmologist. In some states, children who scratch their glasses and have difficulty seeing through them as a result can take the glasses to an optician. The optician then determines the exact prescription with a lensometer, duplicates it, and provides new lenses to the child. However, other states require a new prescription from an optometrist or ophthalmologist for each new pair of lenses that an optician makes.

Unbelievable as it may seem, half of all prescriptive glasses in the United States are *bifocals* and *multifocals*. These glasses are used by persons who require different strengths for near and distant vision and are therefore most commonly used by adults who have presbyopia. However, they are also used by children who have accommodative esotropia or a high accommodative convergence–accommodation ratio. The two main types of bifocals are the progressive additional lens and the two-power lens. The latter is the traditional type that has a line separating the two different lenses. When a child has bifocals, they are usually of the two-power type. The top lens, which is used for distance, may be clear glass. To assess bifocals on a child, determine whether the line separating the lenses bisects the pupils when the child looks straight ahead.

Children's willingness to wear their glasses may be a challenging problem for nurses in selected settings. Although it is tempting to assume that children are being stubborn or vain, it is important to listen to them and assess their complaints.

For example, what is the purpose of the glasses? If the child has a refractive error, how severe is it? Many children with mild refractive errors do not require glasses at all times. To assist you in determining this, request the child's records from the eye examiner, along with the examiner's recommendations for use of the glasses.

Also assess whether the child understands the purpose of the glasses. Sometimes children or their parents may not be convinced of the need for glasses or may have wrong notions regarding their use. For instance, they may feel that the glasses weaken the child's eyes or make the child's eyes dependent on them. Through simple explanations of optics and refraction, you can change these misconceptions.

Also ask how long the child has been wearing this particular prescription. Some children, especially those with hyperopia, need time to adjust to their glasses.

By emphasizing this point, you may convince the child to "give the glasses a chance." If the child continues to complain that the glasses don't help, however, reassess the child's visual acuity both with and without glasses. Then compare your findings to the examiner's report. If you note a beneficial difference between the acuities taken with and without glasses, explain this benefit to the student. If, on the other hand, you find no difference, or your findings do not match those of the examiner, consult the examiner or refer the child for another examination (which may be overdue). There are numerous reasons why a child may have been given a wrong prescription. For instance, a child with diabetes may have fluctuating glucose levels during the refraction but may not share this with the examiner. Sulfa drugs can also cause temporary refractive changes. Although improper lenses won't hurt a child's eyes, they obviously won't help, either.

Another complaint you might hear is that the frames hurt behind the ears, pinch the nose, or do not otherwise fit properly. Often these complaints can be easily remedied in the examiner's office. To determine proper fit, see that the frames keep the lenses parallel before the eyes; if the frames are bent or broken, the lenses may not be precisely parallel. In addition, the child should be looking through the center of the lenses. During fitting, the examiner measures the interpupillary distance (PD) to locate the visual center and then suggests certain frames. However, if the child selects frames that are very fashionable, they may be too large or too small, and the visual center may be off. Some frames have been known to impede driving by blocking peripheral vision. Children from families with limited income who received their glasses either through welfare systems or charity organizations may have had a limited choice of frames and hence dislike them.

If, despite assessment of all of these issues, the child will not wear the glasses, then most likely the change in the child's body image caused by the glasses is the reason for the noncompliance. For children who have poor self-esteem, the addition of glasses is certainly no blessing. Some children have to endure teasing during school hours, then go home to a nonsupportive family environment. If the child or family views the glasses as a sign of weakness, intelligence, or aloofness, the child may assume these roles. So try to coax your uncooperative students into a private discussion about how the glasses interfere with their lives. If the glasses interfere with sports, athletic straps or headbands may alleviate the problem. If children feel unattractive in glasses, collect pictures and articles from various magazines to provide role models.

Be supportive and understanding to adolescent students. You may have to compromise your goals and settle for helping the student decide which situations require glasses and in which situations they are optional. Safety of the wearer and others is the primary purpose for mandatory use of glasses, for example, while driving or operating machinery. The student should also agree to wear glasses while studying. On the other hand, although sitting in the bleachers during a football game may not be very stimulating for someone who cannot see, it may be more psychologically gratifying for the student to do this.

Compliance by infants and young children may initially be no easier to enforce than with adolescents. However, these young children are susceptible to such problems as amblyopia. Hence, they do not have as many options regarding the use of their glasses, and parents may need much support as they pursue the "battle of the spectacles."

Some infants and young children readily accept glasses; they appear to be more influenced by the way the glasses help them see better than by the ways the glasses bother them physically. Others find it initially difficult to ignore the strange new thing resting on their nose and ears but need only a day or two to explore the glasses with their fingers, eyes, and mouths before they readily comply with the wearing regimen. However, still others will require a more ardent approach, and the child's eye examiner may have specific suggestions. One approach is to develop a behavioral modification program, starting with several brief time periods throughout the day. During each of these periods, the parent places the glasses on the child and then tries to distract the child with an age-appropriate activity. Each time the child removes the glasses, the parent places them back on and tries once again to divert the child's attention. Each day these time periods are lengthened until the child adjusts or becomes resigned enough to the glasses to accept them.

A more firm approach is to replace the glasses on the child's eyes consistently, whenever the child removes them. In this manner, the child will often accept the glasses within a 1- to 3-day period; however, these 1–3 days may be quite stressful for the family.

Finally, some parents choose to use a small reward system during the early stages of adjustment, especially for a child of preschool age. For example, the reward may be eating at a favorite hamburger stand. Each day that the child successfully wears glasses, a letter of the word *burger* is written on the family memo board. When the entire word is spelled out, the child is taken out to eat. Whichever method is selected to assist children in wearing their glasses, remind parents that occasionally the child will test parents and teachers by removing the glasses.

Finally, additional interventions that may involve nurses include locating financial resources, such as the Lion's Club, to assist children in obtaining glasses and monitoring a regular follow-up program to see that these children receive any necessary treatment. In addition, you may wish to consider starting a recycling program for glasses that are no longer used; contact your local NSPB office or charity organizations for more information.

CONTACT LENSES

Contact lenses may be desirable for infants and children to provide optical correction of various congenital or traumatic conditions. These include unilateral or bilateral aphakia, aniridia, albinism, severe coloboma, corneal opacities or scars, or high refractive errors. They may also serve as bandage lenses to promote healing or to relieve pain.

Types of Lenses

With the advances in contact lens design over the last decade, there are now various types of plastics and designs available.

Hard lenses are those made from polymethylmethacrylate (PMMA), cellulose acetate butyrate (CAB), and polyacrylate silicone. The last two groups are gas-permeable. Hard lenses are smaller than a dime, being approximately 7.0–10 mm in diameter. They cover only the pupil and iris and may be clear or tinted. They may also be fenestrated, with little ''windows'' in them to allow for increased gas exchange. PMMA hard lenses are the oldest type of contact lenses. They are generally less expensive, more durable, and easier to care for than soft lenses. Hard lenses in general are known to cause more discomfort during their first weeks of use, however. As a result, the user must wear the hard lenses on a regular basis; each time there is a period of nonuse, the corneas must build up tolerance again. In addition, hard lenses decenter more often than soft lenses. They also scratch easily, may shatter, and generally need to be removed during sleep in order to prevent corneal complications. Finally, the use of hard lenses can result in *spectacle blur*, or the temporary modification of one's refractive error.

Soft lenses (both daily and extended wear types) are usually made from the soft polymer hydroxyethylmethacrylate (HEMA). Soft lenses are also called hydrogels or *hydrophilic* (water-loving), as they have a water content ranging from 35 to 85 percent; the higher the content, the greater the amount of oxygen permeability. Soft lenses extend beyond the cornea (Fig. 3-5A) and generally

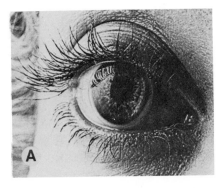

Fig. 3-5A.   A soft contact lens in place. Notice that its border goes slightly beyond that of the iris.

have no tint, unless they are made to cover unsightly parts of a nonseeing eye. Also, soft lenses are more comfortable than hard lenses in the initial wearing period and are frequently preferred for such sporting activities as jogging, skiing, and tennis. Disadvantages include their unsuitability for use by persons with moderate or severe astigmatism and their accumulation of deposits at a faster rate than hard lenses. In addition, soft lenses tend to be more expensive, more difficult to care for, and to have a higher incidence of associated infections and solution sensitivities.

A third category of contact lenses are the newer *silicone elastomer* lenses. These can be hard or soft and have a very high gas permeability. They are designed for extended wear. In recent years silicone lenses have appeared to be quite beneficial for use with children.

Finally, *scleral* lenses are the lens of choice in treating ocular albinism. They cover the entire visible sclera and cornea.

Orthokeratology

As defined by the International Section of Orthokeratology of the National Eye Research Foundation, *orthokeratology* is the reduction, modification, or elimination of refractive anomolies by the programmed application of contact lenses. It is accomplished by prescribing hard contact lenses with slightly different parameters than would normally be prescribed for a patient with the goal of changing the corneal curvature in a way that decreases the patient's refractive error. Normally it takes 6–20 weeks before any corneal change can be noted. When such a change does take place, another contact lens, again with slightly different parameters, is prescribed. This process continues for a 1- to 2-year period until, ideally, the refractive error has disappeared. Then a "retainer" lens is prescribed, to be used several hours a day in order to maintain the results.

Currently orthokeratology is not used for children, as its methods are still controversial. The few studies that have been published in the medical literature point out that the corneas tend to return to their pretreatment state once the lenses are no longer used and that it has a higher incidence of corneal complications. In addition, it is quite expensive and requires high motivation of the patient. It is difficult to predict who will do well; the best results have been with some patients who have a low refractive myopia.

Insertion and Removal

One of the most common nursing interventions regarding contact lenses concerns their insertion and removal. Nurses who wear contact lenses have little anxiety about these procedures. However, those who have never even touched a contact lens may be unnerved by such a request. In either case, obtain a booklet describing a child's specific contact lens whenever possible. These booklets contain explicit information on the insertion and removal of that brand of lens and usually have excellent illustrations. You may also wish to keep a small contact lens care kit available. Travel-size kits for both hard and soft contact lenses are available from manufacturers. Or you may wish to devise your own, including storage bottles labeled *left* and *right* and saline solution to keep soft contact lenses wet once they are removed.

Many children beyond their preschool years are able to insert and remove their own lenses. However, if your assistance is needed, first determine whether the lens is of the hard or soft type. Soft lenses may feel hard if they have been out of the eye for more than 5 minutes; therefore, do not assume a lens is of the hard type just by feel. Also notice whether any tinting is present (a strong clue that you have a hard lens) and size (if the diameter of the lens appears more than the diameter of the child's iris, you usually have a soft lens [Fig. 3-5A]).

Next, wash your hands and assure that the lens is clean (see the section on cleaning contact lenses). Also inspect the lens for tears or scratches. Most people insert or remove the right lens first to avoid confusion.

To insert a hard lens, first apply a few drops of wetting solution on your dominant index finger and also on the lens; tap water may also be used if wetting solution is not available. Then place the lens, with the cupped side up, on the index finger while lifting the upper lid with your other hand. Gently place the contact lens onto the eye over the iris. Have a towel or other object beneath your work area, so that if the lens falls, it can be easily located.

To insert a soft contact lens, determine whether the lens is inside out or not. To do this, either gently pinch the two edges of the lens together (if the edges point outward, the lens is inside out) or turn the lens inside out and note in which position the inner surface is more round (the rounder surface goes against the eyelid). Then place the wetted contact lens, with the cup up, on an index finger. Separate the lids with your free hand, ask the child to look upward, and gently place the lens beneath the cornea. Then let the child blink the lens into place while you gently release the lids.

If a lens becomes decentered, assure the child that there is no place for it to go; much to the astonishment of some children, the lens will not come out of their ears or go into their brain. If the child cannot tell you where in the eye the lens has moved, shine a penlight at the side of the eye as the child looks in several directions. Once you have located it, have the child close the eyes and "look" in the opposite direction. Then, using your fingers over the eyelids, gently slide the lens toward the center. Or, also with the child's eyes closed, hold the lens in place and have the child look toward the lens. Sometimes it is possible for a child to recenter a soft lens simply by gazing quickly in different directions.

Although the directions for inserting a lens may sound simple enough, the process can sometimes be difficult. On the other hand, removing contact lenses is much easier. We often teach children how to remove a lens first, so that they may feel some sense of accomplishment.

The principle behind the removal of all contact lenses is to break the water seal that attaches the lens to the cornea. Before removing any lens, wash your hands and make arrangements to keep the right and left lenses separate and labeled once they are removed.

For hard contact lenses, have the child bend the head forward while keeping the eyes as wide open as possible. Then pull slightly upward at the outer corner of the eye; the lens will usually pop right out. Or ask the child to lie down. Then place your thumbs above and below the child's eyelids as close to the lashes as possible and separate the lids slightly. This will cause the water seal to break; gently pressing the lower lid under the edge of the lens will cause the lens to eject outward.

To remove a soft contact lens, first ensure that the lens is centered and moistened; you may need to add some saline solution and wait a few minutes if it is not. Then, when possible, ask the patient to look upward or toward the nose and simply but gently pinch the lens off the eye with your fingers (Fig. 3-5B and 3-5C). Be careful, however, no to use your nails.

Special suction cups for the removal of scleral lenses are available. Simply wet the end of the suction cup and touch it to the inferior portion of the lens. Then pull this portion out and away from the eye and remove the lens. Suction devices are also available for hard and soft contact lenses; however, unless you are familiar with their instructions, you may prefer to remove the lenses manually.

If you are working with an infant or unconscious child, you will first need to identify the location of the lens before you attempt to remove it. Again, use a penlight at an oblique angle to note the location. Once you have located the lens and are assured that it is centered properly, add a few drops of normal saline and then proceed to remove the lens as above. However, if you have any difficulty or cannot see the cornea clearly, do not remove the lens yourself; instead, contact a physician, as there may be some epithelial damage. Also, do not use your nails or cotton swabs to assist in removal of the lens.

Caution children not to insert or remove their lenses over a sink basin, as many contact lenses have left our visible world at this point. If they must insert or remove the lenses near a sink because of a nearby mirror, they can place a paper towel or one of the specially designed stoppers over the drain.

Cleaning Contact Lenses

Even children who cannot insert or remove their lenses should be taught to clean and care for them as early as possible. Both hard and soft lenses are cleaned according to specific directions that are explained to the child and family when they obtain lenses. In general, both types are cleaned with specific cleaning solutions; be careful not to use solutions designed for soft lenses on hard lenses, or vice versa, and check to see that the brand of contact lens is listed on a specific brand of cleaning or soaking solution.

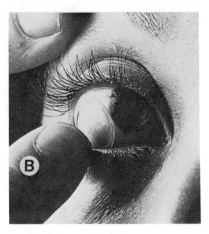

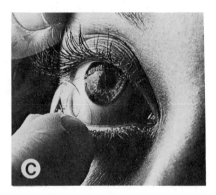

Fig.3-5B and C.   B: Step 1 of removing a soft contact lens: have the patient look to the side and slide the lens off the cornea onto the sclera. C: Step 2: gently pinch the lens off of the sclera. (Figures used with permission of the American Optical Corp., now Reichert Scientific Instruments).

After washing your hands, place a few drops of cleaning solution onto the lens. Then rub the lens gently between the fingers or between the inner surface of the palm and the finger for approximately 20 seconds. Afterward rinse hard lenses well with tap water or rinsing solution and place them into a soaking solution for a prescribed period. The soft lenses are rinsed with a steady stream of saline solution for 10 seconds and are then chemically or thermally sterilized. The chemical procedure involves no heat and requires at least 4 hours. The thermal method may be completed in approximately 1-1/2 hours. Some soft lenses can be cleaned by the chemical or thermal method only; therefore, do not attempt to clean a lens if you are not sure which method is preferred. Also remember to use fresh solutions for every cleaning and to cover soft lenses completely when placing them into their storage containers.

Hard lenses must be cleaned daily. This is also true of soft contact lenses, unless they are of the extended-wear type. Children with soft contact lenses designed for extended use will most likely have their lenses removed and cleaned in their eye examiner's office. Advise all children never to use saliva to moisten or clean their lenses, to prevent contaminating the lens or eye.

Finally, the lens container also needs to be cleaned regularly. Once a week is acceptable, but after each use is preferred. To clean the container, rinse it with hot tap water three times and then allow it to remain open to dry.

Other Care of Contact Lenses

In addition to the cleaning regimen, all children should be taught some basic principles regarding the care of their lenses. For example, they should handle the lenses carefully; soft contact lenses can be ripped or torn easily, and hard lenses may be scratched, especially if cleaned with a paper towel or rough cloth. Children should not rub their eyes while their lenses are in place, since such pressure against the cornea may cause some epithelial damage. Since contact lenses are made from plastic, they should not rest on a television or other warm surface that may change their shape or properties. Unless otherwise advised, children should not wear their lenses while swimming because the lenses may slide out; if soft lenses are kept in while swimming, one should wait at least 30 minutes before removing them because the water bond will be quite strong. In addition, all persons wearing contact lenses should keep a spare pair of regular glasses around, in case they lose their contacts or cannot wear them because of problems.

Adolescent girls should discuss using makeup with their practitioners. Many practitioners prefer that the patient put the lenses in first; in this way, the patient can see what she is doing, and the makeup won't spoil the lenses, and vice versa. Other practitioners prefer that all makeup except mascara be placed on first. Then, after diligent handwashing to remove oils and creams, the lenses are inserted. When a teenager is initially learning to wear contacts, she may have to be conservative in her use of makeup until her skill in inserting the lenses has become adequate. Most practitioners agree that the lenses should be removed before the makeup itself is removed.

Other principles to which children should be alerted include the avoidance of sprays, fumes, or hair dryers when their contacts are in place. In addition, the child should not insert any eye medication while the lenses are in place unless advised by the eye practitioner; otherwise, the medication may have increased duration by being trapped under the lenses or may damage the lenses themselves.

Finally, teach children to be aware of their peers or younger children who may be watching them insert or remove their lenses. Several cases of preschool children who lost their vision after inserting a piece of glass into an eye while imitating an older person have been reported. A contact lens wearer who has an audience should explain the purpose of the lenses carefully and caution young spectators to refrain from any similar activities.

Wearing Schedule

Children should adhere to the prescribed wearing schedule for their lenses as closely as possible, especially in the initial stages of contact lens adaptation. If possible, try to obtain the recommendations for the wearing schedule, as some children without early symptoms may wish to prolong the use of their lenses, causing increased symptoms at a later time. The child may initially wear non-extended-wear lenses for up to 3 hours a day. By the end of 2 weeks the child may be allowed to wear the lenses during all waking hours. Children should also be instructed that, unless the lenses are of the extended-wear type, they should never be kept in place during sleep. If this accidentally happens, some saline or contact lens lubrication should be inserted as soon as possible. If the lenses cannot be removed easily after a brief waiting period, the child's eye practitioner should be called.

Complications of Lens Wear

If a child complains of pain, photophobia, blurred vision, appearance of halos around objects, or excessive tearing or redness of the eye, the lens should be immediately removed and cleaned. Sometimes a foreign body (such as dust) may cause the symptoms, or the lens may be off-center. Usually a lens placed into the wrong eye or inside out does not hurt. If, after cleaning and reinsertion of the lens, the child's complaints continue, remove the lens and notify the child's eye examiner.

During the first few weeks of contact lens use, the child may experience some initial symptoms following their insertion. For example, the eyes may water or burn, the lenses may move around or fall out, or vision may come and go. These reactions are due both to the patient's inexperience with the lenses and to the initial adaptation period. It is not uncommon at this time for children to have small corneal abrasions due to their lack of skill (or that of their parents) in inserting the lenses.

Some children will require additional lubricant in their eyes to maintain adequate tears. For example, if a lens is comfortable immediately after insertion but later in the day causes irritation, the use of one drop, three or four times a day, of a contact lens lubricant may help. Such lubricant may also be useful for any lens wearer on a hot, dry, or windy day or when near a fan. If the child's complaints are excessive, or continue, however, determine whether the lenses need cleaning and are properly in place.

The most common complications of contact lens wear are corneal abrasions, the anoxic overwear syndrome, corneal edema, infection, and irritation. *Corneal abrasion* occurs when the eye is scratched by fingernails or particles held between the lens and cornea during insertion or overwear of the lenses (Chapter 12). The *overwear syndrome,* as its name implies, results when the lens has been in place too long, and the cornea becomes somewhat anoxic. Symptoms and treatment are similar to that for corneal abrasions.

Corneal edema may result if the overwear is significant, or if a contact lens is too tight. The child may complain of rainbows or halos around objects or of blurred vision. When significant edema is present the cornea may actually become cloudy, resulting in possible permanent loss of vision.

Extraocular infections are indicated by an acute red eye or excessive tearing or discharge. They can result from contamination of the lens or eye. However, excess tearing or redness may also indicate a sensitivity to various lens solutions.

Some persons may experience discoloration of their lenses or may develop lens deposits. These may be due to inadequate cleaning or decreased blinking, which is seen in persons who engage in sustained visual work.

Follow-Up

In the initial stages of contact lens wear, the child will need close follow-up by the eye practitioner. It is usually preferred that the child have the lens(es) in place for at least several hours before each follow-up visit. During each visit, the examiner will explore any complaints, check the visual acuity and external eye area, perform a refraction and slit-lamp examination of the anterior eye, and examine the lens. Young children with extended-wear lenses may need to see their examiner on a 2- to 4-week basis, even after the initial period. All children with contact lenses should be seen by their eye examiner at least every 6 months, unless the examiner indicates otherwise.

REFERENCES

1. Spollen JJ, Davidson DW: An analysis of vision defects in high and low income preschool children. J Sch Health 48:179, 1978
2. Nader PR: A pediatrician's primer for school health activities. Ped in Rev 4:83, 1982
3. Havener WH: Ocular Pharmacology (ed 4). Saint Louis, Mosby, 1978, p 246

SELECTED BIBLIOGRAPHY

Binder PS, May CH, Grant SC: An evaluation of orthokeratology. Ophthalmol 87:729–744, 1980

Crom DB: Topical ophthalmic anesthetics. J Ophthalmic Nursing and Technology 1:57–59, 1982

Forman AR: A new, low-concentration preparation for mydriasis and cycloplegia. Ophthalmol 87:213–215, 1980

Gould H: How to remove contact lenses from comatose patients. Am J Nurs 76:1483–1485, 1976

Nursing 78: Eyedrop instillation—patient teaching aid. Nursing 78 8:51, Feb. 1978

Reynolds R, Sanders TL: Contact lenses. Daly City, Calif., *Patient Information Library*, 1981 ($1.00)

Summey PS: Compliance of school children in getting and wearing glasses. Sightsav Rev 48:59–69, 1978

Chapter Four

Amblyopia

A mblyopia sounds strange and ominous to parents and teachers. More commonly known as *lazy eye,* amblyopia is a decrease in visual acuity in an eye despite adequate correction with lenses for any refractive problems. It is estimated that amblyopia effects at least 2 percent of our population; this includes 250,000 children in the United States under the age of four.

Studies with newborn kittens have provided interesting data regarding amblyopia.[1] For example, when a kitten's visual system is blocked by taping its eyelids closed for several weeks, a significant number of cortical neurons lose their ability to be stimulated once the eyelids are reopened. These neurons are obviously quite vulnerable, requiring early and adequate stimulation to activate them.

When a child with normal vision focuses on an object, the visual image is transformed into electrical and chemical signals by the retina. It is then sent along the optic nerve and visual pathway to the visual cortex in the occipital area of the brain (Fig. 1-1). In children with amblyopia, however, these images are essentially ignored by the visual processing centers in the brain; the brain does not "learn" to see with that eye.

The earliest possible detection and treatment of amblyopia is very important; the prognosis is decidedly more favorable in cases that are detected early than for those in which it has existed untreated for longer periods of time. Therefore, a child with strabismus, anisometropia, cataracts, or a history of amblyopia should be followed at regular intervals until about the age of 9, when the visual system becomes mature. This will assure optimal benefits of treatment if and when any amblyopia appears or recurs.

Some parents may question the fuss associated with treatment until they understand the implications of noncorrected amblyopia. First, for children who have a loss of vision in one eye because of amblyopia, there is always the danger of losing vision in their other (better) eye through injury or disease. Second, children with amblyopia often find driving, fast-action sports, and certain jobs more difficult. In fact, many public transportation jobs and certain military positions

NURSING GOALS, OUTCOME STANDARDS, AND DIAGNOSES

The primary nursing goal for Chapter 4 is that *every nurse who works with children aims toward decreasing the incidence and impact of amblyopia in his or her own unique job setting.* This goal is based on several considerations. First, in a number of cases amblyopia is a preventable eye disorder. This is particularly true when children with its primary precursors (strabismus, anisometropia, or cataracts) are identified and referred for treatment shortly after the onset of the precursor. Second, in children with amblyopia below the age of 9, visual acuity can almost always be improved to some degree. However, the earlier the identification of the amblyopia, the better. Third, screening for amblyopia and its precursors is rather quick and painless for the child and the screener and requires minimal training and relatively inexpensive and easily accessible equipment. Finally, since nurses work in such a wide variety of settings, we may be the only health care professionals with whom a child has contact, and hence, may be the only ones with the opportunities to screen for amblyopia.

Outcome Standard 1

Children who do not have access to a professional eye examiner will have a complete amblyopia screening at the ages of 4–6 months, and at 2, 4, 6, and 8 years of age.

Suggested interventions
- The nurse requests appropriate records from the examiner for children who have had a professional eye examination.
- The nurse requests appropriate records for children who have a primary care provider who may have performed an amblyopia screening.
- The nurse performs the screening according to Table 4-1 for children who have not had a recent amblyopia screening. (See also Outcome Standard 1 in Chapter 1.)

Outcome Standard 2

Each child who has failed the amblyopia screening or has documented amblyopia or one of its precursors is seen by an ophthalmologist.

Suggested interventions
- The nurse refers all children who do not pass their amblyopia screening to an ophthalmologist, if the child is not currently being followed by one.
- The nurse follows all children who do not pass their amblyopia screening to assure that each child has had an examination by an ophthalmologist and receives the recommended treatment and follow-up. (These interventions can minimize the *sensory deficit* brought about by the amblyopia, as well as the problem of *noncompliance.*)

Outcome Standard 3

The visual acuity of children under the age of 9 with amblyopia improves with proper treatment and follow-up.

Outcome Standard 4

Parents of all children with amblyopia and older patients explain amblyopia, how and why treatment is administered for a particular child, the frequency and importance of follow-up visits, and the consequences if such treatment and follow-up are not followed.

Outcome Standard 5

Parents and older children verbalize the impact of the diagnosis and treatment of amblyopia on their daily lives.

Suggested interventions

• The nurse clarifies and offers repeated explanations and education about the diagnosis and treatment plan (counteracts *knowledge deficit* and *noncompliance*).

• The nurse provides the patient and family opportunities to discuss any factors that might decrease compliance with the recommended treatment and follow-up.

• The nurse assists in decreasing any financial or other problems that might inhibit proper treatment.

For example, if a family cannot afford the necessary and frequent follow-up visits, or even the patches, or if work responsibilities prevent them from keeping their appointments, you may have to help find solutions to these problems. Or if the child does not like to wear the patch because of discomfort, irritation, body image, or sensory perception alterations, you will need to work with the parents and the child in overcoming these problems. (Remember that patching occludes the child's better eye and hence initially decreases the child's useful vision.) Associated nursing diagnoses include *alteration in comfort, actual or potential impairment of skin integrity, disturbance in body-image, social isolation, sensory perceptual alterations, impaired home maintenance management,* and *noncompliance.*

In addition, be alert for other signs of *ineffective individual or family coping.* For example, the parents of young infants with deprivation amblyopia may not only be dealing with the loss of their fantasized perfect baby because of the presence of cataracts but may also be dealing with the presence of other problems sometimes associated with cataracts, such as Down syndrome or galactosemia (rule out *dysfunctional grieving*). Or the urgency of surgical and medical treatment for the eye or other problems may rudely interfere with the parent–infant bonding process (rule out *potential or actual alterations in parenting*).

Furthermore, the child may have *impaired physical mobility* brought about by the treatment regimen or the decreased visual acuity from the amblyopia and may be more clumsy than usual. Associated with this and the decreased vision is an increased *potential for injury*, so recommend the use of safety glasses at all appropriate times (see Chapter 12).

• The nurse makes referrals as necessary to community or other professional resources that can help in these matters. For example, if both eyes are affected and the child is considered visually impaired, assure that all available resources have been adequately presented to the parents for their consideration (see Chapter 13).

Outcome Standard 6

The child's behavior becomes increasingly more cooperative during subsequent examinations and follow-up visits for amblyopia, as well as for treatment procedures.

Suggested interventions

• The nurse uses play therapy as necessary so that children become increasingly knowledgeable about the office and treatment procedures, while expressing their understanding and feelings through age-appropriate means. (These measures counteract *ineffective individual coping* and *anxiety and fear* about the procedures and treatment.)

• The nurse provides information about behavior modification techniques to parents.

---

are not available to persons with limited vision in one eye, since such limitation interferes with one's ability to perceive depth. Finally, in severe cases, the amblyopic eye may look different from the other, thus influencing the child's self-image.

As a means of preventing these possibilities, mass screening programs for amblyopia detection are being promoted on an international level. The state of Michigan has been a leader in this area for over 25 years, promoting screening programs similar to those used for immunizations. Unfortunately, such programs have not become as widespread as desired.

CLASSIFICATIONS OF AMBLYOPIA

Because many of the mechanisms in the development of amblyopia remain unclear, it has been traditionally difficult to classify. Nevertheless, the following classifications are often used. Just keep in mind that a child may infrequently have more than one type of amblyopia.

Strabismic Amblyopia

Strabismic amblyopia is by far the most common type; 50 percent of children with amblyopia have strabismus, and approximately 50 percent of children with strabismus have amblyopia. In the past the term *amblyopia exanopsia* ("amblyopia from disuse") was used to describe strabismic amblyopia. However,

Table 4-1
Reference Guide to Amblyopia Screening

History

Patching or amblyopia (can recur)

Strabismus (can lead to strabismic amblyopia)

Glasses (may indicate anisometropia or cataracts)

Cataracts (can lead to deprivation amblyopia)

Ptosis (can lead to deprivation amblyopia if visual axis is occluded)

Any ocular surgeries (may indicate a history of strabismus, cataracts, or ptosis)

Obtain consent for any pertinent medical records as needed

Examination

Brief external exam: Look especially for manifest strabismus, complete ptosis, or obvious cataracts

Visual acuity (also see Tables 1-3 and 1-4)

Children 4 months to 3 years: Check their ability to fix and follow, and observe for any behavioral changes

Children 3–4 years: Use any method that presents only one symbol at a time

Children 4 years and older: Use any linear method to help determine the presence of the crowding phenomenon

Stereotests: For children 3 years and older

Corneal reflex and/or cover test for children 3 months and older to help rule out strabismus

In newborns and young infants, if an ophthalmoscope is available, check the red reflex to rule out any significant opacities or cataracts

now this term refers to *deprivation amblyopia*. The amblyopia in strabismic children usually results from a disuse of the deviating eye and is always unilateral. However, occlusion amblyopia can also occur in the child's better eye.

At the turn of this century numerous discussions as to whether amblyopia caused strabismus or strabismus caused amblyopia occurred. It is now firmly established that strabismus precedes amblyopia in the following manner. When an eye deviates, the child initially sees double, as the straight eye relates one set of images to the brain, while the deviating eye sends another. Since double vision is intolerable, causing headaches and confusion, the child quickly learns to suppress or cortically ignore the set of images from the deviating (non-dominant) eye. In some cases (most acquired and some congenital esotropes) this suppression can then develop into amblyopia. Children with exotropia or other forms of alternating and intermittent strabismus do not usually develop amblyopia, however, because the suppression is not constant in the same eye. Contrary to one's expectations, no correlation exists between the severity of a child's amblyopia and the size of the angle of the deviating eye. Thus, a child with a quite noticeable deviation may have little or no amblyopia, although a child with a nonapparent microstrabismus may have a severe case.

Treatment should be started as soon as possible; the older a child is with strabismic amblyopia, the longer it takes to complete treatment. Frequently babies only need part-time patching for several weeks to reverse the amblyopia, but children 4–6 years old may require full-time patching for several months. Upon successful completion of treatment, both of the child's eyes may deviate, instead of one. To many parents, this makes the original strabismus problem appear worse, not better, and they need to understand that their child now has equal vision in both eyes.

Currently, amblyopia treatment precedes any surgery to realign the eyes. This can also be difficult for parents to understand, as their main concern may be the cosmetic appearance of their child. However, if an eye does not function properly—that is, if amblyopia is present—the eye is more prone to deviate again, and the chances of developing fusion are decreased. Sometimes when the strabismus is corrected before the amblyopia, parents believe that the surgery has corrected all of the child's problems and do not return for follow-up to correct the amblyopia. Even when the amblyopia is treated prior to surgery, parents must be reminded that microstrabismus can occur after surgery and may result in amblyopia. Microstrabismus can sometimes be difficult to notice unless special instruments are used; hence, follow-up until the age of 9 years is important.

Refractive Amblyopia

Refractive amblyopia, also known as *passive suppression amblyopia,* can result from anisometropia or, less frequently, from aniseikonia. Anisometropic amblyopia is often identified around the age of 4, when many children receive their first professional eye examination. At that time a refractive error is first noticed and treated with glasses. The child who returns for follow-up several weeks later may still have a decrease in visual acuity. Ultimately anisometropic amblyopia is diagnosed, and a regimen of patching begins. Some children may not comply well with their patching program because the patches significantly interfere with their useful vision, especially if they are school-aged. And much to the confusion of everyone, a few cases have been known to improve over the course of time with glasses alone!

Deprivation Amblyopia

Also known as *amblyopia exanopsia,* or *stimulus deprivation amblyopia,* deprivation amblyopia is caused by such problems as cataracts, complete ptosis, or corneal opacities, all of which can block the transfer of images to the retina.

To prevent deprivation amblyopia, the original eye problem must be surgically corrected as soon as possible. Otherwise, the retina may never learn to transfer images to the visual pathway, and hence a significant loss of vision can occur. Following appropriate surgery, a vigorous patching schedule must be instituted, and the child receives any refractive lenses that are needed. (See Chapters 10 and 11 for detailed discussions on cataracts and ptosis.)

Occlusion Amblyopia

Occlusion amblyopia occurs in a patient's better eye as a result of prolonged patching of that eye. Younger children are especially vulnerable to developing it, because their retinas are immature and are readily affected by withdrawal of stimulation. This type of amblyopia is usually prevented by patching the amblyopic eye for specific periods of time, such as 1 hour a day for infants, or 1 day a week for toddlers and preschoolers. Such alternating of patching allows the better eye a chance to be restimulated.

Organic Amblyopia

Many authorities do not consider *organic amblyopia* to be true amblyopia in the modern sense because in these cases the poor vision is directly related to pathologic processes along the visual pathway, such as optic nerve atrophy. Not all of these processes may be detectable, however, and confusion can result when they are not. For instance, it is estimated that 10 percent of patients with other types of amblyopia must have some form of organic amblyopia, as they cannot reach the appropriate visual acuity for their age despite early and adequate treatment.

Although most causes of organic amblyopia appear to be congenital, the condition can also result from nutritional deficiencies or from toxins in older persons. For example, alcoholism causes a type of reversible organic amblyopia. On the other hand, congenital organic amblyopia is usually neither reversible nor treatable; patching these children only decreases their available useful vision. In fact, some children with organic amblyopia have been known to fall asleep frequently or to withdraw when patched, as the patching becomes a source of sensory deprivation.

OPTICAL PRINCIPLES RELATED TO AMBLYOPIA

Fusion

Fusion, or *binocular single vision,* is the ability to see the same single image from each eye at the same time. Infants develop fusion by the age of 3 months.

Stereopsis

Stereopsis is the ability to perceive depth, or three-dimensional space. It is an advanced grade of fusion and is one of the main advantages in having two eyes. Stereopsis begins to develop when infants are learning hand-to-hand, hand-to-object, and hand-to-mouth skills, around the age of 10–12 weeks. Later, when infants throw toys out of the crib or playpen and watch them drop, they are refining their stereoscopic skills (much to the dismay of their parents!).

We measure stereopsis in terms of minutes and seconds of *arc*, (the viewing angle from the fovea to the object of regard). Smaller degrees of arc correspond to greater refinement of stereopsis. For example, 50 seconds of arc is more refined than 2 minutes. Therefore, the more refined one's stereoscopic ability, the more one is able to determine the relative depth an object is from oneself or from other objects. A person with 15–40 seconds of arc is considered to have excellent depth perception, and certain occupations such as piloting require such sharp stereopsis (although stereopsis is not possible beyond about 2 miles.) In addition, persons who play such fast-moving sports as tennis or baseball benefit from more refined stereoscopic skills. However, persons with only monocular vision (hence, no stereopsis) can learn to drive safely using cues other than depth perception.

During screening of stereopsis in children, 250 seconds of arc is usually the threshold to determine the presence of adequate binocular single vision. A child who fails a stereoscopic screening may have amblyopia and should therefore be referred for a more complete ophthalmic examination.

Diplopia (Double Vision)

Each eye normally transfers the same image at the same time through the visual pathway. However, if one of a child's eyes is misaligned, two different images are relayed. When the brain accepts both images, diplopia occurs. Diplopia is an intolerable sensory adaptation, as it causes confusion and possible headaches. Hence, a child may close one eye to eliminate sporadic double vision (for example, in intermittent exotropia), adopt an abnormal head posture, or develop suppression if the diplopia is constant. Diplopia of sudden onset requires prompt medical attention, as the patient may be experiencing some type of nerve or muscle damage secondary to disease or trauma.

Suppression

Suppression develops when the brain accepts only one of the two separate images from the eyes. It is an active, although unconscious, process by the brain and occurs only if both eyes are open; if the child closes the nonsuppressed eye, the suppressed eye will again relay retinal images. In contrast, a child with amblyopia who closes the better eye will *not* be able to reactivate the transmittal of retinal images immediately. Hence, suppression and amblyopia are different visual problems.

True suppression can only occur in children less than 9 years old, because their visual system is still immature. The suppressed image is usually from the nondominant eye, such as the one with strabismus or greater refractive error. Children who have an alternating strabismus in which the eyes take turns in deviating may have suppression, but they do not develop amblyopia.

SCREENING FOR AMBLYOPIA

Patient Education

Since most people have never heard of amblyopia, one of your first goals should be to provide an education and awareness program whenever possible. In your own unique job setting, determine how you can use the various pamphlets now available on amblyopia, such as *Charlie Brown, Detective* ($5.00/100) or the *Home Eye Test for Preschoolers* ($6.00/100), both by the NSPB; or *A Guide to Understanding Strabismus and Amblyopia* ($1.00 each) from the Patient Information Library; or *Amblyopia—Lazy Eye* ($5.00/100) from the Maryland Society for the Prevention of Blindness. Many parents may be able to use some of these to screen their child at home, allowing any necessary treatment to begin even sooner than if the child waits for a health professional or volunteer to perform the screening.

History

Whenever possible, inquire about a history in the patient of any predisposing factors to amblyopia, such as strabismus, cataracts, or refractive errors (Table 4-1). A history of amblyopia itself is also important, since amblyopia can recur until the visual pathway is mature at approximately age 9.

The history or reports will also help you differentiate the presence of amblyopia from a permanent loss of vision. Remember, though, that a child may have amblyopia in addition to an organic visual loss.

Visual Acuity

For practical purposes, some authorities have defined amblyopia in terms of visual acuity; that is, a child is considered to have amblyopia when no clinically detectable cause is identified for a visual acuity difference of two or more lines between the eyes.

Use the fixation test described in Chapter 2 to screen infants and young children. Those who have moderate-to-severe amblyopia will usually turn their head or fuss when their better eye is occluded because their main source of vision has been blocked. In contrast, occlusion of the amblyopic eye should have no remarkable behavioral effect (unless a child is objecting to the use of a patch). You may also wish to incorporate the cover tests for strabismus (Chapter 5) here and note whether any eye movements occur. Then repeat these procedures on the other eye. Refer any child who has behavioral changes, fails to fix and follow with either eye, or has abnormal eye movements.

In older children the determination of the *crowding phenomenon (separation difficulty)* can also provide information for your amblyopia screening. About two-thirds of children with amblyopia exhibit this phenomenon and therefore perform better with their amblyopic eye when each figure on a visual acuity line is presented individually than when the entire line is presented at once. Although the exact mechanism is still unknown, it appears that linear testing requires more complex cortical functioning than singular testing does. A child's amblyopia is considered to be improved only when improvement in the linear testing occurs.

Therefore, when screening children 4 years and older, always use the linear method first. If the child does not attain age-appropriate visual acuity, use the pinhole test to determine whether a refractive error is present. If no improvement occurs, try pointing to single figures, starting at the last line at which the child was successful. Finally, if there is still no improvement, show only one figure at a time. Record your results, mentioning which method of presentation you used, as well as the name of the particular visual acuity test. Although the use of Allen and single *E* cards and blocks prevents the identification of the crowding phenomenon, information from their proper use along with stereoscopic tests can provide an ample baseline for amblyopia detection.

Stereoscopic Tests

As discussed previously, stereopsis is the ability to perceive depth and requires binocular vision. Therefore, children with significant suppression or amblyopia do not have stereopsis, since their vision is primarily monocular.

The stereoscopic tests described next have been developed to assist in amblyopia screening (Figure 4-1). For each test there is a pass–fail point that determines whether a child has gross stereopsis. In addition, the tests allow examiners to determine various levels of stereoacuity.

The costs of the stereograms range from $30.00 to $60.00, and each includes complete instructions. In general, they should be stored in a cool, dry place, away from direct sunlight, as the dyes can fade with heat and humidity. When administering the tests, select a location that is well lit (at least 10 ft-c) yet glare-free.

If the child has prescription glasses, place the stereo-glasses over them. For children with bifocals, see that the test glasses cover the near vision part. Some children are initially frightened by the stereo-glasses, so it may be helpful to describe them as sun-, movie-star, or magic glasses to persuade the child to wear them. Others will wear them only if you do. Since some glasses are not available in children's sizes, a piece of tape will help hold them in place.

When administering the test, tell children to look straight ahead and present the test directly in front of them, with no tilt. Keep instructions to a minimum, as

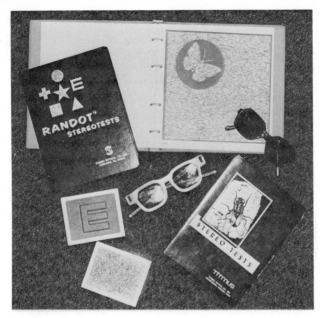

Fig. 4-1. Some popular stereotests. Clockwise from top: the TNO Test; the Titmus Stereo Fly Test; the Random Dot E (RDE) plates; the Randot Stereotest.

too much description will lessen the validity of the test. After the test, clean the plates or glasses with a soft damp cloth as necessary; cleaning fluids may damage the equipment.

Remember that stereoscopic tests are not diagnostic for amblyopia; they only provide additional information upon which the screener determines whether a referral is necessary. However, when administered properly to a cooperative child, they play an important role in the detection of amblyopia.

Random Dot E (RDE)

Wearing polarized glasses, the child looks at two cards. One card is blank; the other has an *E* that appears raised if the child has stereoscopic vision. If the child does not have stereopsis, both cards appear to be the same. Depending on the distance that the cards are held away from the child, stereopsis of up to 52 seconds of arc can be determined.

There are many advantages to the RDE. It is useful for children with language barriers or impairments, since it allows the child to signal responses. It is culture-free, requiring no answers that may depend on a child's experiences.

Because the examiner controls the cards, the child cannot memorize the test responses. In addition, the use of random dots has negated any monocular cues. Finally, it has been used on 3-year-olds with good results. A main disadvantage to the RDE is that lighting in the room tends to bounce off the cards, interfering with the child's ability to see the target.

The designers caution examiners not to rotate the *E* card, as one does when playing the *E* game for visual acuity. Rather, always present the cards horizontally, or the results will be invalid. To pass the test, the child must give four correct consecutive answers when both cards are held at 1 m (250 arc seconds). Do not tell a child during testing whether answers are right or wrong. If the child fails, try the TNO test (see next section) or refer the child for a more complete ophthalmic examination. The RDE is available from Stereo Optical Company, Inc., or other major ophthalmic equipment stores (WCO, Richmond) for an approximate cost of $40.00.

The TNO Test

Also for preschool and older children, the TNO test was first used in the United States in 1974. It employs red–green glasses (available in two sizes) that are used to view seven plates of random red and green dots. The first three plates help determine the presence of gross stereopsis (33 minutes of arc); the last three are used to rate the refineness of any stereopsis (15–480 seconds of arc). The middle plate is a suppression test. To pass the TNO, the child must correctly answer plates I through V, which ultimately equals 240 arc seconds, from a distance of 1 m. (Some people use 120 arc seconds as the pass–fail mark).

As with the RDE, the TNO has no monocular cues to influence a child's answers. In developing the plates, the designers were careful to ensure that a child without stereopsis would not sense failure; a child always sees at least one picture in the initial plates. However, since various plates require different instructions, the test requires more comprehension and cooperation than the RDE does. Nevertheless, the TNO has been used successfully with some 3-year-olds. Simons suggests such concrete instructions as ''Put your finger in the pie where the piece is missing'' to increase testability.[2] In a screening setting, memorization of correct answers is highly unlikely. Depending on one's area, the TNO may have some cultural bias, since some children may not be familiar with butterflies. In addition, children who are color-defective are unable to use it. The TNO may be difficult to obtain, since some ophthalmic companies do not carry it.

Randot Stereotest

Also employing the more advanced random dot techniques to delete monocular cues, the Randot Stereotest is an update of the older Wirt and Titmus stereotests. Three tests are presented on two plates: one test is for gross stereopsis, one for graded difficulty of stereopsis, and the last for fine discrimination. Polarized glasses are included.

Since this test is relatively new to the market, its reliability, especially with younger children, has not been firmly established. However, it appears compatible with the TNO, requiring some language skills that may not be present in all children. The Randot Stereotest is available from Titmus or WCO for approximately $75.00.

The Fly and Associated Tests (Older Titmus Stereotest)

Using older photographic techniques, this test is still widely used today, as it was designed specifically for children. Like its newer counterpart described previously, it presents three tests on two plates and is used with polarized glasses. The Fly Test which determines gross stereopsis (3000 arc seconds) is the best-known component; a child with stereopsis will pinch the wings of the fly above the plate when requested to do so (Fig. 4-2); the child without gross stereopsis will pinch the wings on the plate. Other tests using animals and circles help determine stereopsis from 40 to 800 arc seconds.

This test was developed before random dot pictures became available; hence,

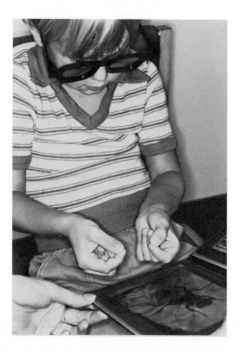

Fig. 4-2. The Fly Test: Children with gross stereopsis pick up the wings of the fly in midair because the polarized glasses give the pictures a three-dimensional look.

it has been faulted because it provides monocular cues. Also, it is felt that children can memorize the answers with repeated administration of the test, although in the screening setting this is not a problem. When using the test, see that the child passes the circle test at least up to number five (100 arc seconds) or gets all three animal answers correct; otherwise, you may be underreferring. In addition, some children may be afraid of the fly at first and may need reassurance that it is only a picture. These tests are also available from Titmus or WCO for $75.00

The Frisby Test

The Frisby Test is composed of numerous triangles of various sizes, divided into four squares. The child is shown a circle that is included with the test and is asked to point to the square that has the circle amidst the triangles. No stereoglasses are necessary. Three different plates come with the test, all of which can be rotated for repeated administration.

Currently this test is most frequently used with children who cannot be tested with other stereograms, as its reliability at the 250 arc second threshold is lower than the other stereotests. As with the Fly test, the Frisby provides some monocular clues; however, the test instructions discuss ways to decrease the clues. The Frisby is also relatively new and is available from WCO for $135.00.

Other Stereotests

More complex instruments to diagnose and treat problems of stereopsis can be found in the eye examiner's office, including haploscopes, stereoscopes, diploscopes, synoptophores, amblyoscopes, and projectographs. Many consist of two moveable tubes attached to a base; for children with strabismus, the tubes can be moved to align with each eye. At the end of each tube are changeable slides or pictures that can be presented in such a manner that no accommodation is necessary. Hence, stereopsis at a distance can also be evaluated.

Suppression Tests

Although suppression differs from amblyopia, tests to detect it sometimes help determine the presence of amblyopia. One of the older and more simpler tests for screening suppression is the *Worth Four Dot Test (W4D)*. A child is asked how many circles he sees while viewing a special grid of four colored dots, arranged as follows:

red
green green
white

During the test the child wears red–green glasses (over prescription lenses, if necessary), with the red lens covering the right eye and the green lens covering the left. This test is commonly performed at near with a special disc placed in front of a flashlight (Fig. 4-3). At distance (where it is more reliable) these circles are often incorporated into a visual acuity machine. A child with no suppression sees a total of four dots: two green and one red, plus the bottom white dot may appear red, green, white, or all three because of retinal rivalry. Other children who may see four dots include those with a constant tropic strabismus. A child who only sees two red dots has suppression of the left eye (the green lens covering the left eye is not seeing the green dots); a child who sees three green dots has suppression of the right eye (the white dot appears green, and the red is not seen). A child who sees five dots has diplopia. (How many dots are you seeing after reading this?) Unlike other tests for suppression, the W4D can be used on children as young as 3 years of age. However, it is only a screening test for gross suppression, and more refined diagnostic tests have decreased its general use among professional eye examiners. The W4D test is available from many ophthalmic companies such as WCO or Richmond for $30.00; the red–green glasses cost $9.00.

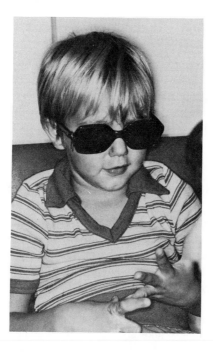

Fig. 4-3. A child, wearing red–green glasses, responds to the Worth Four Dot Test.

TREATMENT

Successful treatment of amblyopia depends on several factors. Most important are the duration of the amblyopia, the child's age at its onset, the child's age at initial treatment, and compliance with treatment. Amblyopia that has persisted for a long time has a poorer prognosis than amblyopia of recent onset. Similarly, if the amblyopia developed in early infancy, the prognosis is somewhat poorer than later-onset amblyopia. It cannot be overemphasized, therefore, that the earliest possible treatment is recommended to reach the best visual acuity and the possibility of fusion. In most cases, treatment after the age of 9 is of questionable value. Other factors to be considered for the child's visual prognosis include the way the child fixates (eccentric fixators have a poorer prognosis than central fixators) and the type of amblyopia.

The two methods of treating amblyopia are occlusion therapy (including mechanical and pharmacologic occlusion) and pleoptics. Occlusion therapy is almost universally tried first, as it is faster, less expensive, and more successful in the majority of patients. Frequently the child will be treated by both an ophthalmologist and an orthoptist.

Occlusion: Patching

Patching, or the mechanical occlusion of vision in one eye in order to help stimulate vision in the other, has been used since the eighteenth century as an effective means of treating amblyopia. Although in theory patching is simple, in reality it is not always so easy. Since it is most effective in children up to the age of 6 years, many children who require patching are infants or preschoolers, probably not the most receptive group to having their source of good vision covered up!

Therefore, the purpose of patching and its regimen must be clearly understood by the parents, caretakers, and the child, depending on age. Once in a while, parents or others think that the purpose of the patch is to straighten an eye or to prevent the need for glasses. Others believe that future surgeries and or glasses will improve the amblyopia. To prevent any misunderstandings, consider using one of the pamphlets listed earlier in the section on parent education. Also suggest sharing these materials with family (grandparents included!) and teachers. We had one child who returned to our practice over several months, with no improvement in vision from the patching regimen. Finally the child said that his teacher made him remove the patch at school; since it was considered a form of treatment it was prohibited without a doctor's order. We had assumed that the parents would inform the school about the patching and tell us whether direct communication with the school was necessary. We no longer make such assumptions and now routinely provide explanatory literature for all interested parties.

The patches are available in many drug stores: Opticlude (3M) and Coverlet (Beiersdorf) have both junior and regular sizes. Some children prefer the "pirate" look of the black patches with the band that goes around their heads, but they may promote peeking. Occlusion is also possible by using micropore tape and moleskin, hard black contact lenses, and soft contact lenses with large refractive errors that obscure the vision; these are all more comparatively expensive and require additional skill in administration.

If a child who needs patching already wears glasses for correction of a refractive error, partial occlusion providing some light and peripheral vision can be attained by using fingernail polish, opaque tape, or transparent contact paper over the appropriate glass lens. However, since patching is most effective when it is complete and constant, it is better to patch the child's appropriate eye first with a regular patch and then put the glasses in place.

Commercial patches are most effective when applied on a slant, with the narrow end pointing toward the nose, and with no peepholes. The child should close the eye before the patch is applied (also to discourage peeking). For full-time occlusion (FTO), the child should only remove the patch at bedtime. Encourage parents and other caretakers to keep a supply of patches in their purse, pocket, or at school, in case one comes off.

Skin care is obviously important during patching. During warm weather or high activity, the patch may come off easily. One pediatric ophthamologist recommends rubbing the appropriate area with cold cream until the area is dry; if the area is not allowed to dry sufficiently, the patch will not stick well. Another suggests the use of tincture of benzoin every morning to help protect the skin and to promote adhesion.

Since parents may unintentionally patch the wrong eye, written instructions outlining the patching routine are strongly recommended. These instructions should describe which eye to patch, the length of patching each day and indicate whether to alternate the patching, when to return to the practitioner for a follow-up appointment, and what to do if this appointment cannot be kept.

As for the patching routine itself, some examiners prescribe 1 week of patching of the better eye for every year of the child's age, followed by an examination to assure that occlusion amblyopia has not developed. Thus, for a child 27 months old, a follow-up examination is scheduled every 2 weeks. More recent studies encourage the use of patching only several hours each day for infants.

Depending on the child's age, the cause of the amblyopia, and its severity, complete improvement may require several weeks to several months. Often rapid changes occur initially and then slow down. If patching does not show any improvement in visual acuity over a 2- to 3-month period, it is discontinued. An alternative method of treatment, such as pleoptics, may be instituted. If the desired results are attained, the patching is decreased gradually. The child is placed on part-time occlusion and seen by the examiner every 3–12 months until the age of 9 years.

Although parents may follow all instructions in detail, one major problem can still interfere with the effectiveness of patching, that is, the child who continually removes the patch for whatever reason. The school-aged child may find that patching interferes with homework, sports, and TV, or the infant may find crawling or eye–hand coordination more difficult. In either case, frustration and irritability may result. In addition, children old enough to have developed a body image and socialization skills know that they look different with the patch. Finally, the patch itself can be uncomfortable.

Initial patching is therefore a trying time for both parent and child. If its purpose is not clearly understood, it can fail from the start. Parents must be forewarned that for a week or two their child will be testing them by removing the patch at various opportunities. Setting limits and maintaining a firm, matter-of-fact approach is difficult yet necessary. In older children, a simple reward system may promote cooperation. As time progresses, the rewards can become smaller, until they are no longer needed. Parents may also wish to role play with their child, reenacting possible comments and questions by the child's peers. Another option is for the parents to wear a patch for a few days, to help the child accept it (and to give the parents some idea of what it is like). The late pediatric ophthalmologist, Dr. Martin Urist, offers a most novel approach: "It takes two grandparents, one holding on to each hand, to walk the child all day to candy stores, supermarkets, zoos, . . . In my last double grandparent case for maintaining occlusion, the vision in a 4-1/2 year old child improved from 20/400 to 20/70 in one week." (unpublished lecture notes).

For younger children and infants, a reward system will obviously have little benefit. In these cases, pure persistance is necessary. Parents should try the initial patching in the familiar home setting, with ample time available. A patch is applied and the child is then engaged in another activity to provide distraction. This routine continues until the child accepts the patch or has been thoroughly unhappy for 5–10 minutes. In these latter cases, frequent sessions involving distraction and immediate reapplication of the patch if it is removed are necessary (as is much support for the parents). Most infants will eventually accept the patch and parents should be informed of this, to help carry them through the initial trying times.

Penalization (Pharmacologic Occlusion)

Blurring of the vision in the nonamblyopic eye is another type of occlusion treatment used on occasion. It is most helpful for hyperopic children who have mild amblyopia, any children with skin sensitivity to patches or latent nystagmus, and those children who continuously remove the patch. To establish penalization, atropine or another cycloplegic is administered daily to the fixating eye. This causes blurred vision in that eye, forcing the child to use the amblyopic eye in a specific manner. After several weeks, if the child can tolerate patching, the cycloplegic is discontinued. Or, in some cases, the penalization is continued indefinitely, with the cycloplegic administered about twice a week.

Parents need to be reminded that the drug is used monocularly, only in the nonamblyopic eye. Since this information may seem confusing initially, repeated explanations may yield better compliance. And as with all medications, parents should be reminded to keep the cycloplegic out of reach when not in use. Since ophthalmic medications frequently come in small vials or tubes, people can underestimate their potency, whether taken internally or topically. (See Table 3-1 for the nursing care plan on administration of atropine.)

Pleoptics

Pleoptics (meaning "full sight") is more commonly used in Europe. It can be particularly helpful for children with eccentric fixation. However, because cooperation is needed from the patient, pleoptics cannot be used in preschool children, nor in many children in the lower elementary grades. In addition, it requires considerably more time, training, equipment, and expense than occlusion therapy. Hence, pleoptics is most often used with those patients in whom occlusion therapy has not been effective.

The purpose of pleoptics is to reestablish central fixation. This can be done in a variety of ways. For example, in Cüpper's method, an after-image is produced by shining a bright light into the real macula, thereby dazzling it for a brief period of time. This causes the patient to see a ring around objects while using central fixation.

Once a patient recognizes how to use the fovea, they can use fine detailed visual tasks to help keep it stimulated. For children, such activities as coloring, beading, tracing, hitting balls, and catching or kicking objects can be quite helpful.

If no improvement is seen after 10 sessions of pleoptics, it is discontinued. Otherwise, several sessions each week over a 4- to 5-month period are usually required for maximum benefit. And as with occlusion, the improvement may not be permanent; additional treatments may be needed at a later time.

The Orthoptist

The diagnostic evaluation of patients with amblyopia or strabismus is frequently performed by an *orthoptist* (meaning "straight eyes"), who is trained in ocular motility. Orthoptists usually see patients after an ophthalmologist has completed a refraction and fundoscopic examination to rule out refractive or organic problems.

In general, the initial orthoptic evaluation involves visual acuity testing; determination of fusion, stereopsis, suppression, diplopia, abnormal retinal correspondence, and type of fixation; and measurement of the angle of strabismus. Appropriate methods of nonsurgical treatment are then instituted, including occlusion, pleoptics, prisms or visual exercises. Close communication with the ophthalmologist allows the patient to benefit from several professionals.

In the United States orthoptists (C.O.) become certified after completing a prescribed 24-month post-baccalaureate program. Currently these programs are offered at 26 different medical institutions around the nation; Britain and other countries also have extensive orthoptic training programs. Nurses who have access to any of these professionals could improve their own knowledge and skills by working closely with them in specific patient treatment programs.

REFERENCES

1. Huble DH, Weisel TH: Single cell response in striate cortex of kittens deprived of vision in one eye. J Neurophysiol 26: 1003, 1965
2. Simons K: Stereoacuity norms in young children. Arch Opthalmol 99: 442, 1981

SELECTED BIBLIOGRAPHY

Simons K: A comparison of the Frisby, Random-Dot E, TNO, and Randot Circles stereotests in screening and office use. Arch Ophthalmol 99:446–452, 1981
Stager DR: Amblyopia and the pediatrician. Pediatr Ann 12:574–584, 1983

Chapter Five

Strabismus

S *trabismus* (squint) describes eyes that are misaligned or not straight (Fig. 5-1). As a result, the visual axes are not parallel, causing the eyes to see two separate images (one from each axis). This is in contrast to children with normally aligned eyes, who see only one image (Fig. 1-1). Double images can lead to the development of suppression or amblyopia in children younger than 9 years.

Although statistics vary, it is estimated that at least 2 percent of the population has a history of strabismus. Children with Down syndrome, cerebral palsy, or a history of prematurity or central nervous system (CNS) disturbances have an even higher incidence. Strabismus normally appears in the early years; 50 percent of all children who develop it do so by the age of 1 year, and 80 percent before the age of 4 years. In addition, about 50 percent of persons with strabismus have amblyopia.

Strabismus can be caused by one or more factors. In some children the cause is anatomic: one or more extraocular muscles are mispositioned or absent or have abnormal mechanical properties. Other children have cranial nerve palsies, involving their third, fourth, or sixth cranial nerve(s) *(paralytic strabismus)*. Still other children have strabismus associated with poor vision. The majority of children, however, have strabismus with no obvious nerve or muscle abnormalities. Children with congenital esotropia or esotropia caused by a hyperopic refractive error fall into this group.

Contrary to popular belief, few children outgrow their strabismus. Hence, children with any kind of strabismus should consult a professional eye examiner regularly.

Early detection and treatment of strabismus are important for a number of reasons. Since children with strabismus have a high incidence of amblyopia their visual acuity can be significantly reduced without any treatment. Even if their visual acuity is equal in both eyes, the ability for stereopsis may be decreased or absent; the longer the presence of the strabismus, the fewer the chances a child has for fusion. Furthermore, strabismus can infrequently indicate an underlying disease, such as retinoblastoma. Finally, children with strabismus look different

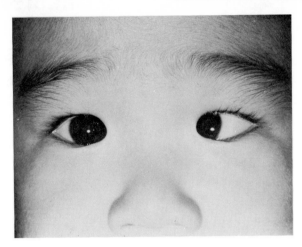

Fig. 5-1.   A child with congenital esotropia and a flat nasal bridge;
note that the light reflex is off-center in the child's left eye.

from other children, and it is sometimes difficult to tell in which direction they
are looking. As a result, they are subject to the social stigmas associated with
these problems.

ANATOMY

Six pairs of eye muscles and three pairs of cranial nerves are responsible for
extraocular movements (the ability of the eyes to look in various directions). Figure 5-2 shows the location of these extraocular muscles (EOMs) in relationship to
one another, as well as their primary function and innervation. The *rectus muscles*
originate in the posterior aspect of the orbit and proceed straight forward to insert
on the sclera at varying distances from the limbus. The *oblique muscles,* as their
name indicates, slant at an angle toward the lateral aspect of the eye.

Similarly to other muscles, the eye muscles within each eye work in pairs;
while one contracts, the other relaxes. The pairs are the *medial* and *lateral rectus
muscles,* the *superior* and *inferior rectus muscles,* and the *superior* and *inferior
oblique muscles.* In addition, when a person looks with both eyes in a certain
direction, one muscle from each eye is activated; these are called *yoke muscles*
and can be identified by their similar locations in Figure 5-2. For example, the
inferior oblique of the right eye and the superior rectus of the left eye are yoke
muscles, which help the patient look upward and to the left.

The three cranial nerves that innervate the EOMs are the third *(oculomotor),*
fourth *(trochlear)* and sixth *(abducens).* Testing of a child's ductions and ver-

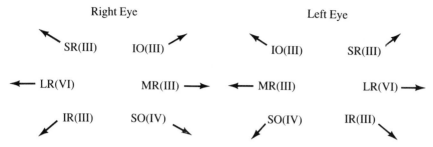

Right Eye   Left Eye

SR(III)   IO(III)   IO(III)   SR(III)

← LR(VI)   MR(III) →   ← MR(III)   LR(VI) →

IR(III)   SO(IV)   SO(IV)   IR(III)

Fig. 5-2. Locations, primary function (designated by arrows), and innervation of the six muscle pairs responsible for extraocular eye movements. The superior and inferior obliques are reversed from their basic anatomic location to indicate their primary function. IO = inferior oblique muscle; IR = inferior rectus muscle; LR = lateral rectus muscle; MR = medial rectus muscle; SO = superior oblique muscle; SR = superior rectus muscle; III = oculomotor cranial nerve; IV = trochlear cranial nerve; VI = abducens cranial nerve.

Table 5-1
Reference Guide to Strabismus Screening

History
The Child's History
(1). Have the parents ever noticed crossed or crooked eyes? If so, at what age? One or both eyes? Any treatment? Is the child still receiving follow-up, if less than 9 years?

(2). Does the strabismus still occur? Always? Only when the child is tired? Sick? Daydreaming? Looking at near or in the distance? When in bright lights?

Family History: (strabismus may be hereditary).

Medical History: obtain a consent as needed for any pertinent medical records.

Examination (for children 3 months and older).
Brief external exam: look specifically for abnormal head postures, overt strabismus, and in infants, a flat nasal bridge.

Visual acuity screening on an age-appropriate basis and stereoscopic testing, if available. (Remember that 50 percent of all children with strabismus have amblyopia.)

Corneal light reflex test: the light should be centered in both eyes.

Cover tests: no eye movement should be detected, and the child should have no behavioral changes.

Ductions and versions: eye movements should be smooth and complete in all directions.

Near point of convergence: the "breaking point" should be less than 6 in.

Fundoscopy: any child with suspected or documented strabismus should be referred for fundoscopy, even if the parents desire no treatment for the strabismus.

NURSING GOALS, OUTCOME STANDARDS, AND DIAGNOSES

The primary nursing goal for this chapter is that *nurses who work with children decrease the prevalence and impact of strabismus in their own unique job settings*. It is not surprising that the goals of chapters 4 and 5 are so similar. Since about 50 percent of all children with strabismus have amblyopia, and about 50 percent of all children with amblyopia have strabismus, identification of one often leads to identification of the other. Both types of screenings are quick, require minimal equipment, and can be done in association with the other. In addition, early identification and treatment of each problem leads to the best results. Finally, it bears repeating that nurses may be the only health professional with whom some children have contact. Therefore, it is important that we perform these screenings and assist in referrals, since a number of children will not otherwise be identified with these problems until much later.

Outcome Standard 1

Each child has a complete strabismic screening or professional evaluation at 4–6 months (preferably at 4 months); at 2, 4, 6, and 8 years of age, and as necessary after that for any suspicious signs or symptoms.

Suggested interventions
- The nurse performs the screening (as shown in Table 5-1) for any child who has not had a strabismus evaluation by either a professional eye examiner (preferable) or the child's primary health care provider.
- For children who have had a screening or evaluation by another professional, the nurse requests reports as necessary for the child's medical or school health record.
- See also Outcome Standard 1, Chapter 1.

Outcome Standard 2

An ophthalmologist examines each child who has failed the strabismus screening or has documented strabismus.

Suggested interventions
- The nurse refers all children who do not pass the strabismus screening to an ophthalmologist. To assist with this, the nurse keeps a list of names of pediatric ophthalmologists in the local or regional area; if none is available, the nurse lists the names of general ophthalmologists who enjoy working with children and provides the list to parents as necessary. Furthermore, the nurse emphasizes to the parents at the time of referral that the initial ophthalmologic evaluation should not be postponed because amblyopia, and less frequently, tumors or neurologic disorders, can be associated with strabismus (thus counteracting *knowledge deficit*).
- The nurse follows all children who do not pass their strabismus screening to ensure that each child has had an examination by an ophthalmologist and

to identify and assist with any problems that might prevent this evaluation from occurring (counteracts *noncompliance*).

• The nurse follows children with a positive history of strabismus to assure that they receive follow-up at least until the age of 9, when they are no longer at risk for developing an associated amblyopia (promotes *compliance*).

Outcome Standard 3

Each child with strabismus has optimal vision.

Suggested interventions:
• If a child has amblyopia, see Outcome Standards 3–6 in Chapter 4.
• If a child has periods of diplopia, instruct parents and teachers not to interfere with any head tilting and to keep the child away from bright lights, if an exotropia is present (decreases *sensory deficit*).
• Also see Outcome Standard 2, Intervention 3 above.

Outcome Standard 4

The parents of all children with strabismus, as well as older patients can define strabismus and can state three reasons why prompt treatment is preferred, as well as the recommended treatment(s) for the particular child.

Outcome Standard 5

Parents and older children verbalize the impact of the diagnosis and treatment of strabismus on their daily lives.

Suggested interventions
• The nurse clarifies and offers repeated explanations and education as necessary about the diagnosis and treatment plan (counteracts *knowledge deficit* and *noncompliance*).
• The nurse provides the patient and family with various opportunities to discuss the impact of strabismus on their daily lives. For example, many older children with strabismus have a *body-image disturbance* because the strabismus affects their appearance. Similarly, occlusion therapy, glasses, or prisms can also cause overt changes in the child's appearance. Children may become so self-conscious that they withdraw, or the remarks or lack of acceptance of peers and family members may force them into *social isolation*. Play therapy and role playing are two helpful interventions at these times, as are allowing the child or parent the opportunity to ventilate and providing support as needed.

Ineffective individual or family coping with the various treatments for strabismus may also occur, especially if repeat surgeries are necessary. In addition, a congenital esotropia may cause *dysfunctional grieving* in parents of a newborn child, or the medical and surgical treatments may interfere with the parent–child bonding process, causing *alterations in parenting*.
• The nurse makes referrals to community or other professional resources to decrease the impact of strabismus on the patient or family, as necessary. For

example, some state-funded crippled children's programs provide financial assistance for the medical and surgical expenses related to strabismus treatment.

Outcome Standard 6

Each child receives the recommended treatment for strabismus.

Outcome Standard 7

Such treatment is performed with minimal risk to the child's psychologic or physical well-being.

Suggested Interventions

• The nurse helps to supervise the proper use of occlusion therapy, glasses, prisms, or medications at the home and community levels (R/O *potential for injury, impaired home maintenance management, noncompliance*) For example, children using phosphate iodine drops should wear some type of identification stating that they are taking this medicine, in case of an emergency requiring anesthesia.

• The nurse refers each child requiring surgery, and the family, to a preadmission program, to familiarize them with the general hospital and surgical routines and equipment. Or, if such a program is not available, the nurse works with appropriate hospital staff in providing an individual program. Either way, the child and family are also informed of the aftereffects of the surgery, using age-appropriate teaching methods for the child (play therapy, cartoons, books.) In addition, the nurse assists the parents in understanding and completing the informed consent form. Related nursing diagnoses include *fears or anxieties* regarding the surgical procedure, hospital environment, or aftereffects; *knowledge deficit; ineffective coping* by the child or parent; potential or actual *alterations in parenting* caused by hospitalization of the child; and *translocation syndrome*, also secondary to hospitalization.

• For children requiring surgery in predominantly adult hospitals (frequently the case for strabismus patients), the nursing education department or other appropriate staff schedules occasional in-service sessions on the special needs of pediatric patients and their families for the operating room, recovery room, and floor staff, as well as for nonnursing personnel in laboratories, radiology department, and so on (to counteract *knowledge deficit.*)

sions (see the section discussing diagnostic tests) in the cardinal gazes is quite helpful in detecting the 10 percent of strabismus cases that are secondary to nerve palsies.

TYPES OF STRABISMUS

Several aspects of strabismus can be used to describe and classify it. The most basic observation, of course, is whether the eyes turn in, out, up, or down. Another is whether the deviation is always present or only present some of the time. These two aspects are usually used in any basic descriptive term.

If the strabismus is always present, it is termed a *tropia*. If it is still readily seen but not always, the description *intermittent* is added. However, if it is only seen when the child is examined with the cover tests, it is called a *phoria*. This latter term refers to a potential strabismus that is currently being controlled by the child.

The direction of the strabismus is added as a prefix to the frequency. *Eso-* refers to eyes that turn in; *exo-* refers to eyes that turn out. Hence, children with *esotropia* (ET) have one eye that visibly turns inward (Fig. 5-1) and are truly cross-eyed because their visual axes likewise cross. Esotropia is three times more common than *exotropia* (XT) or "wall-eyes." Some children may have a *hyper-, hypo-,* or *vertical* strabismus; in these cases, the strabismus is either described according to which eye is higher, or which eye deviates. The prefix *hetero-* refers to an eye that is misaligned in some direction but does not indicate which one. Parentheses around the second letter of the abbreviation indicate that the strabismus is intermittent; whereas, a prime sign indicates that the strabismus is apparent only at near. For example, *E(T)* indicates that a child has an intermittent esotropia, and *X'* indicates that the child has an exophoria at near. (An *E* or *X* by itself implies a phoria.)

Vergence (not to be confused with *versions,* described later) refers to the two eyes moving in opposite directions; that is, while one moves to the left, the other simultaneously moves to the right. *Convergence* indicates that the eyes are coming closer together and hence moving nasally. *Divergence* refers to the two eyes moving away from each other. Usually the eyes have a natural tendency to converge in the young years; around the early school years, however, this tendency changes to divergence.

Strabismus can also be classified according to the type of fixation. Does the child fixate with only one eye *(monocular strabismus)*? Or does he use either eye to fixate *(alternating strabismus)*? This second type is better because it implies that the child has equal visual acuity in both eyes.

Strabismus can also be divided into those cases that have a cranial nerve involvement (paralytic) and those that do not (nonparalytic). The paralytic types are discussed in Chapter 8.

Pseudostrabismus

Some newborns and infants *appear* to have strabismus, especially when they look toward the side. However, if you perform the corneal light reflex test on them, the light will land on the same spot in each eye, indicating that their eyes are straight. This test is discussed later in this chapter. In addition, if you examine their external eyes carefully you will note that these children have a flat nose and prominent epicanthal folds. With time, the skin folds will be pulled up by the growth of the nasal bridge. Other children who may have false strabismus are those with *hypertelorism* (widely spaced eyes) or those with facial asymmetry.

Congenital Esotropia

As the name indicates, children with *congenital esotropia* have an eye that is turned in, either at birth or shortly thereafter. If these children do not have an alternating fixation pattern, they will need occlusion therapy until they have equal visual acuity in both eyes. Preferably, this treatment begins when a child is only a few weeks or months of age. Once equal acuity is attained, surgery is scheduled. However, because of the tendency of the eyes to diverge in later years, repeat surgery for exotropia, development of a vertical strabismus, or recurrent esotropia may be needed. Early occlusion and surgery will increase the chances for these children to develop some binocularity, which cannot be achieved by treatments received at a later age.

Accommodative Esotropia

Accommodation is linked with convergence. Esotropia can therefore result when either excessive accommodation or convergence occurs. For example, some children with significant hyperopia require so much accommodation when looking at near objects that their eyes converge too much. Other children have higher than normal convergence for the amount of accommodation used. This second example is called a *high accommodative convergence–accommodation (AC/A)* ratio. One-half of all children with esotropia have an accommodative component, and it usually appears between 2 and 5 years of age.

Sometimes regular glasses for the hyperopia may relax the eyes enough to prevent the esotropia at near. In other cases bifocals will be necessary, with the top portion correcting the hyperopia at distance and the bottom portion having an even stronger refraction for near work. Children with accommodative esotropia must wear their glasses at all times. Appearance of the esotropia is to be expected when their glasses are off and they are looking at near objects. Some children may take a few weeks to adjust to their glasses, and a few will continue to look over them, requiring the use of cycloplegics. With time, however, the hyperopia tends to decrease, as do the accommodative powers. Hence, some children with *total accommodative esotropia* grow out of their strabismus by their pubertal years and eventually do not need glasses.

However, some children with accommodative esotropia require surgery because their strabismus is only partially due to their hyperopia; in addition, they have a "nonrefractive" component not corrected with glasses. Still, glasses are always prescribed first.

In addition, many children with accommodative esotropia develop amblyopia. However, with proper treatment and correction of their refractive error, they usually develop good visual acuity. They also tend to develop good fusion abilities.

Exotropia

Exotropia is usually intermittent in most children and is first noticed in the pre-school and elementary school years. Visual acuity is often good because constant suppression or amblyopia infrequently develops. However, children with exotropia may have difficulty working in bright lights, as such light causes constriction of the pupils with associated divergence; as a result, their exotropia can appear or increase and can result in double vision.

In the typical intermittent case, the exotropia may be noticed only when the child is fatigued, sick, daydreaming, or exposed to bright light (such as the sun). Distance vision can also promote divergence. The child may otherwise be able to control the exotropia—especially in your office or the night before strabismus surgery! For this reason, parental reports are very important.

Children who are exotropic only at near have a low AC/A ratio. This means that the child does not have enough convergence to promote fusion at near. Exercises or minus lenses to promote convergence may be prescribed.

Intermittent exotropia can remain well-controlled, or it can progress. On rare occasions it will resolve spontaneously or become constant. Therefore, close follow-up is important to indicate whether surgical intervention is necessary.

Vertical Strabismus

Vertical strabismus may be due to any of several causes (nerve palsies, trauma, myasthenia gravis, CNS lesions, thyroid disease), or it may occur in association with other types of strabismus. Abnormal head posturing is common in some children with vertical strabismus, especially when it is associated with cranial nerve palsies (see Chapter 8).

Children with vertical strabismus often complain of diplopia. Because some cases of vertical strabismus, especially those secondary to trauma, may resolve by themselves, examiners may wait 6–12 months before correcting the strabismus surgically. However, all children under 9 should be followed closely in the interim, in case amblyopia develops.

Since these children often have other medical problems or experiences, your interventions may also have to be combined. For example, if the strabismus is secondary to a CNS lesion or trauma, your main efforts will most likely be addressed toward these other problems.

A And *V* Patterns

You may notice in an examiner's report that a child has an *A* or *V* pattern of strabismus. As its name indicates, a child with an *A* esotropia will have a greater esotropia when looking up than when looking down. A child with an *A* exotropia has more exotropia when looking down than when looking up; *V* patterns are just the opposite. If the strabismus is too pronounced, surgical intervention may be needed.

Microstrabismus (Small-Angle Strabismus, or Microtropia)

Microstrabismus may be esotropic, exotropic, or vertical. It is generally difficult to detect in a screening examination. Unfortunately, a small-angle strabismus in a child can create a large degree of amblyopia. Therefore, all children with a history of strabismus should be followed at regular intervals until the age of 9, in order to detect any small-angle strabismus and subsequent amblyopia that may appear.

DIAGNOSTIC TESTS

Measuring Strabismus

In assessments by professional eye examiners, strabismus is measured in terms of *prism diopters* (designated by Δ). Two prism diopters equal approximately one degree of deviation. Persons with normal extraocular muscles have eye deviations of less than 5 prism diopters and can eliminate these with the binocular fusion drive. The deviations in persons with strabismus can change from time to time, and therefore several measurements with prisms are often taken before any treatment is initiated. Depending on their size and placement, prisms can make the misaligned eye appear straight.

History

Some types of strabismus are not constant and may not be apparent during an evaluation. Therefore, always ask parents whether they have ever noticed their child's eyes being crossed or crooked; have a picture or two available in case the parents are not quite sure what you are asking. If there is a history of strabismus, ask about its age of onset, which eye is affected, and whether the child has had any treatment. Momentary inward deviations are normal in infants less than 3 months. In older children, do the eyes ever cross when the child is stressed? Tired? Sick? In bright lights or when playing at near? What about other family members? Refer all children who have a positive history and strongly encourage parents with a positive family history to have their children examined routinely.

External Examination

When possible, observe the child briefly in the waiting area or ask the child to play while you are taking the history. In that way, you can note any unusual head posture that may indicate a possible nerve palsy. After taking the history, determine whether the child has any overt strabismus; or for infants, observe whether the nasal bridge is still flat. (A flat nasal bridge may contribute to pseudostrabismus.)

Fundoscopy

Every child with strabismus should have a complete eye examination with fundoscopy by an ophthalmologist as soon as possible. Rarely, a tumor or other serious pathology can cause strabismus.

Corneal Light Reflex Test (Hirschberg Test)

The Hirschberg Test is one of the basic screening tests used for strabismus. In a darkened room, let the child sit (on a parent's lap, if necessary) about 18 in away from you. Ask him to look straight ahead, or attract his attention with your flashlight. Then shine the light into the eyes (Fig. 5-3) and observe where the light reflex falls. In a child with normal eye muscles (including those with pseudostrabismus) the reflex will fall in the center of the eyes or very slightly nasally. A child with strabismus, however, will have the light centered in one eye but off-center (up, down, or sideways) in the other eye (Fig. 5-1). Any observable deviation requires a referral.

Professional eye examiners use a prism with their "muscle" light (the Krimsky

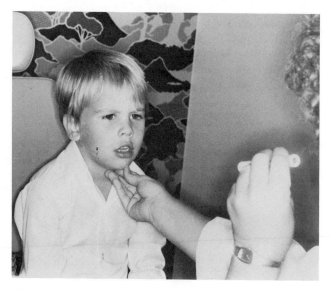

Fig. 5-3. Examiner performing the corneal light reflex test.

test) to center the reflex and measure each deviation. Without a prism, it is estimated that 1 mm of deviation of the light reflex equals 7 degrees or 14 prism diopters of deviation. Since the average cornea is 12 mm in diameter, a light reflex that falls halfway between its center and edge at the limbus represents an approximate deviation of 3 mm, or 20 degrees. Furthermore, the location of the light represents the opposite direction of the strabismus. For example, a reflex that shines in the left eye slightly temporally represents a left esotropia; the light is outward, indicating that the deviation is inward.

The Cover Tests

Cover tests can be quickly performed after the corneal light reflex test or can be combined with the fixation test for visual acuity screening in young children. The easiest and most useful test is the *alternating cover test*. This consists of covering one eye with a 3-by-5 card or commercial occluder (Fig. 5-4) and then moving the cover to the other eye. As the cover is being switched to the other eye, watch the eye that is being uncovered. Repeat this process back and forth. If one eye must move to assume fixation, it must be misaligned under the cover. Professional eye examiners can use a prism to measure how much it is misaligned.

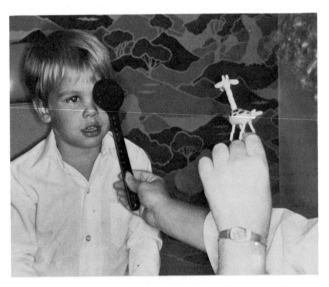

Fig. 5-4. Examiner using a commercial occluder to perform a cover test.

The important feature of the alternating cover test is that one eye is always covered; this allows you to determine whether either eye has a tendency toward being misaligned when binocular vision (fusion) is interrupted. Such a misalignment may be either a tropia or phoria. During the test be careful not to touch the eyelashes or skin with the cover and to continue to maintain the child's attention with an interesting stimulus held in your other hand.

If you want to distinguish between a tropia and phoria, use the *cover–uncover test*. In this test, watch the uncovered eye as the other eye is being covered. Continue to watch the same eye as you remove the cover from the other, so that now neither eye is covered. If the uncovered eye moves in this test, the child has a tropia. If the uncovered eye moves in the alternating cover test but not in the cover–uncover test, the child has a phoria. In either case, refer the child for a more complete evaluation. Also refer any child with behavioral changes when one eye is covered, since they may indicate amblyopia.

Although simple in theory, the cover tests can miss a number of children with strabismus, even when performed by professional eye examiners. For example, unless you repeat the tests by using a distant target (15-20 feet) and also have the child look in the up and down gazes, you will miss children with such problems as divergence excess or *A* and *V* pattern deviations. In addition, microstrabismus may not be detected by these tests. For most screening purposes, however, additional cover test procedures would be impractical or inefficient.

Ductions and Versions (D&V)

Figure 5-5 shows a child with normal eye muscles looking with both eyes in all possible directions. Such free movements in all direction by a child's eye muscles are called *versions*. Children 3 months of age or older should have normal versions. *Ductions* is a similar assessment of one eye at a time. When time is a factor, some examiners test ductions and version only in the primary *(center)* and six *(cardinal)* gazes corresponding to those muscle movements shown in Figure 5-2.

If you use an interesting stimulus, the testing of ductions and versions is usually easy. To test an infant, have the parent gently hold the child's head straight, while you move the stimulus around until all gazes have been tested (the infant can be lying or sitting). Of course, such testing also gives you information about the child's visual acuity.

During your assessment, note whether the eyes move well in each direction and whether these movements are smooth (and together, in versions). The appearance of a few beats of nystagmus when the child is looking in the extreme lateral gazes is normal. Children with strabismus whose angle of deviation is constant in all directions with either eye fixating are said to have *comitant (concomitant)* strabismus; those whose deviation varies in different gazes or with one eye fixating are said to have *incomitant (noncomitant)* strabismus. Finally, note

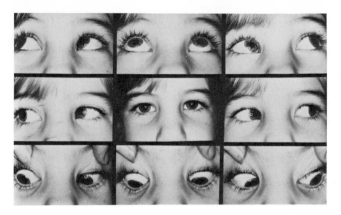

Fig. 5-5. Normal versions in a child (the small white rings are used for photographic purposes). Note how one must gently hold up the lids when assessing the lower gazes.

whether the child moves the head or develops a head tilt during certain gazes. Such assessment may be difficult with toddlers and preschoolers, who may naturally forget to keep their head still. Refer all children with abnormal eye or head movements.

Near Point of Convergence (NPC)

Convergence, that is, the ability of the eyes to turn inward simultaneously, is important for reading and close work. However, some children may have a convergence excess, or high accommodative convergence–accomodation ratio, which can result in strabismus. The NPC test allows you to determine whether the child's convergence ability is too strong. This test is performed by having the child stare at an object of interest held in the center of vision, and then bringing the object toward the child. The examiner notes how the two eyes move toward each other and the distance of the object from the eyes when the movement ceases or changes. The normal ''breaking point'' is less than 6 in.

The Worth Four Dot Test

The Worth four dot test described in Chapter 4 is still used by some examiners as part of their strabismus evaluation. Although this is not a specific test for either strabismus or amblyopia, it gives the examiner additional information regarding the visual capabilities of the eyes.

Office Equipment

Professional eye examiners may use a number of other tools in their office. The amblyoscope, synoptophore, and similar machines have already been discussed in Chapter 4. The *Maddox rod* is a piece of red striated glass that makes dots of light appear as a line. All of these instruments require subjective responses by the child and hence are not used during screening examinations.

TREATMENT

Most authorities feel that the earlier the treatment, the better the prognosis for children with strabismus. Such early intervention increases the chances for binocular single vision (fusion) because the visual portion of the young child's nervous system is still so adaptable.

The initial treatment for strabismus usually revolves around securing equal vision in both eyes. In addition, best operative results occur when the deviation is relatively constant. Hence two to four sets of measurements are taken before any surgery is done. Glasses are used when indicated. For many children with strabismus, particularly of the nonaccommodative type, surgery is the usual mode of treatment.

Occlusion

Occlusion therapy is a treatment for amblyopia, not strabismus. However, since many children have amblyopia secondary to their strabismus, occlusion therapy is often used. Most examiners prefer to correct a child's amblyopia before any strabismus surgery is done.

Glasses

As stated in the section on accommodative esotropia, glasses or bifocals are always prescribed for children with this diagnosis. Children with total accommodative esotropia require no other treatment than glasses, although those with the partial type require surgery at a later date. A few children with exotropia may be treated with minus lenses. Children with nonaccommodative strabismus may require glasses for refractive problems that are unrelated to their strabismus.

Prisms

Prisms have been successfully used with a few children for correction of their strabismus. However, in many cases the prisms only neutralize the deviation, and the eye may misalign further to compensate for their presence. When used, prisms are usually pasted onto glasses.

Exercises

A few children, particularly those with small-angle intermittent exotropia and double vision, can benefit from eye exercises prescribed by a professional eye examiner. These exercises help the child learn to use the eyes in a way that can eliminate double vision.

Medications

One of several anticholinesterase drugs may be used on a short-term basis to treat children with accommodative esotropia and high accommodative convergence–accommodation ratios. These drugs act on the ciliary muscles and change the neural response linking accommodation and convergence. As a result, convergence is decreased.

Phosphate iodine (PI, echothiophate iodide) is available in various strengths, and is administered once or twice a day or on alternating days. It loses its potency quickly, whether kept at room temperature or refrigerated, so patients must remember to keep bottles tightly sealed and not to use them for more than 4 weeks. The more potent demecarium bromide (Humorsol Sterile Ophthalmic Solution [Merck Sharp & Dohme]) and the older isoflurophate (Floropryl Sterile Ophthalmic Ointment [Merck Sharp & Dohme]) may also be used.

Families should be taught that these medications interfere with anesthesias containing succinylcholine, and they should stop using them 2–3 weeks before any surgeries. Otherwise, severe respiratory depression will result. These children should also carry a card or wear a plastic hospital bracelet or Medi-Alert necklace stating that they are using these medications, in case of an emergency.

These drugs also effect smooth (but not striated) muscles. Patients may complain of increased sweating, increased salivation, nausea, vomiting, diarrhea, and bradycardia. In addition, they can have ciliary spasms, with associated brow and head aches, blurred vision, myopia, and decreased night vision secondary to miosis. Atropine may alleviate the smooth muscle effects, and the ciliary spasms may spontaneously decrease in a week or so. Iris cysts and even cataracts can occur in children taking PI or Humorsol for long periods; the cysts usually disappear once the medication is discontinued, and their incidence may be decreased with the simultaneous use of phenylephrine.

Another drug that is being studied for its use in strabismus is purified botulinum A toxin. It is injected over the muscle(s) of the deviating eye causing a temporary paralysis that results in normal movement. However, use of botulinum toxin is still experimental.

Surgery

Pre- and Postoperative Care

Adequate preparation is most important for children about to have surgery for their strabismus. Sometimes young children worry that their eyes will come out, or that they will go blind. Unfortunately, we often forget to tell them otherwise because "they're too young." You may alleviate many of the child's fears or misconceptions by encouraging the use of hospital preadmission programs that inform both parents and children about general routines. In addition, numerous books are now available that can prepare children for surgical procedures and hospital experiences. You can supplement these general tools with specifics about the strabismus surgery.

For example, children have a very red eye for 1–2 weeks after surgery; depending on their their age, they should expect to see this when they look into a mirror. Many children go home the day of the surgery or the day after, so separation from family and home is less of a problem now than in the past. Few children complain of pain, but the family may wish to use warm compresses to make the eye area more comfortable. The tiny scars may feel like sand or fine dust in the eye, and the child should be told to avoid rubbing the area until it has been well healed. The fine, absorbable sutures that are used today prevent the catgut reactions seen in previous years. In addition, finer instruments reduce postoperative inflammation. However, to assist in the healing process, antibiotics and anti-inflammatory medications (Maxitrol Suspension and Ointment [Alcon Laboratories] has both properties) are administered for varying lengths of time. Some children have double vision for a few days after surgery, but usually do not have any discharge.

Parents also need to realize that about one-third of all strabismic cases need repeat surgery because the process of altering the extraocular muscles is not an exact science; even the most experienced surgeon can under- or overcorrect a muscle. A few children will even require a third or fourth surgical correction.

General anesthesia is used for all children having strabismus surgery, and parents naturally have concerns about this. Again, the hospital preadmission program can often decrease some of these concerns, while introducing some equipment and procedures when the child's anxiety level is low. Interestingly, many eyes temporarily straighten when general anesthesia is administered.

During the procedure, a child may experience bradycardia because the vagus nerve has branches in the extraocular muscles. When the surgeon manipulates these muscles, the vagus nerve is stimulated. Intravenous atropine usually reverses the bradycardia.

Following surgery, the conjunctiva helps cement the area together. If additional operations are necessary, or if a child has congenital esotropia or a paralytic strabismus, the conjunctiva may also need to be recessed. Repeat surgeries may be slightly more difficult because the scarring from the original surgery cements the area together.

Surgical procedures used to correct strabismus include the following:

- *Resection:* By removing a piece of the appropriate muscle(s), the surgeon can increase the strength of that muscle by increasing its contractability.

- *Tucking:* Tucking is also a strengthening procedure; the surgeon shortens the muscle by folding it. Tucking has less predictable results than resecting, however, because the tuck sometimes adheres to adjacent parts of the eye, decreasing the desired effects.

- *Recession:* In the recession procedure, the surgeon detaches the muscle at its normal insertion and reattaches it further back on the eye. This procedure causes the operated muscle and its yoke muscle to weaken. Recession of the lateral rectus is often done in children with intermittent exotropia; recession of the medial rectus (often in combination with resection of the lateral rectus) is done for children with esotropia. Not more than 6 mm of muscle is usually recessed at any one time.

- *Myotomy and Tenotomy:* Myotomy and tenotomy are also weakening procedures, used infrequently in children. The appropriate muscle or its tendon is severed completely or partially.

- *Adjustable Sutures:* In recent years adjustable sutures have been developed in an effort to decrease the need for further surgeries. During the initial surgery several sutures are loosely knotted and left available for further manipulation. Within the next 24 hours, after the patient has awakened, the results are observed. If any under- or overcorrection is present, the surgeon unties the sutures and gently moves the muscles in the proper direction. For younger children, nitrous oxide is given a few minutes before the measurements are taken, as the procedure is painful. Older patients remain awake, to provide the surgeon with additional feedback. Adjustable sutures are not used on children below the age of 1 year and are not preferred for any children by a number of ophthamologists.

ADDITIONAL RESOURCES

You may wish to obtain patient education pamphlets on strabismus. The NSPB prints *Crossed Eyes: A Needless Handicap* ($7.00/100), and the Patient Information Library publishes the excellent *A Guide to Understanding Strabismus and Amblyopia* ($1.00 each). Harriet Langsam Sobol has written *Jeff's Hospital Book,* a short illustrated book about a young boy's experiences in the hospital as he undergoes strabismus surgery (New York, Henry Z. Walck, 1975).

In addition, the Denver Eye Screening Test by LADOCA Publishing Foundation includes the corneal light reflex and cover tests, as well as screening forms and training films.

SELECTED BIBLIOGRAPHY

Barker J, Goldstein A, Frankenburg WK: Denver Eye Screening Test. Denver, LADOCA Publishing Foundation, 1972

Crawford JS, Morin JD (eds): Strabismus, in *The Eye in Childhood*. New York, Grune & Stratton, 1983

Hiles DA: Strabismus. Am J Nurs 74:1082–1089, 1974

Martonyi EJ, Iacobucci IL: *Strabismus and Amblyopia Screening of Infants, Toddlers, and Preschoolers*. Ann Arbor, University of Michigan Hospital, Ophthalmology Associates, 1981

O'Neill JF: Strabismus in childhood. Pediatr Ann 6:10–45, 1977

Reinecke RD, Miller D: *Strabismus: A Programmed Text* (ed 2). New York, Appleton-Century-Crofts, 1977

von Noorden GK: *Von Noorden-Maumenee's Atlas of Strabismus* (ed 3). St. Louis, Mosby, 1977.

Chapter Six

Color Vision

When I was a school nurse, I used to be fascinated every time a child failed the Ishihara Color Plates. I could see those numbers so clearly, yet the child didn't even know they were there. However, in advising the teachers, parents, and students of the implications of the results, I was at a loss for words. With the exception of some broad generalities regarding possible career difficulties I wasn't sure what color deficiency really meant.

Deficiency in color perception has been described since the time of the ancient Greeks. The eighteenth century scientist John Dalton became so well-known for his deficiency that it has often been called *Daltonism*. Unfortunately, the term *color-blindness* has also been used extensively in the past; yet as this chapter shows, the term is usually inappropriate and may cause a negative self-image in the person so labeled. As a result, use the terms *color vision deficit* or *color perception alteration* instead. In scientific circles, the term *dyschromatopsia* may be used to refer to all persons with color deficiency, although in Europe this term is frequently restricted to persons who have the acquired type.

INCIDENCE

The incidence of congenital color deficiency varies among different populations. Eight to ten percent of white males are said to be congenitally color deficient,[1] as are 0.5 percent of white women.[2] In addition, approximately 2 percent of American Indian males, 3.7 percent of black males, and 5 percent of Oriental males are affected.[2] The reason for the significantly higher incidence of congenital color deficiency among males is that most of these defects are inherited through a sex-linked (X) recessive gene.

SOME PRINCIPLES OF COLOR VISION

"Color" vision occurs when one has the ability to discriminate between light waves of various energy levels. These are usually written in nanometers (nm). For humans, the visible spectrum ranges from violet (400 nm) through the blues,

114

NURSING GOALS, OUTCOME STANDARDS, AND DIAGNOSES

This chapter's primary nursing goal is that, barring unassociated problems, *every child with a color vision defect is a fully functional person, integrated into his or her social and physical environments.* Most children with color vision defects have the congenital types, for which no treatment is available. Fortunately, the majority of these defects are mild and present only minor inconveniences or problems for the child. The impact of the more severe types can be reduced, often to significant degrees, with proper counseling and support.

In many locales, school and occupational nurses have traditionally been the primary screeners for color vision defects in their respective environments. Aside from these individuals, however, assessment of color vision has rarely been incorporated into the nursing process. Yet many nurses are in key positions not only to assess a child's color vision but to provide appropriate recommendations and follow-up, so that the impact of the defect on the child's life can be minimized.

Outcome Standard 1

All children (boys and girls) are screened for congenital color vision defects once between the ages of 5 and 10.

Suggested Interventions:
- The nurse asks parents and older children whether each child has been screened for color vision in the past, realizing that many parents are not aware that a screening has occurred unless their child has failed it *(knowledge deficit)*.
- The nurse requests records from the child's elementary school if the parent or child is uncertain whether a screening has occurred. In many cases, color vision screening is a routine part of the elementary school services.
- The nurse screens children who have not yet received a color vision assessment and who are not enrolled in school systems where an assessment is part of the routine school procedure; or the nurse screens all appropriate children in those schools where color vision screening is mandatory (R/O *sensory deficit*).

Outcome Standard 2

Children at risk for acquired color vision defects are screened at 6- to 12-month intervals, depending on the degree and length of their risk.

Suggested interventions:
- The nurse identifies which children are at risk and screens or refers them appropriately (R/O *sensory deficit*). Children particularly at risk include those on certain medications (Table 6-1) and those with fundus changes or diseases. If you do the screenings yourself, remember to screen each eye separately for these cases only.

Outcome Standard 3

Each child who fails a color vision screening has the degree of the defect determined.

Suggested interventions:

• The nurse uses verbal or written communication to inform children and their parents that the child has failed the color vision screening (Fig. 6-1) (to counteract *knowledge deficit*).

• The nurse uses a valid and reliable method of determining the degree of a child's color vision defect or refers the child to the primary care provider, ophthalmologist, optometrist, or school psychologist for such determination. However, children with suspected acquired color vision defects should be referred only to a medical doctor, in case associated changes occur in the fundus (establish *level of sensory deficit*).

Outcome Standard 4

Each child with a color vision defect, as well as his parents and teachers, defines *color deficiency* and the type, degree, and implications of the color deficiency that the particular child has.

Outcome Standard 5

Each child with a color defect, parents, and teachers verbalize the impact of the defect on the child's current and future life.

Suggested interventions:

• The nurse provides verbal and written information about the child's color defect or supplements the information given by another provider (to counteract *knowledge deficit*).

• The nurse explores with the child and family the daily problems (if any) that the defect causes and assists in providing solutions to minimize these problems (to counter *knowledge deficit, sensory deficit,* and *potential for physical injury*). For example, some children may need help in marking their clothes so that they can select those that match. Others may have difficulty in determining when to cross the street at a stop light. If the defect is so severe that it is associated with a loss of vision, and the child is visually impaired as a result, the nurse refers that child to appropriate resources (see Chapter 13). Finally, the nurse provides appropriate supportive and counseling measures to the occasional child who has a subsequent *altered self-concept* or to the child or family experiencing *ineffective coping*.

• The nurse assures that the child's educators are aware of the existence, degree, and implications of a particular child's color vision defect or any associated visual acuity changes and assures that such information appears on the child's medical, school-health, and cumulative educational records *(knowledge deficit)*.

• The nurse assures that adolescents and young adults with color vision defects and parents of all children with such defects can verbalize possible limitations in vocational goals secondary to the presence of a particular color defect (rule out *knowledge deficit*).

Table 6-1
Acquired Color Vision Defects Associated With Various Drugs

Drug	Chromatopsias	Type I Acquired r-g Defect	Type II Acquired r-g Defect	Type III Acquired b-y Defect
Antidiabetics (oral)			+	
Chlorpropamide			+	
Tolbutamide			+	
Antipyretics			+	
Ibuprofen			+	
Phenylbutazone			+	
Salicylates	+			
Nitrofurane derivatives	+	+	+	
Furaltodone		+	+ ?	
Nalidixic acid	+		−	
Phenothiazine derivatives		+ ?		+
Thioridazine	+			
Quinoline derivatives	+	+	+	+
Atebrin	+			
Chloroquine derivatives			+	+ +
Clioquinol			+ +	+
Quinidine			+	
Quinine	+	+	+	
Sulfonamides	+		+	
Salazosulfapyridine		+		
Tuberculostatics			+	
Dihydrostreptomycin			+	
Ethambutol			+	
Isoniazide			+	
PAS			+	
Rifampin			+	
Streptomycin	+		+	
Adrenalin	+			
Amoproxan			+	
Amyl alcohol	+			
Arsenicals	+		+	
Barbiturates	+			
Cannabis indica	+			
Chloramphenicol			+	
Chlorothiazide	+			

(continued)

Contraceptive agents (oral)		+	+ +
Cyanide		+	
Digitalis	+	+ +	+	+
Disulfiram		+	
Ergotamine	+	+	
Erythromycin			+
Ethanol	+	+	
Hexamethonium		+	
Indomethacin			+
Lead	+	+	
MAO inhibitors		+	
Mercaptopurine		+	
Penicillamine		+	
Strychnine	+		
Thallium		+	
Tobacco amblyopia		+	+ +
Trimethadione	+		+
Vincristine		+	

By permission from *Congenital and Acquired Color Vision Defects* by Joel Pokorny et al., Grune & Stratton, New York, 1979.

Table 6-1 summarizes the occurrence of chromatopsias as described by Sloan and Gilger (1947), Laroche (1967), Henkes (1968), Haut, Haye, Legras, Demailly, and Clay (1972), Dubois-Poulsen (1972), Hermans, Le Jeune, Van Oye, Watillon, Robe-Van Wyck, Dralands, and Garin (1972), Lyle (1974), and Saraux (1975).

greens, yellows, oranges, browns, and finally to the reds (700 nm). This spectrum is well demonstrated by using sunlight prisms and a darkened room. Rainbows also provide a similar illustration.

White results when an object reflects all wave lengths. For this reason, white is often the preferred color of clothing used by religious or military groups in tropical areas; since these persons are not accustomed to the tremendous heat, the white clothing allows maximum reflection of the sun's rays from the person. In contrast, black results from the complete absorption of light waves with no resulting reflection. White, black, and gray are sometimes referred to as *achromatic* colors.

Unlike horses, dogs, or cattle, which have little or no color perception, primates (including humans) are said to have *trichromatic* color perception. Our color vision is based on three primary colors that, when combined, result in all other colors. Artists and scientists differ in their definition of the three primaries, with artists using red, yellow, and blue, and scientists exchanging green for yellow.

In the 1960s, three different types of *photopigments*, which demonstrate sensitivity to different colors in the visible spectrum, were identified in the cones of primates. *Alpha* receptors correspond to blue light. A person who has a deficiency in these "blue cones" will have difficulty discriminating colors in the blue end of the spectrum. Similarly, *beta* receptors correspond to green light; and *gamma* receptors correspond to red light. Deficiencies in the beta and gamma cones will cause the patient to have difficulty discriminating green and red colors, respectively. A person who has only two functioning neuroreceptors is said to be *dichromatic;* a person with only one functioning neuroreceptor is said to be *monochromatic,* and a person without any functioning neuroreceptors is called *achromatic*.

Cones are located throughout the retina but are most densely packed in the fovea, the area on the retina responsible for sharpest vision. Animals such as hens and falcons, which are active primarily in the daylight hours, have a much higher proportion of cones to rods; in humans, however, cones provides only 5 percent (7 million) of the total retinal makeup.

In contrast, the *rods* are located in the retinal periphery and are the only photoreceptors functioning during scotopic or night vision. They help discriminate form and motion. Numbering 120 million in humans, rods comprise 95 percent of the total retinal makeup and are much more sensitive to light rays than the cones. Yet, because of their location in the retinal periphery and their anatomy, they provide a visual acuity of only about 20/200, at best. Owls and other primarily nocturnal animals have a predominance of rods.

Color is best perceived by humans from the ages of 16 to 35. After this time, the lenses begin to lose some of their clarity, and light rays are therefore absorbed differently. With a "yellowing lens," there is a decrease in the perception of violets and blue-greens.

TYPES OF COLOR DEFICIENCY

Congenital Color Deficiency

Congenital color deficiency, also known as *hereditary* or *stationary color deficiency,* is a nonprogressive, irreversible defect.

The terms describing the various types of congenital color deficiency are derived from Greek words and were developed by Von Kries in 1897. *Trichromats* are persons who use the three primary colors of red, green, and blue as the basis of their color perception; from these three primaries, trichromats can mix and match variations of all other colors. Persons with trichromatic color vision can be divided into two groups: those who have normal color perception and those who have difficulty shading one of the primary colors *(anomalous color vision)*. People who have difficulty with shades of red have *protanomaly*. They often confuse gray with pink or pale blue with green and account for 1.5 percent of all white males. Persons with *deuteranomaly* have a green weakness and may confuse gray with pale purple or green. They represent an overwhelming 5–6 percent of all white males.[1] Both deficiencies are X-linked recessive. Finally, persons who have a blue weakness are said to have *tritanomaly,* an extremely rare congenital color defect whose inheritance mode is unknown.

In general, persons with trichromatic anomalous color vision can state the color of an object, but have difficulty matching its shade. As a result, they show more of a color alteration than color deficiency. They may fail or pass a screening, depending upon which tool is used. For accurate professional diagnosis, an *anomaloscope* is preferred.

The second major category of congenital color deficiency involves those persons who have *dichromatic* (also known as *bichromatic*) color vision. This is considered a severe color defect; these persons can use only two primary colors to match what they see because only two of the cone systems are working properly. Dichromatics also can be divided into those who have protanopia, deuteranopia, and tritanopia. *Protanopia* is red deficiency and has a 1 percent incidence among white European males. Persons with this defect see black for red and therefore have great difficulty in noticing brake lights on highways. A well-known example of this black–red confusion concerned John Dalton, who belonged to a family of strict Quakers. One day, much to the horror of Dalton's congregation, he inadvertently purchased and wore a scarlet overcoat to the service; Dalton had thought the cloak was black!

Deuteranopia is the terminology used to describe green deficiency and has the same 1 percent incidence as protanopia; both are X-linked recessive inheritance. *Tritanopia* is quite rare as a congenital color defect. It usually results from the use of certain medications or toxins or is secondary to the loss of clarity in the lens, especially after the fourth decade. Persons with tritanopia show a blue deficiency and often confuse yellow with violet or blue with green.

The *monochromatopsias* are the other major category of congenital color deficiency. They are usually inherited through an autosomal recessive gene, although a few may be chromosome-linked recessive. The overall incidence of the monochromatopsias is extremely rare, equaling 0.003 percent of all color deficiencies. Persons with a complete color vision deficit are called *monochromatics* because they have a single cone system functioning, usually the blue cones. They have no perception of color whatsoever but have normal vision because the one functioning system allows good foveal function. If there is no functioning cone system, however, *achromatopsia,* or *rod monochromatism,* results. Rod vision is poor, and daylight dazzles the rod system. Such persons have photophobia and nystagmus.

Although there is no treatment for congenital color deficiency, attempts have been made to alter the brightness of objects to provide additional clues for the subject. For example, a change in the illumination from daylight to night will increase the brightness of an object for persons with certain color deficiencies, as the rods that are normal are now at their maximum functional level, whereas the cones that have the deficiency are functioning minimally. This explains why it is important to use daylight illumination when screening for color deficiencies, since an examiner may have false positives if the lighting is too poor. Attempts have also been made to use green or red filters or contact lenses to alter the brightness of objects for persons with specific color deficiencies; however, this method is beneficial only in selected cases.

Acquired Color Deficiency

Acquired color deficiency is rare in children. When it does occur, it can result from medications or toxins (for example, excessive alcohol intake), head trauma, systemic diseases such as diabetes, and any other ocular or systemic problem that causes damage to the retina (which houses the cones and rods) or optic nerve. Table 6-1 lists the possible acquired color vision defects that can result from the use of various medications.

Unlike congenital color deficiencies, those of the acquired type may progress or regress. In addition, persons with acquired color deficiencies may have other ocular symptoms, such as decreased visual acuity, decreased visual fields, or difficulty with dark adaptation. Furthermore, the two eyes of a person with acquired color deficiency may have different shadings of color perception, whereas those of a person with congenital color deficiency will have the same shadings.

Acquired color deficiency can be divided into three types. Types I and II involve red–green deficiencies, may be mild to severe, and are usually accompanied by moderate to severe reduction of visual acuity. However, Type I is usually caused by cone changes, and Type II results from damage to the optic nerve. In addition, the person with a Type II color defect may have an associated blue–yellow defect. Type III is by far the most common of the acquired color defects and involves a deficiency in the blue–yellow range. The associated visual acuity loss may be mild to severe. Type III also results from aging of the lens, especially after the age of 55.

Chromatopsia is the perception of white appearing as a color. For example, when the white is seen as blue, the condition is called *cyanopsia;* when it is seen as green, it is called *chloropsia.* Chromotopsia is temporary and can be caused by many of the medications listed in Table 6-1.

The best device for diagnosing acquired color deficiency is the Farnsworth–Munsell 100-Hue Test (discussed in detail later in this chapter). Unfortunately, it is difficult to administer to children under the mental age of 12 years or to those persons whose visual acuity is less than 0.2 (20/100). The Lanthony Tests are also helpful for assessing acquired color vision defects.

IMPLICATIONS OF COLOR DEFICIENCY

Throughout history, numerous unfortunate incidents have occurred in the workplace as results of a person's color deficiency. For example, in 1875, a Swedish rail disaster occurred because the engineer had a red–green deficiency. As a result, Sweden developed the first systematic color testing for railway personnel, and to this day many public transportation agencies exclude persons with red–green color deficiencies. In the United States the Armed Forces, Civil Aviation, and Railway Boards have similar exclusionary standards, especially for aviation and navigation.

Securing a driver's license may also be a challenge. The majority of color-deficient persons—those with anomalous defects—usually have no problem. However, persons with protanopia or deuteranopia may be excluded altogether. *Protans* usually have difficulty with red brake lights, *deutans* often confuse red and orange traffic lights, and both groups must rely on other clues, such as the flow of traffic or the position of the brightness of the light to assist them.

Other occupations from which the person with dichromatic color vision may be excluded include textiles, electronics, photography, pharmaceuticals, interior decorating, police work, printing, and agriculture. Such incidents as a color-deficient person picking unripe tomatoes too early because the green looked like red or of a huge batch of green textiles being the wrong shade because the dye assistant and quality control supervisor had the same defect no doubt have cast a shadow over opportunities in these fields. However, employers are gradually beginning to realize that such general exclusion of persons with color deficiency is discriminatory and that specific color deficiency tests must be developed for each specific job.

In the school setting, colors are widely employed in remedial education and in such courses as geography, geology, chemistry, and art. Preschoolers are often asked to match colors as a method of learning, and an increase in intensity of one color may be used to show an increase in magnitude. Yet most studies continue to show that the school performance of children with color defects does not differ from that of children who have normal color perception.[3] What does create problems is the students' career plans. Of 355 students between the ages of 10 and 15 who had a color deficiency, 62 percent had plans for a career in which their color deficiency would be a severe handicap. However, with proper counseling, 50 percent of those students changed their career plans to more suitable vocations.[4]

GUIDELINES FOR COLOR VISION SCREENING

The selection of color vision screening tools is frequently determined by the agency with which you are affiliated. Since only one or two tests are usually selected, the administration of color tests becomes significantly easier than that of vision screening tests. Nevertheless, it may be helpful to review some general guidelines concerning color vision screening.

Authorities differ in their opinion of the age at which a child should be color screened. Some feel that the earlier a child is screened and identified as color defective, the less chance that child has for developing a negative self-image.

Armed with this knowledge educators and family can work together to ensuring that it does not create a handicap. In contrast, others feel that color vision testing around grade three or four is quite satisfactory for early vocational guidance. In addition, they feel that since most children with congenital color deficiency are conditioned to name colors in the same manner that persons with normal color vision do, little, if any, effect is made on the child's self-image secondary to the color defect.

Most authorities agree, however, that both males and females should be tested for color vision. Despite the greater incidence of this defect among the male population, both sexes can significantly benefit from vocational counseling.

Once you have selected your population and tools, pay special attention to the lighting requirements. Most tests for color vision recommend 25 ft-c of light or more. This is the equivalent of what is termed *average daylight,* with the source coming preferably from the north sky. Special "daylight" lamps are also available; these may be of the tungsten, xenon, or fluorescent types and tend to be less variable than ordinary window light. When using these other lights turn off the regular incandescent lights in the room. Such measures will provide you with the desired lighting composed of all spectral wave lengths, rather than an incomplete spectrum that may negate some colors. Finally, remember to keep the color screening devices closed or covered when not in use, since repeated exposure to light can change their chemical properties.

Other guidelines include paying careful attention to the distance of the tool from the child, as recommended in the instructions. Also, if a student wears tinted contact lenses or glasses, they may interfere with the colors of the test itself. In addition, children who are screened to rule out congenital color defects can be tested with both eyes at once, since if any defect is present, it will be equal in both eyes. On the other hand, if it is suspected that a child may have an acquired color vision defect, you may wish to screen each eye individually; in acquired color defects, the defect may be greater in one eye than the other. Also try to assure privacy for the child, both to ensure better performance and to ensure that the other children do not memorize or learn the test ahead of time. Be careful not to mention any color names or differences or to provide clues in any other manner. Most authorities agree that a child need only be screened for congenital color deficiencies once during the school years, unless the findings are questionable.

When a child fails a test, measures to inform the child, parents, and educators are necessary. Figure 6-1 shows the form used by the Arizona Department of Health Services for parent notification of color deficient tests. A referral to an ophthalmologist is recommended if an acquired color vision defect is suspected or if other visual problems are noted during the screening. In addition, the parents may wish to inform their child's pediatrician or general practitioner. Finally, it is important that you tell the child's current teachers about the deficiency and note it on the cumulative record and health card.

Whenever possible, try to determine the severity of the child's defect. One

Recommended form for reproduction and use by schools

SCHOOL DISTRICT NAME AND ADDRESS

PARENT NOTIFICATION REGARDING COLOR DEFICIENT TEST

Date ______________________

Student's Name ____

Address ____

Grade ________ Teacher ______________________________________

To Parent or Guardian:

During a recent vision screening, results indicate that your child has some degree of color deficiency. Although this problem cannot be corrected, and does not affect how a person sees, it is important that the student and people close to the student are aware of this color deficiency.

The main reason for color deficiency testing is to alert the student about his color deficiency and that in the future there may be implications in planning or preparing for certain jobs or careers.

Information regarding results of the color deficiency test will be recorded on his health record, and education record, to alert school personnel who work with, or counsel, your child.

If you have any questions regarding results of this screening, please feel free to contact the school nurse or to consult an eye specialist about further testing.

Additional remarks:

Sincerely,

____

SCHOOL NURSE

Fig. 6-1. Parent notification regarding color deficient test, a recommended form for reproduction and use by schools (Reprinted with permission of the Arizona Department of Health Services).

authority has stated that failure to do so is similar to screening children only at the 20/20 vision line; if they pass, one knows that they have good vision, but if they fail, one has no indication of how much they see.

Career guidance is much more beneficial when such severity is determined early. Unfortunately, a great debate exists over who should do the actual career guidance. Several clinics in the United Kingdom and Japan have been developed to perform this function, but no similar service in the United States could be located.

Finally, even with all these measures taken, color vision screening tests can still be frustrating for children who have color defects. Sensitivity to each child's needs and adequate knowledge of the implications can be critical in assisting these children in adjusting to their defect.

TOOLS USED TO DETECT COLOR DEFICIENCY

Wool Tests

Wool tests have been around for quite some time and are among the oldest methods of screening for color defects. The Holmgren Wool Test uses 40 various colors and 3 master swatches and is available with directions from WCO or Richmond for about $16.00. Because the dyes in the wools tend to change in response to handling and exposure, their results are not always reliable.

Pseudoisochromatic Methods

Pseudoisochromatic tests use dots in specific colors and arrangements as a means of causing color confusion for persons with color deficiency. Usually the background consists of closely related shades of one color, and a numeral, letter, or other pattern is presented in closely related shades of another color. Pseudoiso-chromatic test plates are most often used to test congenital red–green deficiency; the manufacturing of such plates for the determination of blue–yellow deficiency is considerably more difficult.

Pseudoisochromatic plates have therefore been criticized for this. In addition, they do not always differentiate between protans and deutans, and it is sometimes difficult to determine the severity of a person's color deficiency. Nevertheless, because the pseudoisochromatic tests are so sensitive, are portable, require no trained personnel, can be administered quickly and easily, and are relatively inexpensive, they remain the mainstay for color deficiency screening.

Ishihara Plates

Although the first pseudoisochromatic tests (the Stilling plates) were developed in 1877, the Ishihara Color Plates developed in 1918 remain the oldest unchanged pseudoisochromatic test still in use today. The test is now available in several versions. The original 38-plate version comes with two introductory demonstration plates, 24 pages using numerals and 12 plates allowing persons who are illiterate to trace a pattern. In addition, there are versions with 8, 14, 16, and 24 plates that vary in cost from $45.00 to $85.00. (Most ophthalmic companies, such as Goodlite, Richmond, and WCO offer some type of the Ishihara Test Plates.)

The Ishihara Color Plates continue to be recommended as a rapid, sensitive method of screening for congenital protan and deutan defects, especially among children who are 6 years of age or older. Younger children may confuse the double digit numbers used in the Ishihara and should be offered the tracing patterns if they do not have problems with manual dexterity.

Although the Ishihara Plates cannot distinguish persons with dichromatic vision from those who have severe anomalous trichromatic vision, it is sometimes possible to differentiate persons with less severe forms of anomalous trichromatic vision. This can be done by counting the number of plates missed; depending on the edition used, up to two partial errors are allowed for persons with normal trichromatic vision.

Children who fail the Ishihara should be retested with another method, such as the City University Test, AO-HRR, or Farnsworth D-15, to determine the severity of their deficiency.

American Optical HRR and American Optical Company Plates

The Hardy, Rand and Rittler (AO-HRR) Pseudoisochromatic Test was developed in 1954. Although out of print at the present time, it is still one of the most popular color screening tools among those who have access to it. It includes testing for red–green and for blue–yellow defects. In addition, it has a number of grading plates to help classify the defects as mild, medium, or strong.

Unlike the Ishihara, the HRR Plates employ three symbols (a triangle, circle, and cross) in place of numerals. Its use of such symbols allows the test to be used among even younger children, such as those 3–5 years of age, especially when these symbols are placed on a sheet before the child and the child is asked to match any symbol seen on the plate with that on the sheet. A score sheet is provided with the HRR Plates to assist one in identifying the specific color defect.

In 1965, the American Optical Company manufactured another (now discontinued) pseudoisochromatic test simply referred to as the *American Optical Company (AOC) Plates*. It contains 15 plates with numbers, some of which are taken from the Ishihara Test, and some from other pseudoisochromatic plates. It is intended to be used for the determination of persons with red–green deficiency. The AOC Test is not recommended for children in preschool or kindergarten because they may be confused by the double-digit numbers.

Guy's Color Vision Test

The Guy's Color Vision Test was developed by Peter Gardiner in 1973 and is based on the Sheridan-Gardiner Vision Screening Test (STYCAR). Six plastic uppercase letters *(P, A, M, G, S,* and *D)* are placed before the child (Fig. 6-2).

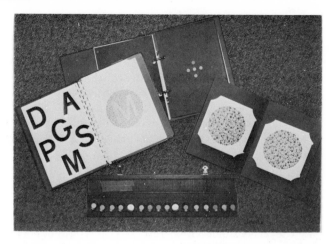

Fig. 6-2. Various tools for color vision. From top, clockwise: the City University Test (TCU Test); the Ishihara (the figures normally in the center of each page are not visible in this black-and-white illustration); the Farnsworth Panel D-15 Test, with the 5th and 10th caps turned upside down to show how each cap is marked; the Guy's Color Vision Test, with the black letters used for matching placed to the side for illustrative purposes.

The screener then holds a book containing eight pseudoisochromatic plates 2–4 feet in front of the child. The child looks at each plate and points to a matching symbol (if the child sees one). The Guy's Color Vision Test is currently difficult to purchase.

The Guy's Color Vision Test was developed in order to screen young children of school-entry age for color deficiency. Similar to the STYCAR, it requires no literacy, knowledge of numbers, manual dexterity, or language skills. Other benefits include portability and easy implementation, even by untrained personnel.

On the other hand, it only screens for red–green deficiencies and doesn't allow one to determine the kind or depth of color defect. Since its pages are glossy to promote easy cleansing, light can be reflected from its surfaces; therefore, remember to hold the book vertically before the child and be sensitive to any possible reflections. Few evaluative results concerning its usefulness have yet been published, but some authorities feel that the colors of the dyes are not as good as those of the Ishihara. If you use the Guy's Color Vision Test, remember to have the child point to, not say, the corresponding letters.

Other Pseudoisochromatic Plate Methods

A number of other pseudoisochromatic plate methods for the determination of color vision exist. The Dvorine Color Vision Test was introduced in 1944. Consisting of separate plates for those who are literate and those who are not, it was designed to determine red–green deficiency. The severity of such deficiency can be estimated by counting the number of errors. It includes a manual and score sheet and can be obtained from the Psychological Corporation for approximately $75.00.

Since the Ishihara, the Japanese have developed other pseudoisochromatic test plates. The Matsubara was specifically designed in 1957 for use by young children but contains some pictures (such as cherry blossoms) that may be culturally biased. More experience is needed to determine its validity among children of other cultures.

Nonpseudoisochromatic Color Vision Tests

The City University Test

The City University Color Vision Test (TCU Test) was developed in London in 1972. It consists of 11 pages, arranged in book format; each page contains five dots, four in a diamond pattern around one center dot (Fig. 6-2). The subject is asked to select a dot in the diamond that most closely resembles the one in the center. Depending on the dots selected, a determination of normal trichromatic vision, protanopia, deuteranopia, or tritanopia can be made. The color matches are taken from the Farnsworth Panel D-15, which is described in the next section.

Among the advantages of the TCU Test are that it is based upon the principle of matching, making it appropriate for testing children, and that blue–yellow deficiencies can be determined, as well as those of the red–green type. In addition, it also allows determination of the severity of the color deficiency by counting the number of errors made. Finally, it provides no brightness clues. Disadvantages include the fact that about 20 percent of all color deficient persons pass it; as a result, it is not an ideal screening tool. Also, some subjects find that none of the outside circles is similar to the center one or that more than one of the outside circles appear quite similar. The TCU Test is available from Keeler or WCO for approximately $160.00.

The Farnsworth Panel D-15 Test

The Farnsworth Dichotomous Test for Color Blindness (otherwise known as the *Panel D-15*) was developed in 1947. It consists of a wooden box containing 16 plastic caps; each cap has a color on the top that varies slightly from the others and a numeral on the bottom of the cap, not visible unless the cap is turned upside down (Fig. 6-2). The subject is asked to place the caps in order of hue and is timed while doing this. Usually the task can be completed within 2 minutes. The order of the caps is then plotted on a special graph to determine whether any color deficiency is present, and if so, of what kind. The Panel D-15 Test is useful in determining blue–yellow deficiencies, in addition to the red–green type. A persons who fails initially should be retested.

The single most common error for normal trichromats on the Farnsworth D-15 Test is placing the number 15 cap next to the number 7 cap. Young children may initially comply well with the test procedure and then in the middle place their favorite colors next to each other. Therefore, until a child understands the concept of ordering well, usually around the age of 8, pseudoisochromatic color tests should be used. Finally, like the TCU Test, the Farnsworth D-15 is not considered a screening tool for color vision. It can be obtained from the Psychological Corporation or WCO for an approximate cost of $185.00.

A variation of the Farnsworth D-15 Test is designed expressly for persons with acquired color vision defects. Initially developed in 1973, it is known as the *Lanthony Desaturated Panel D-15*.

The Farnsworth–Munsell 100-Hue Test

Also known as the *FM 100-Hue,* the Farnsworth–Munsell 100-Hue Test was developed in 1943 and modified in 1949 and 1957. The original version employed four wooden boxes, each containing 25 caps with colors of slight variability. Modifications have since reduced the total number of caps to 93, 85 of which are moveable and 8 of which are reference caps. Abridged versions use every second or third color.

The FM 100-Hue Test is decidedly more sensitive to color vision defects than are pseudoisochromatic plates. It is useful for determining both congenital and acquired defects, including the red–green and blue–yellow types. In addition, this method is often used in occupational settings for determining the color discriminatory ability of persons with normal trichromatic vision. The time required for total administration of the test is usually 10 minutes; however, the recording of the test results is done by hand and can be quite tedious.

This test is not recommended for persons who lack manual dexterity, such as the elderly or physically impaired, and may be boring for students who are not yet in their junior high school years. The FM 100-Hue Test is available from the Psychological Corporation, WCO, or Munsell Colors for approximately $400.00. As with the other nonpseudoisochromatic color tests, it is not recommended as a screening device for color vision but it may be used to test those who have failed a screening method.

Color Tests Associated With Visual Screening Devices

If your facility has purchased a machine for visual acuity screening, chances are the machine may also have the means for some color vision screening. For example, one or two plates from the Ishihara may be included. However, the color reproduction and necessary lighting are sometimes not adequate in these methods. Therefore, try to employ more lengthy and accurate methods of color vision screening whenever possible.

Anomaloscopes

Anomaloscopes are quite expensive optical instruments used for the accurate determination of color vision defects. Because of their expense they are not frequently used in clinical practice but are used more often in research.

REFERENCES

1. Pokorny J, Smith VC, Verriest G, et al (eds): *Congenital and Acquired Color Vision Defects*. New York, Grune and Stratton, 1979, p 184
2. Voke J: Seeing is not always believing. Nurs Mirror 150:49, 1980
3. Lampe JM, Doster ME, Beal BB: Summary of a three-year study of academic and school achievement between color-deficient and normal primary age pupils: phase two. J Sch Health 43:309–311, 1973
4. Taylor WO: Effects of employment of defects in colour vision. Br J Ophthalmol 55:753–760, 1971

Chapter Seven

The Retina

T he retina has frequently been compared to camera film because each converts light into electrochemical energy. Since many of us are familiar with the consequences of having the wrong film (or worse, no film) in our camera, the implications of an ill-functioning retina become quite clear: the "pictures" are distorted, often to a significant degree. Fortunately, retinal problems are statistically rare in children and adolescents.

ANATOMY THROUGH THE OPHTHALMOSCOPE

Until a decade or so ago, few nurses had the skills required to perform a basic retinal assessment. Now the ophthalmoscope has been introduced into many educational programs, allowing nurses the opportunity to study retinal anatomy on a firsthand basis. As a result, this section will use the ophthalmoscope as the means of discussing retinal anatomy. Keep in mind, however, that skill with the ophthalmoscope comes only with much practice and continued association with an experienced supervisor. If you do not have access to an ophthalmoscope, this section can at least introduce you to some of the principles behind its use, in addition to the basic anatomy of the retina.

Types of Ophthalmoscopes

Ophthalmoscopes provide the means of examining the *fundus,* or visible inner structures of the eye. Therefore, the terms *fundoscopy* and *ophthalmoscopy* are often used interchangeably. Two types of ophthalmoscopes are widely used, both of which provide a light source and magnification. Most nurses are familiar with the hand-held direct ophthalmoscope (Fig. 7-1), which is the focus of this section. It provides magnification of up to 15 times and is usually available in office, clinic, and hospital settings. The other type, the *indirect ophthalmoscope* includes head gear and a separate hand-held magnifying lens (Fig. 7-2). Although the indirect ophthalmoscope is more costly ($800.00 versus $225.00 for the direct type), it provides increased illumination, a wider field, and binocular and stereoscopic views. In addition, it can sometimes be used with uncooperative children. Therefore,

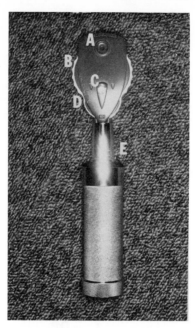

Fig. 7-1. A direct ophthalmoscope: A, Viewing window (lens);
B, lens dial; C, lens setting; D, light beam dial; E, on–off control.

it is often preferred by professional eye examiners, especially if scleral indentation is necessary.

Handling a Direct Ophthalmoscope

In a relaxed and private atmosphere, allow yourself one or more "play" sessions to become comfortable in handling an ophthalmoscope. First, become familiar with turning the instrument on and off (usually by depressing and rotating the red button) and determine from which side the light shines. Then identify and manipulate the various dials. When two dials are present, the smaller one monitors the various light beams. For example, the smaller white circular beam is used to examine undilated eyes, and the larger circular one is used for dilated eyes. Many instruments also have a white slit beam, in addition to a green filter to provide contrast and a white grid to help measure selected findings. Because the use of these other beams is usually restricted to advanced examiners, they will not be discussed further here. Practice shining the circular beams at objects near you.

The larger dial determines the actual lens being used to examine the eye. By

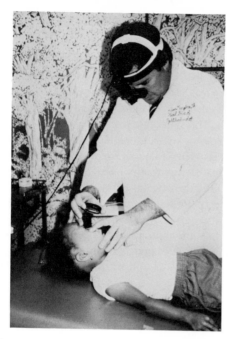

Fig. 7-2. A child being examined with an indirect ophthalmoscope.

placing your index finger on it you can change the lens settings. Most settings on direct ophthalmoscopes range from −20 (red numbers, which minimize what you are viewing) to +20 (black numbers, which magnify the field).

Once you can move the dials comfortably with both hands, locate the lens. Then, while looking through the viewer, practice moving your head and the instrument together. This unison movement is most important, as it will give you better control of the instrument, especially when examining squirming children. From the beginning, learn to keep both eyes open and to use your right hand and eye to examine the patient's right eye, and your left hand and eye to examine the left. Don't become discouraged if you have a dominant eye and find it initially difficult to use your other eye; just keep practicing.

If you normally wear glasses, learn your correction and modify the lens setting as needed. As a result, you can remove your glasses while using the ophthalmoscope and have better viewing because of the closer proximity.

After you have become comfortable with handling the ophthalmoscope and have viewed objects near and far, select a staff member, spouse, or friend for your first exam. If the subject wears glasses, remove them, again to allow for

NURSING GOALS, OUTCOME STANDARDS, AND DIAGNOSES

The primary nursing standard for this chapter is that *each child with a retinal disorder has the best possible vision and overall health status, in view of his or her own particular medical history.* Although nurses as a group are minimally involved in the assessment of retinal disorders, many of us have the opportunity to become involved with children who already have or hold the potential for developing such a disorder. This is because many retinal disorders in children are associated with other illnesses or health problems. For example, diabetic retinopathy is associated with a disease well known for its many systemic manifestations. A diagnosis of retrolental fibroplasia indicates that a child was probably quite premature and had a difficult neonatal period. Retinoblastoma threatens not only vision but a child's very life because of possible or actual metastases. Therefore, the goal regarding children with retinal disorders is not just to preserve their vision as much as possible but also to promote their general health and well-being.

Because of the differences among the various retinal disorders seen in children, the nursing outcome standards and diagnoses for this chapter will be listed separately.

Outcome Standard 1

Each child who has, or is at risk for developing, a retinal disorder is followed at recommended intervals by an ophthalmologist, as well as by any other necessary medical specialists.

Suggested Interventions:

- The nurse follows all children with known retinal disorders, to ensure that each has received the recommended follow-up by the ophthalmologist, primary physician, and medical specialist, as necessary. This often implies that the nurse has verbal or written communication with these practitioners (with parental consent) to document the status of the child's health and to determine how often follow-up is necessary.
- The nurse identifies children at risk for developing retinal disorders and ensures that they have an initial visit with an ophthalmologist. Children at risk include (but are not limited to) those with strabismus (R/O retinoblastoma); young children who were less than 1500 grams (g) at birth (R/O retrolental fibroplasia [RLF]); those with a positive family history for such retinal disorders as retinoblastoma, retinitis pigmentosa, or other inherited retinal disorders; children with diabetes (especially if they have had diabetes for 3 years or more); children with a history of a TORCH infection; those with a history of blunt or internal eye trauma; and children on selected medications that can effect the retina (Table 6-1). The nurse then has verbal or written communication with the parent, ophthalmologist, or medical specialist to determine the frequency of any additional ophthalmic follow-up.

- The nurse assists in identifying and decreasing any financial, psychosocial, or other problems that might otherwise inhibit a child from receiving the recommended follow-up and treatment.

Outcome Standard 2

Each child receives the recommended treatment(s) for the retinal disorder and any associated health problems.

Outcome Standard 3

The child's behavior becomes increasingly cooperative during subsequent examinations and treatment procedures.

Outcome Standard 4

Examinations and treatment procedures are performed with minimal risk to the child's psychosocial and physical well-being.

Suggested Interventions:
- The nurse assists in increasing the child's and family's knowledge regarding the fundoscopy process and other diagnostic and office treatment procedures (electroetinograms [ERGs], ultrasounds, laser, fundus photography) and in decreasing their fears and anxieties regarding these through such age-appropriate preparatory interventions as the use of dolls, puppets, or stuffed animals, hospital and house play equipment, story books, pictures, or preexam visualization of actual equipment.
- The nurse makes every possible effort to decrease the discomfort associated with the administration or side effects of mydriatic eyedrops or topical ophthalmic anesthetics, or from the use of any ophthalmic equipment or instruments.
- For children requiring surgery, see Outcome Standard 7, Chapter 5 and the sections on treatment at the end of this chapter. In addition, if staff are not experienced with retinal patients, ensure that they receive in-service training before the child's surgery. For example, they should understand that it is preferable for a child to deep breathe rather than cough after surgery.

Outcome Standard 5

Older children with retinal disorders and the parents of all children with retinal disorders define *retina,* its function, the child's particular retinal problem and its implications, and the frequency and importance of any recommended treatment and follow-up.

Suggested Interventions:
- The nurse clarifies and offers repeated explanations and education about the diagnostic and treatment plan. When possible, the nurse provides written information and illustrations to supplement the teaching. In addition, the nurse reviews with the family any home-care instructions (such as the avoidance of contact

sports or heavy lifting) or the necessary safety measures to protect the child's remaining vision.

Outcome Standard 6

Older children with retinal disorders and the families (siblings included) of all children with retinal disorders verbalize the impact of the disorder and any associated illness on their daily lives.

Suggested Interventions:

- The nurse offers the older child and all families ample opportunity to discuss the effects of the child's retinal disorder and any associated health problem on their lives.
- The nurse assesses whether the child has any sensory perception alterations secondary to the retinal disorder and, if so, explores with the child and family ways to minimize these alterations when possible.
- The nurse makes referrals as necessary to outside resources. These may include parent groups, disease-related organizations (for example, the National Retinitis Pigmentosa Foundation or the American Diabetic Association), genetic counselors, family counselors, psychologists, clinical social workers, public health nurses, low-vision centers, early child educators, and vocational rehabilitation centers.

Relevant Nursing Diagnoses

- *Anxiety:* of parents or children concerning diagnostic or treatment procedures (ophthalmoscopy, fluorescein injections, fundus photography, ERGs, ultrasounds, laser, hospitalization, surgery, enucleation) or about possible sensory deficits and general health outcomes.
- *Alteration in comfort: Photophobia* (after mydriatic eyedrops or from ophthalmoscopy); *pain* (from topical ophthalmic anesthetic eyedrops, scleral indentation, speculums, surgery, or any associated glaucoma).
- *ineffective individual or family coping:* during diagnosis or treatment. If the disorder is inherited, such as retinitis pigmentosa or some cases of retinoblastoma, parents or other family members may experience feelings of guilt. For children who have had a previous or associated illness, such as those with RLF or diabetes, the retinal disorder may exceed the family's coping abilities.
- *Diversional activity deficit:* for children who are newly or temporarily visually impaired.
- *Alteration in family processes:* especially possible for families with inherited disorders, such as retinitis pigmentosa (RP) or retinoblastoma (RB).
- *Fears:* regarding blindness, loss of an eye, pain, sickness, side effects of treatment, surgery, hospitalization, injury, death.

- *Anticipatory or dysfunctional grieving:* regarding possible or actual loss of vision, an eye, health, or life.
- *Impaired home maintenance management:* concerning financial coverage for diagnosis or treatment, eye safety precautions, avoidance of contact sports or lifting of heavy objects, care of prosthesis.
- *Potential for injury:* coughing, heavy lifting, and contact sports can lead to retinal detachment for some patients; decreased visual functioning generally increases a person's potential for injury; remaining vision must be adequately protected; other family members (for example, new siblings of patients with retinoblastoma) of a child with an inherited disorder can also develop the problem; staff may be uninformed about the special needs of pediatric or retinal patients.
- *Knowledge deficit:* of patient, family (including siblings), significant others, and/or staff about eye disorder, any associated illness, diagnostic process, treatments, safety precautions, home care, referral resources, hospital care and process.
- *Impaired physical mobility:* the patient must avoid contact sports; if newly and severely visually impaired; preceding or following retinal surgery; during any radiation treatment; with selected sensory perception alterations, such as decreased night vision for RP patients.
- *Noncompliance:* with initial or follow-up appointments for patient or family members; with treatment for any associated illness.
- *Actual or potential alterations in parenting:* parents especially vulnerable for this are those with an infant with RLF, persistant hypoplastic primary vitreous, TORCH infection, or retinoblastoma; can also occur with hospitalization of child.
- *Self-care deficit:* if newly and severely visually impaired.
- *Disturbance in body image:* enucleation, microophthalmia, or the presence of a chronic illness can lead to problems; also can result from the temporary edema and ecchymoses brought about by surgery.
- *Sensory deficit:* can include decreased visual acuity (see Chapter 13 if the child is visually impaired); decreased night vision; photophobia; color perception changes (see Chapter 6); double vision (especially after laser therapy); spots or floaters (also after laser therapy or may indicate retinal detachment); bilateral patching (before or after surgery); tunnel vision or other visual field changes; deafness for some patients with RP.
- *Actual or potential impairment of skin integrity:* for children receiving radiation treatment.
- *Social isolation:* children most susceptible to isolation are those with an altered appearance, those with a chronic illness such as diabetes or cancer, or those who cannot participate in contact sports.
- *Spiritual distress:* any child or family member is at risk.
- *Alteration in tissue perfusion:* applies to the underlying pathology of many retinal disorders, such as RLF or diabetic retinopathy.

closer inspection. Keep the room lights dimmed so that the pupils will enlarge. Then instruct the person to look straight ahead at a fixed object; if the subject looks at you, he will naturally use his maculas, and the light from the ophthalmoscope will momentarily blind him, causing squinting and tearing. Initially most new examiners feel uncomfortable using the ophthalmoscope because of the close proximity to the patient and the feeling of infringing on another's territory. However, the more relaxed and comfortable you are, the more your patients will be.

Normal Retinal Anatomy

Most examiners begin a fundus exam by eliciting the red reflex. This is done by moving the lends dial to + 6 (black) and holding the ophthalmoscope about 15 inches directly in front of the patient's eye. Then slowly move in closer to the patient until you see an orange glow, more commonly called the *red reflex*. When you see this you know that the patient does not have any significant corneal, lens, or vitreous opacities that may interfere with vision. Refer any child who has an absent, partial, or abnormal reflex.

Now move about 15 degrees to the patient's side and bring your ophthalmoscope even closer while you simultaneously change the lens setting into the minus (red) numbers so that you can clearly focus on a retinal vessel. Once you see a vessel (and this alone may take some practice), follow it centrally until you come to its end; this is the *optic disc,* where the optic nerve and blood vessels enter and exit the eye (Fig. 7-3). The optic disc is located in the half of the fundus nearest

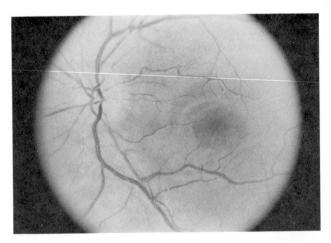

Fig. 7-3. A normal retina of the left eye. Note the macula and darker fovea centralis at 3 o'clock, and the optic disc about 10 o'clock. The optic cup is not visible in this picture.

the nose and is round or slightly oval with well-defined margins (except on the nasal side, which may have blurry margins). The optic disc is normally yellowish in color. Most discs measure about 1.5 mm in diameter, and disc diameters (DD) is a frequent unit of measure for identifying the location or size of abnormal fundus findings.

Within the disc is an even lighter colored area (yellowish-white) called the *physiologic cup*. As its name implies, its center is depressed like a cup. If you cannot see the cup, do not be alarmed; this is normal in some patients. The diameter of the cup is normally less than one-half the diameter of the disc. If this ratio is equal to or greater than 1:2 the child may have glaucoma, as the increased intraocular pressure is flattening out the cup.

Other features of the disc include scleral (light) and pigment (dark) crescents (which are normal) and blurred cup or disc margins combined with a reddish tint, indicating possible papilledema and requiring immediate referral (see Chapter 8). The disc is also the location of the *physiologic blind spot:* the only area of the normal fundus from which no vision is possible.

Once you have completed your assessment of the disc, follow a vessel outward and up and begin observing the retinal blood supply. (If you have spent considerable time examining the disc and cup, allow subjects some time to rest their eyes.) The optic arteries are narrower and lighter in color and have a much better light reflex than the veins; they carry oxygenated blood away from the disc to other parts of the retina. Unlike other arteries, however, those in the retina do not pulsate; instead, the veins, which are wine-red in color and have a decreased or absent light reflex, pulsate. Try to compare the diameters of the arteries to the veins, which should be a ratio of 2:3 or 4:5.

When viewing normal optic vessels, carefully note the way vessels smoothly cross each other, progress in a fairly straightforward fashion toward the periphery, and are free of any blemishes. Persons with hypertension may have nicked or tapered crossings and may have small dark hemorrhages or white or yellow exudates on the vessels.

Sometimes vessel changes are more noticeable in the peripheral retina. The *ora serrata* is the most peripheral border of the retina, and it is actually located in the anterior portion of the eye. Only professional eye examiners can examine this area, since a special instrument (scleral indentor or depressor) must be gently pressed into the anterior portion of the sclera at various locations. Then, with the use of the indirect ophthalmoscope, the peripheral retina can be brought into view. Scleral indentation can be painful. Parents may become upset at the sight of pain or of a speculum in their child's eye (see Fig. 3-3). A little preprocedural preparation, using photographs if possible, can decrease some of this anxiety.

To complete your assessment of the retinal vessels, return to the disc and follow the other vessels in their various directions.

Next focus your attention on the retinal background. Its color is similar to the red reflex and results from the choroid and retinal layers and the natural skin color of the patient. Patients with lighter skin have a more orange background, those with darker skin tones have a more reddish hue. Observe whether the background is consistent. The background should be free of spots, streaks, or crescents that may indicate hemorrhage; and without any white or yellowish patches from lipid exudates. A gray color with sudden cessation of the red reflex may indicate a retinal detachment.

To complete your fundus examination, have the patient look directly into the ophthalmoscope so that you can view the macula. Keep this part of the examination quite brief, however, as the patient may begin to tear or complain of seeing spots. The macula is a deep red oval area about the same size as the disc (1.5 mm), located about 2 DD to the side of the disc. Since it is supplied by minute capillaries, you will not see any vessels crossing it. The darker circle inside the macula indicates the *fovea centralis,* the area responsible for sharp vision. Any abnormalities seen here or nearby have serious implications.

OTHER DIAGNOSTIC TESTS

In addition to ophthalmoscopy and testing of a child's visual acuity, examiners may order one or more of the following diagnostic tests when a retinal disorder is known or suspected.

Color Vision

Many retinal disorders can cause an alteration of color vision. In addition, a number of medications can also cause retinopathy with color vision changes. See Chapter 6 for details on color vision testing.

Fundus Photography and Illustrations

Figure 7-4 shows a child whose fundus is being photographed. Such photographs allow the examiner to compare the status of the retina from one visit to the next. Other examiners may draw diagrams of the retina during a fundus examination, measuring and marking specific findings with great care.

Fluorescein Angiograms

Fluorescein angiograms involve a fast intravenous injection of fluorescein dye. As the dye reaches the retinal vessels (within 10–20 seconds), photographs of the fundus are taken at a rapid rate. During this process children must keep their head still on a chin rest, a procedure that can be difficult. Once the photographs have been processed, fragile vessels can be distinguished from normal

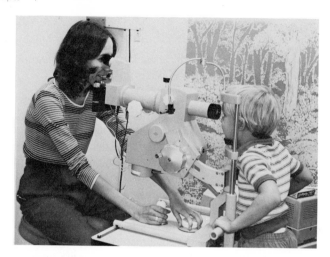

Fig. 7-4. A 4-year-old child whose fundus is being photographed. Young children may initially be frightened of the equipment, so prepare them accordingly.

ones because they leak fluorescein into the surrounding areas. Fluorescein angiograms are especially helpful for patients with diabetic retinopathy or other retinal vascular diseases.

Before administration of the dye, the eyes must be adequately dilated. Then read the package insert for the recommended dosage of fluorescein for the child's particular body weight.

Many examiners obtain consent from the child's parents before performing a fluorescein angiogram because the test carries some risks. Expected side effects include bright yellow urine for a day or so following the test and less commonly, some transient yellowing of the skin. Infrequently, some children will become nauseous for a few moments as the fluorescein is injected into the blood; a few will vomit. Although examiners debate whether informing the patient of these possibilities may increase their incidence by the power of suggestion, it is helpful to stock some towels and an emesis basin in a nearby cabinet, just in case. When the children complain of nausea, assure them that it will pass quickly and tell them to take several deep breaths. Other patients may complain of associated dizziness or headaches.

Quite rarely a child will have an anaphylactoid reaction to the fluorescein. For this reason, you may wish to obtain baseline vital signs and a weight (in case emergency medications must be given) prior to the test. Also take a brief history of any allergies and any current medical problems. In case a child complains of itching or hives, have oral diphenhydramine hydrochloride (Benadryl; [Parke-Davis]) available. In addition, have an emergency cart with adrenalin in the vicinity.

If someone else is injecting the dye, advise that person to tape down the intravenous (IV) apparatus and keep it in place until the entire procedure is completed; this procedure will ensure a patent line, should any severe reactions occur. Finally, keep in mind that fluorescein is painful if it extravates.

Electroretinograms (ERGs)

An ERG measures the electrical response of the entire retina to flashes of light. Under appropriate conditions both rod and cone activity can be stimulated. ERGs are particularly helpful for infants who have questionable retinal functioning (R/O retinal problems versus CNS problems), for patients taking medications that can cause retinopathy, and for children with hereditary retinal degenerative diseases, such as retinitis pigmentosa.

Normally a specially trained ophthalmic technician or professional eye examiner carries out this test because the equipment is complex. Once the eyes have been dilated, several drops of a topical eye anesthetic are inserted, and then a special contact lens is placed in one eye; some brief discomfort may result. A wire is then connected from the ERG machine to the contact lens, and an electrode is attached to the child's forehead. The machine is activated, and rapid lights of various strengths are flashed before the patient. Children less than 5 years old may be frightened by the insertion of the contact lens or the flashing lights, and hence, the administration of chloral hydrate or another sedative may be necessary. Sometimes, however, a little therapeutic play before the procedure and the presence of parents and a favorite toy or blanket may relax some of these younger children. The actual test takes about 30 minutes, and children should refrain from rubbing their eyes until the topical anesthetic has worn off. Sunglasses are also recommended until the pupils have resumed their normal size.

Electrooculograms (EOGs)

The EOG measures the activity of the retinal pigment layer to light adaptation and is usually performed with an ERG. However, because of the cooperation needed with an EOG, this test can seldom be done on children who are less than school age.

To begin an EOG, the technician will place a number of electrodes near the child's eyes, which have been previously dilated. The child is then asked to look back and forth between two fixation lights. The first 15 minutes of the test is conducted in the dark, and the second 15 minutes is conducted with ample lighting. A normal response is a light/dark ratio (L/D) of 2.0 or more.

Ultrasound

Ultrasound is based on the principle of impedance mismatch; that is, different tissues reflect sound waves in different ways. In ophthalmology, the ultrasound technique has proved particularly useful as a nonsurgical method of examining the posterior portion of the eye, especially to determine the status of such retinal problems as diabetic retinopathy, retinoblastoma, congenital defects, or trauma.

To obtain a B-scan ultrasound of the orbit, a penlike transducer is applied over the closed lid, to which methyl cellulose or another substance is first applied. The transducer sends sound waves into the orbit, which are then reflected back. The transducer converts the sound waves into electrical energy, and a two-dimensional picture appears on the screen. Instant photographs can be taken of these results for the patient's chart. A-scan ultrasounds provide a one-dimensional linear reading. No cooperation is needed from the child for either type, but preparation of both parents and the child, depending on age, is recommended.

The Slit Lamp

The slit lamp is an ophthalmic microscope that can magnify items up to 40 times. It is often used for examining the anterior portion of the eye. With a mirrored contact lens the ophthalmologist can also view the retina and its periphery. A topical eye anesthetic and a contact medium such as methyl cellulose are needed for retinal exams.

Visual Fields

A decrease in visual fields is often seen in patients with retinal problems. With a detached retina, the loss is usually in the sector opposite to the detachment. Characteristic changes are also seen with hereditary and metabolic diseases of the retina (see Chapter 8).

COMMON PEDIATRIC RETINAL DISEASES

Retinopathy of Prematurity (Retrolental Fibroplasia)

Retinopathy of prematurity (ROP) is an alteration in the immature retina's circulation system. The term *retrolental fibroplasia (RLF)* actually describes the final stage of this retinopathy. However, because of historical events leading to the identification and etiology of ROP in the 1940s and 1950s, the term *retrolental fibroplasia* has become entrenched in medical vocabulary.

Development of Retinal Circulation

Circulation within the retina starts to develop gradually at 16 weeks gestation. By 28 weeks gestation, only about 10 percent of babies have fully developed retinal circulations (Fig. 7-5A). By 40 weeks gestation, however, almost 100 percent have. Once this vascular network is complete and mature, it cannot be effected by ROP.

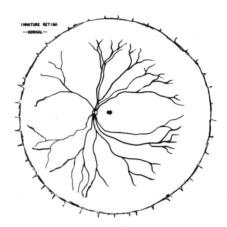

Fig. 7-5.   A, A normal immature retina of the left eye. Note that retinal circulation does not yet reach the edge of the retina (the ora serrata), especially on the temporal side; B, active stage II RLF (Reese system). Notice the shunt on the right, the branching of vessels near the shunt, and the tortuous, dilated vessels.

Pathology of ROP

In any baby with immature retinal circulation, exposure to greater than normal levels of oxygen can cause a constriction or spasm in the larger retinal vessels. In addition, such exposure can destroy or severely alter the smaller capillaries. This is called the *vaso-obliterative,* or *primary phase,* of ROP.

The second, or *vasoproliferative,* phase occurs after the termination of supplemental oxygen to the baby. Although new vessels grow in abundance, they begin to shunt blood through the damaged capillaries, rather than growing farther out to complete the retinal circulation. Retinal examination reveals a yellowish arteriovenous (A-V) shunt at the edge of branching blood vessels. The central vessels leading into the shunt can become tortuous and dilated (Fig. 7-5B).

In about 80 percent of infants who develop proliferation (arborization, neovascularization) and a shunt, the vessels will eventually cross the shunt and proceed to vascularize the rest of the retina in a normal or near-normal fashion. This process may take months, however. In the remaining patients a scarring process known as *cicatrization* occurs. The optic disc may become "dragged," and infrequently the retina may become partly or fully detached if abnormal vessel growth causes enough traction on it. These problems are most common in infants who weigh less than 1000 g at birth.

A number of ophthalmologists have proposed various classification systems

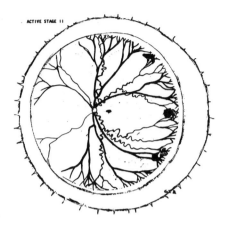

in an attempt to assess the degree of severity of the ROP and to predict possible visual outcomes. All of them divide ROP (RLF) into the active and cicatricial processes and, in turn, divide these into various stages according to severity. Table 7-1 shows the standard classification system, developed by Reese. (A new classification of retinopathy of prematurity has recently been proposed for international use.)*

Treatment and Implications

Because most cases of ROP regress spontaneously, medical treatment usually consists of close observation by an ophthalmologist and communication with the child's parents and pediatrician. It is important that children who have a history of ROP that has not fully regressed continue to see an ophthalmologist at prescribed intervals because they have an increased incidence of myopia, amblyopia, strabismus, retinal detachment, and other eye disorders.

Some surgical interventions are now possible for children with advanced vessel proliferation, significant scarring, or retinal detachment. These procedures have only been used since the early 1970s, however, and their results have been variable.

The visual potential for any infant with a history of ROP depends on whether the retina has been damaged from the ROP process. It is important to remember that no two cases are alike. In general, the early grades of ROP that regress spontaneously have little detrimental effect on vision. As retinopathy increases, however, so does the possibility of developing some visual problem. The old adage "Only time will tell" is frequently true for the baby with advanced ROP.

Finally, some experimental evidence has shown that vitamin E (tocopherol) may inhibit the ROP process, at least by decreasing its severity.[1]

---

*Ad hoc committee: An international classification of retinopathy of prematurity. Pediatr 74:127–133, 1984.

Table 7-1
Modified Reese Classification of Retrolental Fibroplasia (RLF)*

Active RLF

Grade I: Early proliferative stage, as evidenced by arborizing vessels

Grade II: Vascular dilation stage, including dilated and tortuous vessels and a
              prominent arteriovenous shunt

Grade III: Retinal traction stage, with neovascularization into the vitreous, dragging
              of the disc, and local traction on the retina

Grade IV: Advanced proliferative stage, with less than one-half of the retina detached
              and vitreous hemorrhages

Grade V: Total retinal detachment

Cicatricial RLF

Grade I: Minor changes, such as retinal pigment epithelium mottling

Grade II: Dragged disc into vitreous membrane

Grade III: Retinal fold to peripheral mass, dragging some vessels

Grade IV: Incomplete retrolental ("behind the lens") mass

Grade V: Complete retrolental mass

Modified from Reese AB, King MJ, Owens WC: A classification of retrolental fibroplasia. Am J
Ophthalmol 36:1333–1335, 1953
*Kingham, McCormick and others have developed similar systems.

Selection of Infants for ROP Examinations

In 1971 the Committee on the Fetus and Newborn of the American Academy of Pediatrics (AAP) recommended the following:

A person experienced in recognizing retrolental fibroplasia (retinopathy of prematurity) should examine the eyes of all infants born at less than 36 weeks or weighing less than 2,000 grams (4.2 pounds) who have received oxygen therapy. This examination should be made at discharge from the nursery and at 3 to 6 months of age.[2]

In all studies, birth weight appears to be the most outstanding primary risk factor, especially for babies less than 1000 g at birth. For infants weighing 1500 g or more at birth, the incidence of ROP appears to decrease significantly.

Other possible risk factors for ROP are the length of time and amount of oxygen therapy, incidence of apnea, length of mechanical ventilation, number of exchange transfusions, and occurrence of sepsis. However, studies differ regarding the amount of risk for these and other factors. Finally, a few full-term infants, premature infants with cyanotic conditions, and infants with no history of oxygen therapy have been known to have ROP or a condition clinically very similar to it.

The Examination

In conjunction with the AAP directive of examining at-risk infants prior to discharge, most neonatal centers have an ophthalmologist who makes weekly "RLF rounds." A list of infants for the week's rounds can be kept at the unit desk.

Dilation of the eyes is necessary for an adequate examination. One recommended dilating solution consists of 0.5 percent cyclopentolate (Cyclogyl [Alcon Laboratories]), 0.5 percent tropicamide (Mydriacyl [Alcon Laboratories]) and 2.5 percent phenylephrine (Neo-synephrine [Winthrop]). It can be prepared in one bottle by mixing 3.75 cc of 2 percent cyclopentolate, 7.5 cc of 1 percent tropicamide, and 3.75 cc of 10 percent phenylephrine.[3] Then the drops are usually given twice, 5 minutes apart, starting about 40 minutes before rounds are scheduled. Such a combination dilates the pupil well for an adequate examination of the vessels in the retinal periphery, while having negligible systemic effects on the babies.

When the examination begins, one or two drops of a topical ophthalmic anesthetic are placed in each eye, followed by the insertion of a wire speculum to separate the lids and to aid visualization (Fig. 3-3). The indirect ophthalmoscope is used for the examination because it provides a wider field, better illumination, and a stereoscopic view.

Usually the ophthalmologist looks at the retinal vessels in a clockwise fashion, sometimes using a scleral depressor or cotton applicator to move the eye so that the entire periphery may be seen. More attention is given to the areas at the lateral aspect of each eye; for anatomic reasons the retinal circulation at this location may not be as complete as in other areas. Despite the use of the topical anesthetic most babies cry while the speculum is in place, becoming even more agitated while scleral depression is occurring.

Examining both eyes requires approximately 10–20 minutes. Bradycardia, possibly from pressure on the globe, has been noted to follow an ROP exam directly on infrequently occasions.

If vessels are complete and mature, either no follow-up or a 3- to 6-month check is usually indicated. For babies with identified ROP or immature or questionable vessels, examinations are repeated at 1- to 6-week intervals, depending on the findings.

Additional Nursing Interventions

The diagnosis of ROP is frequently made a few days prior to discharge, when the discontinuance of any oxygen therapy and the baby's improving condition allow for a more adequate eye exam. For parents who have weathered the complications of respiratory distress syndrome, necrotizing enterocolitis, and so forth and are now eagerly anticipating their baby's discharge, the diagnosis of ROP can be a devastating blow. As one mother of a baby who developed advanced ROP stated, ''I couldn't believe it. We had been through so much; I thought the worse was over. But it wasn't.''

Nurses can play a significant role in bridging gaps of communication and providing support and information. Recommended interventions begin with incorporating the examination into the baby's discharge program and telling parents about the examination and its purpose before it occurs. The nurse should then see that the parents are told of the results, and notified of any need for follow-up. If the parents desire, have a set of pictures available to show them how the examination is done. Furthermore, for babies with a normal examination, provide a brief note to give to the parents when the results are presented to them (Fig. 7-6).

For babies who do not have a normal examination, you may want to develop a pocket-size book (20-frame, 3 by 5 photo books work very well) and insert illustrations of immature and mature retinal anatomy, the various stages of ROP, and so on, to use as a teaching tool. You can then select appropriate frames on an individual basis. In addition, you may wish to call the parents after the baby's discharge to see whether the necessary follow-up has been arranged. Such liaison between inpatient and outpatient services can greatly enhance compliance.

Persistent Hyperplastic Primary Vitreous (PHPV)

PHPV is characterized by a small eye with a white membrane behind the lens that is actually the remnant of an embryologic ocular membrane. Because of the presence of leukokoria (white pupil), the differential diagnosis includes retinoblastoma, cataracts, and advanced ROP. However, a history of a full-term pregnancy, the involvement of usually only one eye with associated microophthalmia, a shallow anterior chamber, and the findings from the fundus examination usually confirm the diagnosis of PHPV.

Surgery, if necessary, often consists of a lensectomy and vitrectomy to reduce the incidence or complications of cataracts or glaucoma and to remove the membrane from the vitreous. As discussed in Chapter 10, children who have had their

---

Dear Parent,

As part of our neonatal program, your baby's eyes were examined today by a pediatric ophthalmologist (eye doctor). The reason for this examination is that some small babies who need oxygen in their early days of life can develop an eye problem to the back of the eye. This problem is commonly called "RLF" for short; its longer names are retrolental fibroplasia or retinopathy of prematurity.

We are happy to tell you that the results of today's examination show that presently your baby's eyes do not have any evidence of RLF. If you have any questions about the examination, please do not hesitate to ask your doctor or the nurses. In addition, the following is recommended:

    _____ Have your baby see an ophthalmologist in _____for
           another check-up;
    _____ No further follow-up for this problem is needed. Contact an
           ophthalmologist if other eye problems develop or a routine eye
           examination is desired.

Sincerely yours,

Fig. 7-6.   A letter given to parents regarding their baby's normal retinopathy of prematurity exam.

lens removed should be treated immediately with a contact lens. However, in cases of PHPV, a significant improvement in vision may not always be possible. PHPV can also be associated with strabismus or retinal problems, and infrequently, an eye may have to be removed because of continued problems secondary to glaucoma.

Fortunately, PHPV is not very common. When it does occur the parents will need much support, as their baby may have an altered appearance (white pupil, microophthalmia), pain from glaucoma, or decreased vision in the involved eye. The fact that PHPV is usually unilateral and that the other eye will see normally may be of little comfort to the parents in the early stages of diagnosis and treatment. Therefore, allow them ample time for grief and possibly direct them to a family who has been through a similar experience and has successfully coped with it. Finally, if the child has a significant loss of vision in the eye with PHPV, remember to inform the parents of proper safety methods at an appropriate time (Chapter 12).

Retinoblastoma

Retinoblastoma (RB), a solid intraocular tumor of childhood, may appear at any time during the first 4 years of life. Its incidence in the United States is approximately 1:18,000. As a result, most pediatric clinicians rarely see children with this condition. Yet when it does occur, it creates concern and uncertainty for parents and health care providers alike.

Diagnosis

Any time that a white pupil, strabismus, or unexplained ocular inflammation is seen, RB must be considered. To assist in the diagnosis, the ophthalmologist will perform a complete fundus examination, using the indirect ophthalmoscope and scleral indentation. Some children will need sedation with chloral hydrate or general anesthesia so that an adequate exam can be performed. Other procedures will include the assessment of the child's visual acuity, orbital x-rays, orbital ultrasound, and computerized tomography (CT) scan. The latter three tests may show calcium deposits, which strongly suggest RB. In addition, parents and siblings less than 5 years must be examined. The findings of an unsuspected regressed tumor or retinoma in one of the parents defines a positive family history of the disease. Retinoblastoma affects male and females equally.

Biopsy of the suspected tumor site is not performed because tumor cells can be released in the process. However, affected children will have a complete oncology exam. This may include bone and liver scans; x-rays of the chest, skull, and bones; lumbar puncture; and bone marrow aspiration. A banded chromosome karyotype and esterase D assay have recently been recommended to define the 2–3 percent of affected patients with a deletion of chromosome 13. The finding of this chromosomal change is more likely in patients with delayed mental or physical development or other congenital anomalies.

Classification

Retinoblastoma can be classified in several ways. For example, unilateral and bilateral cases must be distinguished.

Unilateral RB comprises about 70 percent of all cases and usually consists of one tumor. Since the majority of these cases are not inherited, however, the tumor is unsuspected and the child may be 2 or 3 years of age before any symptoms appear. By that time the tumor is often so large that enuculeation of the eye is necessary.

All *bilateral* RBs and a small percentage of unilateral tumors are dominantly inherited. Of these, about 8 percent have a positive family history for RB, and the remainder are new genetic mutations. Any offspring of a bilaterally affected parent is at 50 percent risk for developing the tumor. Because of this, newborn children in families with a positive history should be examined shortly after birth and followed closely thereafter.

Retinoblastoma can also be classified as germinal, somatic, or chromosomal. These divisions are based on the current theory that RB is a tumor of genetic etiology and that at least two mutations are needed before it can develop.

Germinal, or *hereditary,* RB is thought to be the result of one genetic change present in the germ cell and expressed in all cells of the body. The second mutation or genetic change occurs in the retina. The mutation present in all cells of the body in these patients makes them more susceptible to other primary malignancies, such as osteogenic sarcoma. In addition, children of these patients have nearly a 50 percent chance of developing RB through an autosomal dominant pattern, and siblings likewise have an increased incidence. This type of RB comprises about 35 percent of all cases.

On the other hand, in most children with unilateral RB, both mutations most likely occur after conception in one single cell in the retina. Hence, they involve only that eye. This is called *somatic RB* and is considered to be sporadic rather than inherited. The risk for siblings or offspring to develop the tumor is zero. However, there is currently no proven way to differentiate somatic mutations from the germinal kind when only one eye has a tumor. Unpublished data from Childrens Hospital of Los Angeles suggest that direct tumor chromosome analysis may separate the subgroup of unilateral tumors that are hereditary.

Another classification system for RB is based on tumor size and involvement of other structures. Table 7-2 lists the system developed by Reese and Ellsworth which is widely used today.

Treatment

Group 1 patients may benefit from laser therapy or cryotherapy, depending on the location of the tumor(s). Usually radiation therapy is initially used for children with group 2 or 3 tumors. This can be in the form of cobalt, ruthenium or

Table 7-2
Modified Reese-Ellsworth Classification of the Ocular Lesions of Retinoblastoma

Stage I:	Confined to the retina and optic disc	
	Group 1a:	Solitary tumor less than 4 DD at or behind the equator*
	Group 1b:	Multiple tumors, none more than 4 DD in size
	Group 2a:	Solitary tumor, 4–10 DD in size at or behind the equator
	Group 2b:	Multiple tumors, 4–10 DD in size behind the equator
	Group 3a:	Any tumor anterior to the equator
	Group 3b:	Solitary tumor greater than 10 DD behind the equator
	Group 4a:	Multiple tumors, some greater than 10 DD
	Group 4b:	Any lesion extending to the ora serrata**
	Group 5a:	Any tumor involving half the retina
	Group 5b:	Vitreous seeding
Stage II:	Extraretinal but intraocular	
Stage III:	Extraocular, regional spread	
Stage IV:	Distant and metastatic disease	

*An imaginery line separating the anterior and posterior portions of the eye.
**The edge of the retina, located in the anterior portion of the eye.

iodine plaques, or external beam radiation, preferably with a linear accelerator. For the beam radiation, a total of 3500–4500 rads is given. This is divided into approximately 400 rads per session, two to three times a week. The child's head must be kept completely still during this treatment, and hence ketamine or other general anesthesia is often administered. Children receiving radiation therapy need appropriate skin care near the site of the radiation. Laser treatment may also be used with these children, once the tumors have been reduced in size, or if they recur.

Enucleation is preferred by many ophthalmologists as the method of treatment for children with tumors of group 4 or 5. This is especially true in unilateral cases where the tumor has destroyed any useful vision. In bilateral cases the worse eye is often enucleated, and radiation, possibly in association with chemotherapy, is used to try to maintain any useful vision in the remaining eye while preventing tumor spread. During the enucleation procedure, 10–15 mm of optic nerve is removed along with the eye to determine whether the tumor has spread outside the eye.

Chemotherapy is used for children who have actual metastases, or an increased probability for such. Of course, these children and their families will need assistance with its side effects (nausea, vomiting, alopecia, increased risk for infection, hemorrhagic cystitis, and so on) as well as with its psychosocial issues.

About 1–3 percent of tumors regress spontaneously. For example, one mother thought that she only had unilateral RB, which required enucleation during her childhood. However, when RB was diagnosed in her newborn baby, a closer inspection of the mother showed that she had an old regressed site in her other eye.

This example also shows that all persons with RB that has been successfully treated should see their ophthalmologist at regular intervals. During each visit the eyes will be dilated, and a thorough fundus examination will be done. Most parents rapidly comply with these follow-up appointments, but others may need reminding. The appearance of new tumors is extremely rare after age 3.

Additional Nursing Interventions

At the time of diagnosis, most families have never heard of retinoblastoma. When they concurrently hear the words *tumor* and *cancer,* however, they frequently remember little else of the information presented by the physician. Therefore, you will need to repeat and clarify information many times, even long after the diagnosis has been made. In addition, parents may have little time to adjust to the diagnosis before any treatment is begun, and they can remain in a state of denial, shock, or anger for some time. If symptoms have been present for a while (which is unfortunately true in a number of cases), the parents may feel guilty about not seeking treatment sooner. Your support and active listening will be valuable interventions. For children who require an enucleation, the section at the end of this chapter discusses appropriate nursing interventions for the child and family. Similar principles, such as the use of therapeutic play, illustrations, or a role model are also helpful for children who need radiation, laser, or chemotherapy treatment. Needless to say, double enucleation is a tragic complication of RB, and the affected children and their families will need even greater amounts of support and interventions. They should be referred as soon as possible to educators who specialize in working with children with visual handicaps.

Once the crisis period has passed, parents and other relatives may be interested in attending meetings with a few other families. Older RB patients can also be invited. For example, at one of our meetings none of the parents initially realized that one woman had had RB herself with an enucleation at age 3. It was helpful for the other parents to hear that she had completed college, married, and had obviously adjusted well. We have also found that parents are much more able to comprehend facts and features about RB at these meetings than they are during their crisis period. You can use these meetings and office visits to review the concepts of chronic grief, fear of death, and overprotection of the child.

Retinitis Pigmentosa (RP)

The term *retinitis pigmentosa* applies to a group of inherited progressive retinal degenerative disorders that have a similar retinal picture of small, scattered patches of pigment that look somewhat inflamed. The *-itis* in the name is misleading, however, as no inflammatory process has ever been observed in these patients. Hence, some authorities prefer to call RP *pigmentary degeneration of the retina*. At least 16 varieties of retinal degenerations and syndromes have or mimic the retinal changes of RP. Among these are Usher's syndrome (congenital deafness and RP that often develops in a person's teens or twenties) and Leber's congenital amaurosis (nystagmus and significant decreased visual acuity at birth.)

Retinitis pigmentosa can be inherited in any one of the three genetic patterns; it can be sex-linked or transmitted as a dominant or recessive gene. It is estimated that 1 out of every 80 Americans carries the RP recessive gene.

Usually the first symptom of RP is decreased night or dim-light vision. Although it is common for young children to be afraid of the dark, such fears may also represent a decreased ability to see when lights are turned off. Another common symptom is decreased peripheral, or side, vision. One patient commented that she had been labeled "clumsy" as a child because she was always bumping into objects. Years later, however, when she could identify that she had tunnel vision, she requested an eye examination and was diagnosed with RP. Occasionally RP patients also develop posterior lens cataracts or macular cysts. The cataracts can be removed to produce a significant increase in vision.

The symptoms of decreased night and peripheral vision implicate the rods as a source of retinal degeneration. Such degeneration may take years or occur rapidly. Fortunately, in many cases the cones degenerate much more slowly. Since the cones are located in the *macula*, the area responsible for central visual acuity, a patient may retain some valuable central vision for years.

Although there is still no cure for RP, unproven treatments abound. Probably the most famous is the yeast RNA method, made popular in Russia. Also known as *ENCAD*, this substance is given to the patient in hopes that the RNA— which is responsible for protein synthesis and is diminished in the retina of RP patients—will resynthesize. Unfortunately, no scientific studies have proved this helpful. Megadoses of vitamin A and vitamin D have also been tried without success, as have DMSO, snake venom, and placental transplants.

If you have a student or patient with RP under your care, consider the following interventions. First, ensure that all family members have had thorough eye examinations, since RP is inherited and other members may also be affected. Diagnostic tests may include ERGs, dark adaptometry, and visual fields. Also ask the family whether they are interested in genetic counseling and assess whether such resources as low-vision centers and the department of vocational rehabilitation have been used to the fullest extent. The family should also be encouraged to contact the national or local Retinitis Pigmentosa Foundation for literature, equipment information, and emotional support. For example, the Texas Association for RP offers a hotline and publishes the *RP Messenger,* a bi-monthly publication available in both large-print text and cassette. Finally, many patients can benefit from the use of treated sunglasses when in bright lights and from night vision aids when in dim lights.

Retinal Detachment (RD)

Although one may initially believe that a retinal detachment is a separation of the entire retina from the choroid, it is actually a separation of one layer of the retina (the *sensory layer*) from another retinal layer that lies beneath it (the *pigment epithelium*). For anatomic reasons, it is more difficult for the retina to become detached at the ora serrata or (rarely) at the optic nerve.

Retinal detachments can be classified in two ways. *Primary* or *secondary* refers to the cause of the detachment, with the former implying a spontaneous retinal degenerative process, and the latter occurring from other problems such as trauma or inflammation. Detachments can also be classified by their mechanism. *Rhegmatogenous* detachments involve a tear or break in the retina (*rhegma* is the Greek word for "rupture or tear"). In contrast, nonrhegmatogenous detachments may result from exudates or excessive traction on the retina.

In general, retinal detachments are not very common in children. When they do occur, they can be associated with advanced or cicatricial retinopathy of prematurity, retinitis pigmentosa, retinoblastoma, aphakia, severe myopia, a history of intraocular surgery, inflammation, or trauma.

Patients with a retinal detachment may have a variety of complaints or they may have none at all until a severe loss of vision occurs. Light flashes, especially in dim light, may occur, or the patient may see vitreous floaters. These symptoms may come and go and are next to impossible to ascertain in young children. Eventually hemorrhages or the detachment itself may cause shadows ("curtains," "veils") or smoky, blurred vision. No pain is associated with primary retinal detachments. Once a detachment is suspected, the fundus is examined for grayish areas, which indicate the site of the detachment. Visual field studies may show a loss of vision on the opposite side of the detachment.

The ultimate prognosis for children with retinal detachments varies. For example, peripheral detachments have a better prognosis than do macular ones, since the macula is the area responsible for sharp central vision. Similarly, detachments in the inferior portion of the retina pose less of a threat to the macula than do superior detachments.

As for treatment, surgery or photocoagulation (laser) is performed as quickly as possible for primary detachments to provide the greatest opportunity for the sensory retinal layers to remain well-nourished and hence functional. In contrast, surgery is less commonly indicated for secondary detachments. Instead, treatment is directed at the underlying pathology. If the detachment is due to an inflammatory process, steroids (topical or systemic) may be used.

Retinal Inflammations (Posterior Uveitis, Chorioretinitis)

The *uveal tract* consists of the choroid, iris, and ciliary body. Inflammation in one of these parts can ultimately lead to inflammation along the entire tract. Since the retina is located so close to the choroid, inflammation can quickly spread there also, hence the term *chorioretinitis. Anterior uveitis (iridocyclitis)* refers to inflammation of the iris and ciliary body only; while *posterior uveitis* indicates that the choroid is involved.

Toxoplasmosis

In children, toxoplasmosis is one of the leading causes of chorioretinitis, particularly in Central America. In the United States, the incidence of congenital toxoplasmosis is roughly 2.7/1000 live births. It is caused by a protozoan parasite and is transmitted by contaminated cat feces. Toxoplasmosis can only effect an unborn child if the mother becomes infected for the first time during pregnancy.

A newborn with classic severe congenital toxoplasmosis usually has bilateral chorioretinitis, as well as hydrocephalus, intracerebellar calcifications, hepatosplenomegaly, and convulsions. If the child survives, severe visual loss and mental retardation can occur. Although approximately 70 percent of other infants with congenital toxoplasmosis are asymptomatic at birth, a number of them show evidence of visual or neurologic sequelae years later, secondary to either recurrent infection or latent manifestations of earlier inflammation. Acquired toxoplasmosis can rarely cause a unilateral chorioretinitis.

As for treatment, practitioners debate over the use of steroids for ocular involvement. Recent studies, however, indicate that pyrimethamine (Daraprim [Burroughs Wellcome]) and sulfa drugs may decrease visual and neurological problems. (Children taking pyrimethamine need to take folinic acid concurrently to decrease side effects.)

Toxocariasis (Visceral larva migrans)

Toxocara canis and *T. cati* are roundworms commonly found in the intestines of dogs and cats. Should a child become infected with one of these, the larvae can migrate to the child's eye or visceral organs; rarely do both locations become involved. Ocular manifestations include a unilateral chorioretinitis, endophthalmitis, or inflammation occasionally presenting as a white mass in the eye that is confused with retinoblastoma. An enzyme linked immunosorbent serum assay (Elisa test) may help differentiate between the two.

Rubella

Many children with congenital rubella infections have a pigmentary (''salt and pepper'') retinopathy that usually does not affect their vision.

Diabetic Retinopathy

Although visual problems from diabetes rarely occur in the childhood and adolescent years, persons with insulin-dependent (formerly called *juvenile-onset*) diabetes have a higher risk for developing such problems in their later lives. This higher risk results from the close correlation between the presence of visual problems and the length of time one has had diabetes. Retinopathy is the most common cause of visual impairment in persons with diabetes, although other visual problems (cataracts, glaucoma, eye muscle paresis, refractive errors, iritis, and optic neuritis) can also occur. Although statistics vary, estimates show that approximately 50 percent of persons with diabetes for 15 years or longer develop some retinopathy. After 30 years of diabetes, a person has a 95 percent chance of developing retinopathy.

Diabetic retinopathy is divided into the nonproliferative and proliferative phases. The *nonproliferative* (background) phase begins when the small vessels within the retina become involved and eventually become beaded or sausagelike from the appearance of microaneurysms. The vessels may leak exudates or rupture and cause hemorrhages into the surrounding retina. The patient may complain of a reddish tint, blurred vision, or little dark streaks from the hemorrhages, especially if they occur near the macula. As the hemorrhages and lipid deposits are absorbed, vision can return to normal, often on the same day that the complaints are first noticed. Finally, capillary closure (nonperfusion) may occur, causing specific areas of the retina to become deprived of blood.

In some unknown manner the nonperfused areas stimulate new blood vessels to grow nearby. Such growth starts the second phase of diabetic retinopathy, called the *proliferative (neovascular) phase,* or *retinitis proliferans.* Unfortunately, these new vessels are abnormal; being fragile, they can easily rupture from small changes in blood pressure, such as from straining or lifting, or from sheer stress in the eye. In addition, they grow in an abnormal fashion and may appear on the retinal surface or in the vitreous, rather than in the retina. Finally, if this vessel growth is abundant, it can pull on the retina itself, promoting additional hemorrhages. Scar tissue may form, and ultimately retinal detachment can occur.

The majority of diabetics only develop background retinopathy and rarely have any permanent visual loss. However, the prognosis for normal vision is definitely poorer in persons with proliferative retinopathy, especially if the retinopathy occurs near the optic disc or macula. Sudden blindness in this phase is not uncommon. Persons who have had juvenile-onset diabetes for 15 years or longer are especially at risk for developing proliferative retinopathy.

As for treatment, the use of laser therapy in the last decade has shown promising results in many cases of proliferative retinopathy. Vitrectomy has also been used with some success in patients with advanced proliferative retinopathy. In addition, although not a specific treatment for retinopathy, insulin pumps have proved beneficial in decreasing the incidence of retinopathy and other microvascular changes caused by diabetes.

When counseling your students and patients who may already have some background retinopathy, encourage them to express their anger or depression at having been dealt the double blow of diabetes and retinopathy and to discuss their possible fears for the future. One fear may be that blindness will occur immediately after background retinopathy appears. Although diabetic retinopathy is the main cause of new adult blindness in the United States, and a rapidly progressive type (the florid type) occurs in about 1 percent of all patients with diabetic retinopathy, most patients stay in the background phase without permanent or significant visual loss for many years.

In follow-up, ensure that the patient with diabetes has a dilated fundus exam by an ophthalmologist at least once a year, especially if the diabetes has been present for 3 years or more. If background retinopathy is present, visits at 6 months or less may be in order. Fluorescein angiograms may be done at each visit, depending on the findings.

Teach patients with juvenile diabetes to call their ophthalmologist if any unusual symptoms occur. To reinforce your teaching, consider using the new slide program by the NSPB, *The Effects of Diabetes on the Eye* (also available in booklet form for $4.00).

Finally, see the list at the end of this chapter for references treating the special needs of persons who are blind from diabetes (for example, how to do urine or blood testing).

TREATMENTS OF RETINAL PROBLEMS

General Medical Management

Depending on the child's particular retinal problem, various measures may be prescribed to decrease the chances of retinal detachment. For example, most patients with retinal disorders will be advised to refrain from contact sports, to use suppressant cough syrups when needed, to avoid lifting heavy objects, and to pick objects off the floor by bending one's legs, rather than bending over at the waist. In addition, all are taught to immediately report any sudden decrease in visual acuity or change in visual fields, as well as any floaters, light flashes, red tints, or halos, since any of these symptoms can indicate a recent or impending retinal detachment. Finally, patients with retinal problems should be seen at least yearly by their ophthalmologist.

Laser Treatment (Photocoagulation)

The introduction of laser therapy into ophthalmology during the past two decades has allowed many patients with retinal disorders the benefit of successful treatment without an invasive surgical procedure. During laser therapy, an intense beam of light temporarily delivers energy in the form of heat to halt the growth of new fragile vessels or to seal a retinal hole. The heat creates an inflammatory process (choroiditis), and within a few weeks a scar forms over the retinal hole or at the site of vessel proliferation. For example, in diabetic retinopathy the laser is used to make myriads of small "burns" that scar and no longer require oxygen. As a result, there is less demand for oxygen by the retina and a lower tendency to form neovascular tissue. In general, laser therapy does not improve vision. Instead, it helps to arrest the process that is causing the vision to deteriorate.

Several kinds of light delivery systems now exist. The original ruby red laser has been replaced with the xenon arc white light and the argon green laser. The xenon arc has a larger light spectrum and can be used for larger retinal holes or areas with much vessel proliferation. The argon laser, however, remains the most widely used laser method because it has decreased side effects on one's visual acuity and it is easier to use. Other lasers are being developed.

If the child is old enough to cooperate, the laser treatments are usually done on an outpatient basis in the examiner's office, with the child awake throughout the procedure. Following dilation of the eyes, the child is given a topical eye anesthetic (occasionally this may be an injection of anesthesia into the retrobulbar area), and a gonio (contact) lens is placed on the eye. Since these procedures may cause some brief discomfort, the child should be prepared accordingly. Then the child is seated behind the laser machine (which looks like a big microscope), and the room lights are dimmed. Short and painless bursts of light begin to enter the eye and continue for a 10- to 25-minute period. During this time it is important that the child stay very still. Several treatments may be needed for optimum benefit.

Following this procedure, the eye is patched or sunglasses are used until the pupils return to their normal size. Some patients will complain of double vision for 6–8 hours after the treatment. Others will see spots before their eyes or have blurred vision for one or two days. Aspirin or acetaminophen may alleviate any secondary headaches. Laser treatments near the macula can cause decreased central vision for several weeks, and treatments in the retinal periphery can temporarily reduce night or peripheral vision.

Surgical Interventions

Preoperative Care

If a detachment has occurred or appears imminent, bilateral patching may be ordered to promote decreased eye movements. (Since both eyes work as a team, uniocular patching of the involved eye would not decrease these movements.) If patching is necessary, orient the child to the environment, keeping everything in the same place, and visit the child frequently (at least 5 minutes every 1/2 hour), to prevent sensory deprivation or disorientation. A family member should be encouraged to stay with the child. Children who require postoperative patching should also be prepared for it and perhaps have several brief practice sessions prior to their surgery.

Special positioning can also decrease or inhibit the detachment by allowing the retina to flatten against the choroid. For example, if the detachment is in the temporal portion of the right eye, the child will be instructed to lie on the right side, except when using the bathroom. Children with inferior retinal detachments (a less urgent surgical case) will have the head of their bed elevated. In these latter cases, bilateral patching will not be used because the macula is in a relatively safe position from the detachment. Finally, if the macula is already detached, patching and positioning will not be ordered, as they cannot prevent any further damage.

Cryotherapy (Cryopexy/Diathermy)

Cryotherapy (cold treatment) and *diathermy* (heat treatment) are also noninvasive procedures used in the treatment of retinal tears and proliferation. Currently cryotherapy is used more frequently than diathermy. Unlike photocoagulation, these treatments cannot be used for posterior retinal problems. Instead, they are applied to lesions in the peripheral retina. This is usually done with the use of a topical anesthetic, except for young children, who require general anesthesia. Cryotherapy involves the use of a probe that transmits cold to freeze the conjunctiva or sclera on the outside of the eye, in diathermy, heat is transmitted. As with laser treatment, a choroiditis is produced, and within a few days a scar forms. Side effects include blurred vision, a numbing or tingling sensation from cryotherapy (such as when ice is applied to one's skin), and perhaps some edema of the eyelids for several days. Normally the child is discharged on the same day.

Vitrectomy (Pars Plana Approach)

As its name implies, a *vitrectomy* is the surgical removal of vitreous fluid. This type of procedure has only been done since the early 1970s, when a special instrument was designed to grind up and aspirate hemorrhages, membranes, and scar material in the vitreous, while maintaining intraocular pressure with the infusion of selected solutions. Traction on the retina can be alleviated through this clearing of vitreal debris, and vision can be improved by allowing light to reach the retina through a clear(er) vitreous medium once again.

Pediatric candidates for vitrectomy include infants with proliferative retinopathy of prematurity, adolescents with advanced diabetic retinopathy, or children who have had a penetrating ocular injury. The child's ophthalmologist may wait several months to see whether the vitreal hemorrhages can be reabsorbed spontaneously. Vitrectomies are not performed in patients who have increased intraocular pressure (for instance, from hemolytic glaucoma) or who have no light perception preoperatively.

During a vitrectomy the child's eyes are well dilated, and general anesthesia is administered. Then the special instrument (Ocutome [Cooper Vision Surgical/ Systems Division]) is inserted behind the lens into the vitreous near the ciliary muscles, and the grinding and aspirating begin. Possible complications include retinal detachment or retinal holes, recurrent vitreal hemorrhage, or corneal problems secondary to the insertion of the cutter. Patients are usually discharged within a week of the procedure.

Scleral Buckles (Scleral Implants/Explants)

The scleral buckle is a procedure designed specifically to treat retinal detachments. When a "buckle" (silicone band or donor fascia lata) is permanently applied partly or entirely around the sclera, the retina and choroid can be pressed close together so they can reattach. For example, a silicone plate (implant) may be inserted under the sclera over the exact area of the detachment. Or a circle or band (explant) may be placed over the entire sclera (under the extraocular muscles) to provide further pressure. You may wish to reassure parents and older children that the buckles cannot be seen or felt after insertion.

Postoperatively the eye is usually patched for a day or so to help the extraocular muscles rest and adjust to the buckle. Lid ecchymoses and edema often occur and can be somewhat alleviated with the application of a cold compress for 15 minutes, four times a day. Upon discharge the child should be fairly sedentary, although ambulation is encouraged. Light activities can be resumed at 3 weeks after surgery, and by 6 weeks full activities (except for contact sports) can safely by reinstituted.

The results of the surgery may take several weeks to be fully realized. Unfortunately, buckles that are initially successful may fail later, requiring repeat surgery.

Additional Postoperative Care

Children who have had a vitrectomy or scleral buckle procedure should refrain from any activities that may increase intraocular pressure in the immediate postoperative period, since such pressure can cause the retina to redetach. For example, if vomiting occurs, antiemetics should be ordered. In addition, the child should be taught to deep breathe rather than cough to maintain respiratory status and to avoid straining, bending, or lifting heavy objects. If intraocular pressure does increase, acetazolamide (Diamox [Lederle]) may be ordered.

Other postoperative care includes the administration of dilating, antibiotic, and anti-inflammatory eyedrops. Keep the room lights dimmed to decrease light sensitivity from dilating drops. Also remember to teach the family how to administer eye medications if the child will be discharged home with them. Immediately after surgery, the surgeon may prefer that activities involving rapid eye movements (such as reading, coloring, or watching television from near) be avoided. Finally, the family and child should be taught the symptoms of retinal detachment in case the surgery fails at a later time, and reminded of the need for follow-up, since these patients have an increased risk for developing glaucoma and cataracts.

Enucleation and Artificial Eyes

The most common causes for removing a child's eye are glaucoma, trauma, and retinoblastoma. In addition, a few children develop *phthisis,* which is a shrunken, nonfunctional eye, often resulting from trauma or congenital defects.

Needless to say, adequate preparation of both the child and family before the enucleation is an essential part of the nursing plan. In cases such as retinoblastoma, however, the time for such preparation may be markedly limited: perhaps only a day or two.

In preparing toddlers, a doll may be helpful for a simple demonstration of the surgical and postoperative routines. Some older children or parents may wish to talk with someone who has had an eye removed during childhood and has made a successful adjustment. When this is not possible, picture books showing other children or famous people with an artificial eye may be quite beneficial in decreasing any fears the children and parents may have (Fig. 7-7).

Clarification is also important. For example, parents may ask about the possibility of an eye transplant, not realizing that this is the popular term for corneal transplants and therefore not helpful for their child. The parents also may have concerns about their child's vision. If the other eye has normal vision, you can assure them that the child will have good vision. The difference will be in depth perception (stereopsis), and the child will gradually learn to use other cues to help determine distances.

The actual enucleation procedure is simple, consisting of cutting the extraocular muscles and the optic nerve and removing the eye in toto. Then a silicone ball is usually placed with stitches behind the conjunctiva to help the socket maintain its

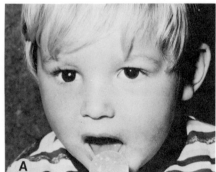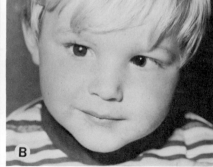

Fig. 7-7. A child with an artificial eye: A, It is initially difficult to determine which eye is artificial. B, When the child looks to the side, the artificial eye does not move.

shape. Parents should be instructed to call their ophthalmologist if during home care the stitches begin to separate, or the ball comes out.

Postoperatively the child recovers quite rapidly and is often playing around the ward the day after surgery. Initially a dressing covers the eye to collect drainage and allow healing. Antibiotic and anti-inflammatory ointments will be administered, often by the surgeon during dressing changes.

Viewing the child's socket postoperatively can be traumatic for parents (or the child, depending on age), particularly since it is swollen and ecchymotic for several weeks. You may wish to use pictures or suggest that the parents only glance at the site initially, until they adjust to its appearance. After several weeks, the inside of the socket will be similar in appearance to the buccal area of the mouth.

Once some of the swelling has decreased, a clear or white plastic conformer will be placed into the front of the socket to also help maintain its shape. Some conformers have holes in them to help in the administration of ointment into the socket and to assist with drainage.

Approximately 4–6 weeks after the surgery, the child will be referred to an ocularist (a technician who makes or supplies artificial eyes). Until 1941 prosthetic eyes were made of glass. Now, however, they are made from hard plastic. Stock eye prostheses cost about $200.00. In contrast, custom artificial eyes cost $700.00 or more but are handmade to fit and match each child individually. Initially it often takes several fittings until a close match can be obtained, and the lids can close adequately.

The care of the artificial eye is taught by the ocularist. The schedule for its cleaning will depend on the amount of secretions that a child has; some children will need to remove their eye daily for adequate cleansing, and others need to do so once a week. In between, the prosthesis remains in the eye, including during hours of sleep. Although special products are commercially available for cleansing the prosthesis, many families use only mild soap and water. Alcohol is contraindicated, as it warps the plastic and can possibly irritate the socket once the prosthesis is reinserted. To remove only mucous or small secretions, keep the prosthesis in place and use a tissue to wipe towards the nose.

To remove the eye, pull the lower lid down, and gently press under the prosthesis; this will create a vacuum and cause the prosthesis to pop out. Then clean and rinse the eye and reinsert it.

Sometimes it is initially difficult to tell how the eye goes back in correctly. However, look for clues (such as more space on the temporal side and a more pointed edge on the top and nasal aspects) or ask the child or family.

To insert the eye, moisten it with water, and then raise the upper lid. With your other hand insert the prosthesis under the upper lid until the pupil is barely visible. Then pull down the lower lid, and it should fall into place.

The child and family should be instructed to contact the ophthalmologist should any pain, redness, swelling, or unusual discharge occur. In addition, the prosthesis can become scratched, and it is advisable to have it repolished every 6 months by the ocularist. At this time, the ocularist can also check the fitting of the prosthesis, especially in young children who will need fairly frequent changes to allow for growth.

It cannot be stressed too often that the family must take adequate precautions in protecting the child's remaining eye, especially during contact or rough sports. Also, a child who swims should use a patch or goggles to prevent the prosthesis from coming out of the eye.

Needless to say, children quickly become sensitive to the reactions of others to their artificial eye. One 3-year-old boy was renowned for quietly removing his eye in the middle of Sunday church services, much to the surprise of the people in the pews behind him. Although he probably did this out of playfulness or boredom, it is possible that he was also testing the reactions of others around him.

In general, children who have an eye removed at an early age tend to adjust to it well. If their families treat them normally and consistently, this adjustment will continue into their later years.

To minimize drawing attention toward the artificial eye, older children may want to practice in front of a mirror or family member to determine when their artificial eye becomes increasingly noticeable because of its inability to move to the side. As a result, they can learn to turn their head frequently, rather than moving their eyes to view peripheral objects.

Finally, you may wish to describe the concept of chronic grief to parents and older children, so that they can realize that occasional periods of grief, even years after the enucleation, are normal. In addition, siblings should be incorporated into the preparation and follow-up programs, as they can play a significant role in the patient's adjustment.

REFERENCES

1. Hittner HM, Godio LB, Rudolph AJ, et al: Retrolental fibroplasia: efficacy of vitamin E in a double-blind clinical study of preterm infants. N Engl J Med 305:1365–71, 1981
2. Graven SN: Oxygen therapy in the newborn infant: A Statement of the Committee on Fetus and Newborn by the American Academy of Pediatrics. Wis Med J 70:224, 1971
3. Caputo AR, Schnitzer RE, Lindquist TD, Suns S: Dilation in neonates: A protocol. Pediatrics 69:77–80, 1982

SELECTED BIBLIOGRAPHY

Boyd-Monk H: Retinal detachment and vitrectomy: Nursing care. Nurs Clin North Am 16:433–451, 1981
Brown MM: Retinal vascular disorders: Nursing and medical implications. Nurs Clin North Am 16:414–432, 1981

Carr RE: Retinitis pigmentosa. Sight Sav Rev 49:147–154, 1979–1980
Cavender JC: *The Retina Book*. Daly City, Calif., Patient Information Library, 1982
Char DH: Current concepts in retinoblastoma. Ann Ophthalmol 12:792–804, 1980
Crom DB, Pratt CB: Care of retinoblastoma patients and their families. J Ophthalmic Nurs Tech 1:16–20, 1982
Eddy DM: Vitrectomy. Am J Nurs 78:608–609, 1978
Herget M: For visually impaired diabetics. Am J Nurs 83:1157–1560, 1983
Kingham JD: Retrolental fibroplasia. Am Fam Physician 20:119–125, 1979
MacFadyen JS: Caring for the patient with a primary retinal detachment. Am J Nurs 80:920–921, 1980
Mechner F: Patient assessment: Examination of the eye, pt 2. Am J Nurs 75:P.I.1–P.I.24, January 1975
National Retinitis Pigmentosa Foundation, Baltimore: Answers to your questions about retinitis pigmentosa and other degenerative diseases
National Society to Prevent Blindness: *The Effects of Diabetes on the Eye*. New York, 1982
Oehler JW: Self-management of diabetes mellitus following vision loss. J Ophthalmic Nurs Tech 1:20–27, 1982
Perrin ED: Laser therapy for diabetic retinopathy. Am J Nurs 80:664–665, 1980
Schulz JM, Williams M: Blind diabetic. Nursing 76 6:19–20, 1976
Schumann D: Assessing the diabetic. Nursing 76 6:62–67, 1976
Smith JF, Nachazel DP: Diabetic retinopathy, in *Ophthalmologic Nursing*. Boston, Little, Brown, 1980, pp 178–191
Smith JF, Nachazel DP: Retinal detachment. Am J Nurs 73:1530–1535, 1973
Stagno S: Toxoplasmosis. Am J Nurs 80:720–722, 1980
Tasman W: Late complications of retrolental fibroplasia. Ophthalmology 86:1735–1738, 1979
Wong DL, Dornan LR: Nursing care in childhood cancer—retinoblastoma. Am J Nurs 82:425–431, 1982
Zucnick M: Care of an artificial eye. Am J Nurs 75:835, 1975

Chapter Eight

Neuroophthalmology

NURSING GOALS, OUTCOME STANDARDS, AND DIAGNOSES

This chapter's primary nursing goal is that *each child with a neuroophthalmologic disorder has the best possible sensory and motor functioning, in view of his or her own particular medical history.* It is related to the fact that neuroophthalmologic disorders often extend beyond the eyes. Therefore, the effects on a child's function can be quite varied.

For many nurses, pediatric neuroophthalmology is often associated with sad or difficult moments. Memories may come to mind of a baby who is blind because of brain damage at birth or of a child in the intensive care unit (ICU) with minimal pupillary responses secondary to a car accident. Yet neuroophthalmology can also be fascinating and rewarding. For example, the discovery of a visual field loss may lead to the identification and successful treatment of a central nervous system (CNS) tumor.

The techniques for neuroophthalmologic screening are not complex, nor do they require much equipment. Through regular practice of the various techniques you will become comfortable in identifying any abnormalities and making appropriate referrals. However, because the incidence of neuroophthalmologic disorders in children is so small, the components of such a screening are usually deleted during mass screening programs.

Outcome Standard 1

Each child who is at risk or has a documented neuroophthalmologic disorder is seen by an appropriate physician at recommended intervals and receives any recommended treatment.

Suggested Interventions:

• The nurse identifies children at risk for having or developing a neuroophthalmologic disorder. These include children with a recent history of head trauma or CNS insult, those with positive findings in the neuroophthalmologic screening (Table 8-1), and those with recent behavioral changes, such as increased clumsiness or dynamic mood changes.

• The nurse immediately refers all children at risk for a neuroophthalmologic disorder to a physician. However, in view of other nonocular signs and symptoms that a child may have, one may be uncertain as to which physician (the ophthalmologist, neurologist, or pediatrician) can best meet the needs of the child. In these cases, time may be of the essence, so refer the child to the most accessible practitioner.

• The nurse follows all children with suspected or documented neuroophthalmologic disorders to ensure that each child is followed as necessary by a physician (decrease *noncompliance*). Treatment will vary for each child. For example, a child with nystagmus, pupil coloboma, or optic nerve hypoplasia may require no other treatment than routine follow-up after the initial examination(s). In contrast, children with CNS lesions may require surgery, chemotherapy, or radiation.

• The nurse assists the family in identifying and removing any financial, psychosocial, or other barriers that might prevent the child from receiving adequate follow-up and treatment (counteracts *impaired home maintenance management, ineffective coping, anxiety* or *fears* about the diagnostic or treatment process or results).

• The nurse has verbal or written communication with the physician and any other health care providers (physical or occupational therapists, social workers, and so on) to promote continuity of care (reduce *impaired communication* or *knowledge deficit* between health team members). In addition, the nurse notes relevant information in the school or health record.

Outcome Standard 2

Each child with a neuroophthalmologic disorder becomes increasingly cooperative during subsequent examinations.

Suggested Intervention:

• The nurse uses age-appropriate play therapy (puppets, dolls, play or actual hospital equipment, story books, pictures and such) as necessary to decrease the child's fears and anxieties regarding diagnostic and treatment procedures and equipment (counteracts *knowledge deficit, anxiety,* or *fears*).

Outcome Standard 3

Older patients and the parents of all patients name and define the child's neuroophthalmologic disorder, its implications, and any recommended treatment or follow-up appointments.

Outcome Standard 4

Older patients and the parents of all patients verbalize the impact of the neuroophthalmologic disorder on their daily lives.

Suggested Interventions:

- The nurse clarifies and offers repeated explanations as necessary about the diagnosis, treatment, and related procedures, using written remarks and illustrations whenever possible to supplement the teaching program.
- The nurse provides families and older patients several opportunities to discuss the impact of the neuroophthalmologic disorder on their daily lives and provides support and guidance as necessary. For example, a child may have such *sensory perceptual alterations* as nystagmus, decreased visual acuity, or decreased visual fields. These alterations may in turn cause a *deficit in diversional activities, self-care, or physical mobility,* especially if the child is newly or severely visually impaired. A change in the child's sensory or motor functioning can likewise increase the child's *potential for physical injury.* Furthermore, a *disturbance in a child's body-image* or *social isolation* from peers may result from such overt problems as nystagmus, strabismus, ptosis, facial asymmetry, head tilting, or altered motor functioning. Finally, the few children with associated CNS problems may have *alterations in their thought processes.*

Parents and older patients can experience *dysfunctional grieving* or *ineffective coping* regarding the child's altered vision, motor functioning, or treatment, or regarding a potential or actual threat to the child's life. There may be associated *alterations in parenting or family processes,* with increased family conflicts or overprotection of the child being two ways in which such alterations are manifested. Or the patient or family members may experience *anxiety* or *fear* about the long-term implications of the disorder.

- The nurse makes referrals as needed to related agencies and community services, such as Crippled Children's Services, low-vision centers, and special educators.

VISUAL ACUITY

As with any ophthalmic evaluation, the neuroophthalmologic assessment starts with a visual acuity screening. Children who continue to have a visual loss despite correction of any refractive errors should be referred to an ophthalmologist for the possibility of a neuroophthalmologic or other organic disorder.

THE PUPILS

The observation "pupils equal, round, and react to light and accommodation" *(PERRLA)* is sometimes written quite casually, after only a cursory look at the pupils. Yet when written after a thorough pupil examination, this notation provides much information about the subject's neuroophthalmologic status.

Table 8-1
Reference Guide for Assessing a Child's Neuroopthalmologic Status*

History: Recent head trauma: denied
Recent CNS insult: denied
Recent behavioral changes: denied

Visual Acuity: Normal, with corrective lenses if necessary

Pupils: Shape: round
Size: 2–5 mm
Equal: Yes
Direct light response in each eye: Yes (constriction)
Consensual light response in each eye: Yes (constriction)
Near reflex response: constriction

Cranial Nerves: Ductions and versions: normal
Facial expressions: normal
Head tilting or turning: absent
Ptosis: absent
Strabismus: absent
Diplopia: denied

**Optic Nerve: Color: yellowish
Margins: clear

Nystagmus: No spontaneous nystagmus present, except in extreme lateral gaze

Visual Fields: Confrontation test: normal
**Perimetry: normal
**Tangent screen: normal

**Visually Evoked Potentials: normal

**X-Rays: normal

---

*A child who has any different responses than those listed may have a neuroophthalmologic problem
and should be immediately referred for a more complete work-up.
**This technique requires special equipment.

All pupillary reflexes occur subcortically. The second (optic) cranial nerve
serves as the sensory or afferent link, transmitting the appropriate stimuli to the
brain. Autonomic outflow accompanies the third (oculomotor) cranial nerve, carrying out the brain's response; hence it is the efferent pathway.

To examine the pupils you will need a flashlight, a ruler calibrated in
millimeters, and a room with subdued light. A card with pupil sizes imprinted on
it can also be helpful (you can make one yourself).

Before the examination, note the child's history and any medications taken
within the last few days. For example, atropine or some motion sickness medications will cause pupillary dilation. If the child is hospitalized or recently traumatized,
also note the level of consciousness.

Begin your examination by inspecting the shape of the pupils. If you must use a flashlight in order to see the pupils clearly, shine it at an oblique angle from below the eyes. In children, irregularly shaped pupils can be caused by a *coloboma* (congenital ocular defect), iritis, midbrain lesion, recent injury, or recent surgery to the anterior of the eye. Refer any child whose pupils are not round.

Next, note your first impressions about pupil size. Are they small? Pinpointed? Dilated? These first impressions are important and should always precede their actual measurement and comparison. Normal pupil size is 2–5 mm in diameter. As a group, newborns and elderly people have small pupils, and adolescents have the largest. In addition, pupil size usually decreases during sleep.

The size of the pupil is controlled by the sympathetic and parasympathetic nervous systems. The sympathetic system controls the iris dilator; when this muscle contracts, the pupil dilates and *mydriasis* occurs. Such emotions as fear and anxiety can also cause dilation of the pupil by their stimulation of the sympathetic nervous system. On the other hand, when the parasympathetic nervous system becomes activated, it causes the iris sphincter to contract. In turn, the pupils constrict *(miosis)*.

Anisocoria is the term used to describe pupils which are unequal in size. Infants up to 1 year of age often have unequal pupil sizes. In addition, approximately 20 percent of the normal population has a 0.3- to 1-mm difference in their pupil sizes. The differentiation of this normal variant from a pathologic problem can sometimes be difficult to determine but may be assisted by the use of close-up pictures taken from the child's younger years. Refer any child with suspicious findings.

In *Horner's syndrome* (sympathetic paresis), the child has anisocoria that is most noticeable in dim light, as well as miosis, ptosis, and lack of sweating, all on the affected side of the face. These symptoms can be caused by birth trauma to the cervical sympathetic nerve or brachial plexus or by a mediastinal or other tumor. Horner's syndrome that appears before the age of 2 years is also accompanied by hypopigmentation of the iris (heterochromia).

Third nerve palsy can also cause anisocoria, as well as abnormal eye movements on the side of the larger pupil. Children with *Adie's,* or *tonic, pupil* (usually a benign disorder) have a unilateral accommodation defect, a weak or absent light response, and a slow near response in addition to their anisocoria.

Once you have determined the pupils' size, use your flashlight to observe their response to light. Remember to keep your room light settings constant during any subsequent examinations on the same child. Start by holding the light 8 in away from one eye (be careful not to shine it into the other) and observe the responses of both pupils. Normally, both pupils quickly become smaller when either eye is exposed to light. The response of the pupil that is actually being exposed is called the *direct response:* the response of the other pupil is called the *consensual response.* An easy way of observing the direct and consensual responses is through the "swinging flashlight" test. Have the child look at a distant object (to decrease the accommodative response of the pupils) and move the flashlight slowly back and forth from one eye to the other. Sometimes examiners use numbers to indicate the response of the pupils to light, with, for example, 4 being a brisk response, and 0 being no response at all. Refer any children who have an abnormal pupillary light response.

A child is said to have a positive *Marcus Gunn pupillary response,* or *afferent pupillary defect,* when the pupil dilates as the flashlight is switched to that eye. This response is often seen in atrophy, hypoplasia, neuritis, or tumors of the optic nerve.

When a child has a sluggish or absent pupillary response with continued dilation of the eye(s), question the child or parents about any recent administration of homatropine, adrenaline, or Neo-synephrine (Winthrop). If none of these has been given recently, the lack of response may be due to a congenital or traumatic third nerve palsy, botulism, tumor, aneurysm, or inflammation. A child with a fixed dilated pupil who is also comatose may have a severe CNS disturbance or recent episode of hypoxia. A fixed constricted pupil may be due to encephalitis, meningitis or orbital inflammation, or to the recent administration of pilocarpine, morphine, echothiophate, or other organophosphate compounds, such as insect poisons. In addition, some children, such as those with juvenile rheumatoid arthritis, may have constricted pupils secondary to iritis.

Once you have assessed the pupils' response to light, you can finish your examination with an assessment of the *accommodative,* or *near-reflex, response* of the pupils. To do this, turn the room lights back to normal and hold an interesting stimulus nearby. Then ask the child to look from the distant stimulus to the near one. Normally, the pupils will become constricted when the eyes converge and accommodation increases as the child looks at the near stimulus. If this is not the case, the child may have diphtheria, Parinaud's syndrome, or other midbrain lesion. Rarely, a child may have an accommodative pupillary response but have a decreased or absent response to light. Such pupils that are also small and perhaps irregular in shape are called *Argyll-Robertson* pupils and are strongly suggestive of CNS syphilis.

Some children may have a constant rhythmic constriction with redilation of their pupils, regardless of light or near stimuli. This is called *hippus* and is usually considered normal.

If you work in an intensive-care or trauma setting, assure that there is a policy regarding the dilation of eyes in these settings. Whether the request for dilation is part of an ophthalmologic consultation or is part of the general work-up, it is generally recommended that the permission of the patient's attending physician first be obtained.

Once such permission is obtained, record the date, hour, and medicines used for dilation on the front of the chart, and in some cases, taped onto the patient's forehead. In addition, the status of the pupils before dilation should be carefully noted. Such measures will prevent any confusion about the patient's pupillary response that may still be present long after a consultation has been completed. Furthermore, some attending physicians may prefer that patients with increased intracranial pressure or in very critical stages not have their eyes dilated, because the natural pupillary responses are so important at these crucial stages.

CRANIAL NERVES (CNs)

''On old Olympus' towering top, a Finn and German viewed a hop.'' Remember that? It's one of the several mnemonics still in use to help one remember the 12 cranial nerves. The sensory or afferent nerves include the olfactory (I), optic (II), and auditory (VIII). The remaining ones are the efferent or motor nerves: oculomotor (III), trochlear (IV), trigeminal (V), abducens (VI), facial (VII), glosspharnygeal (IX), vagus (X), accessory (XI), and hypoglossal (XII). In pediatric neuroophthalmology, evaluation of the second through the seventh cranial nerves can provide valuable information.

Cranial nerves III, IV, and VI innervate the extraocular muscles (EOMs). Any *palsy* (complete paralysis) or *paresis* (partial paralysis) of these nerves can be assessed by checking the child's ductions and versions (Fig. 5-5).

You may have difficulty in determining whether abnormal eye movements are secondary to strabismus or cranial nerve defects, however. The presence of abnormal *head posturing* is a frequent clue to the diagnosis of a cranial nerve problem, especially when the third or fourth cranial nerve is involved. It is the child's way of avoiding diplopia. It contrasts with that of the child with strabismus who often develops suppression and/or amblyopia to alleviate double vision. Any child who turns or tilts the head abnormally should first be referred for a complete ophthalmic work-up, since the incidence of cranial nerve palsies is much greater than pure *torticollis* (head turning secondary to abnormal neck muscles, usually the sternocleidomastoid). Head turning resulting from ocular problems will disappear if one of the child's eyes is patched for 1–2 days, as the diplopia will likewise disappear. However, if the head turning is secondary to torticollis, it will not decrease with this measure. Head tilting can also accompany spasmus nutans (see the discussion of nystagmus) and brain tumors.

Depending on whether the damage is partial or complete, *third cranial nerve* damage can affect the superior, medial, and inferior rectus muscles (Fig. 5-1), as well as the inferior oblique muscle, the sphincters of the iris, and the levator muscle. It also governs accommodation, convergence, and the pupils' ability to respond consensually. The congenital type is more common in children than the acquired type and is characterized by exotropia and tilting of the head. In addition, these children may be unable to adduct, elevate, or lower their involved eye. Acquired third nerve palsy can result from tumors, aneurysms, or trauma. As a result, an immediate referral is necessary for any child who does not have a previous history of nerve palsy and displays ptosis, dilated pupil(s) and/or decreased eye movements. If the source of the palsy is benign, surgery may be indicated to treat the exotropia or ptosis; patching may be used for amblyopia or any complaints of diplopia. Of interest is that an untreated acquired third nerve palsy often disappears by 6 months after its arrival with minimal or no residual damage.

Children with *fourth cranial nerve* problems may have vertical strabismus, diplopia, or head tilting to the opposite side with the chin depressed. These signs and symptoms result from palsy or paresis of one or both superior oblique muscles, permitting the inferior oblique muscle of the same eye to overact. It may be caused by closed head trauma, tumor, aneurysm, or congenital defect. The injury may be very minor, often unnoticed. In congenital forms, eye muscle surgery is desired as soon as possible to help prevent torticollis and facial asymmetry. Surgery in acquired cases is postponed until 6 months after onset, to see whether spontaneous improvement occurs.

Pure congenital *sixth nerve* palsy is rare, and is often confused with *Duane's retraction syndrome* (one eye retracts on adduction, causing a narrowed palpebral fissure), Moebius syndrome, or congenital esotropia. More often, sixth nerve palsy is acquired, caused by tumors; aneurysms; viruses; toxins (lead, for example); or meningeal irritations (after a lumbar puncture). The characteristic sign of sixth nerve palsy is esotropia, caused by lateral rectus muscle paresis. These children also develop head turns, with the face turned toward the side of the affected muscle. A number of cases are transient, especially if the source of irritation is removed.

The fifth and seventh cranial nerves are not as closely related to the eyes as the third, fourth, and sixth, but they can still provide additional information during your assessment. The *fifth nerve* provides sensory innervation in the head. Since any pain in the head may often be referred to various facial areas, a patient with eye pain may also complain that the jaw, for example, hurts. You can test the outer ocular portion of this nerve through tactile stimulation of the cornea. If the cornea is properly innervated, the edge of a cotton wisp should elicit the blink reflex when lightly applied to the cornea. (Some agencies require a physician's order before this test can be done.)

The *seventh cranial nerve* governs facial expression. Therefore, any asymmetry seen in the face can often be connected with a palsy of this nerve. Children with *Moebius syndrome* have palsies of the sixth and seventh cranial nerves and have facial asymmetry combined with esotropia. Children with *Bell's palsy* have a damaged seventh nerve in the area that governs lid closure. These children need to have their eyelids closed for them during rest and have artificial tears inserted at frequent intervals to prevent corneal damage (which can happen quite rapidly).

OPTIC NERVE DISORDERS

The optic disc, or *papilla,* is the head of the optic nerve, located in the retina. It is responsible for the physiologic blind spot, which measures 15 degrees in height and 7 degrees in width and is located about 15 degrees temporally to the patient's point of fixation (Fig. 8-1).

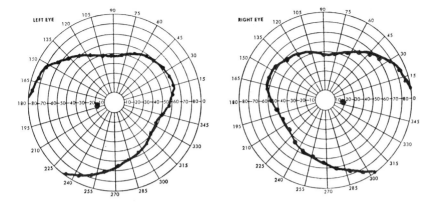

Fig. 8-1. A set of normal visual fields, obtained through perimetry. Note the physiologic blind spot near the center.

Color and size are the two main characteristics for which the optic nerve is observed. Normally it is yellowish in color. A paler or whitish color often implies nerve damage, and a reddish color may indicate inflammation. However, premature and full-term babies often have paler discs, as do children who are moderately myopic. In contrast, a child with moderate to severe hyperopia may have elevated and reddened discs, which are not to be confused with papilledema.

Disc Edema

Papilledema

Papilledema implies swelling or edema of the optic disc secondary to increased intracranial pressure *only*. Both discs are involved and are quite swollen and reddened, with engorged veins. In addition, there may be retinal edema and wrinkling near the disc, and the disc margins are quite blurred.

An important feature of children with papilledema is that they have normal visual acuity and normal pupillary responses to the swinging flashlight test (negative Marcus Gunn pupillary sign). In addition, the visual fields are usually normal, except perhaps for an enlarged physiologic blind spot.

Papilledema represents an immediate medical emergency, not because of potential ocular damage, but rather because of the increased intracranial pressure causing it. However, the diagnosis of papilledema must be made with extreme caution, as it can easily be confused with drusen of the optic disc, pseudopapilledema, or papillitis.

Other Causes

Other causes of disc edema in children are hypertension, leukemia, or uveitis. As in papilledema, the patient has normal vision acuity and consensual pupillary responses. Frequently a CT scan helps in the differential diagnosis. The term *pseudopapilledema* refers to an anomalous elevation of the optic disc but implies no pathology.

Drusen

Drusen represent the development of hyaline bodies in the optic nerve and must be differentiated from disc edema. They are frequently inherited as an autosomal dominant trait and are much easier to identify in adults by their appearance as yellowish-white nodules. Hence, when it is difficult to determine whether a child has drusen or papilledema, the parents may be examined. Other signs and symptoms of drusen include progressive field loss, elevated optic nerve, and blurred disc margins. In the child's younger years the visual acuity is normal, but it may decrease later.

Optic Neuritis

In contrast to papilledema, children with *optic neuritis* (inflammation of the optic nerve) experience a relatively rapid decrease in visual acuity, have a central visual field defect, and may have some eye pain. Only one eye may be involved. The child may also have decreased color perception and a positive Marcus-Gunn pupillary sign.

If the inflammation occurs in the visible portion (the optic disc), it is termed *papillitis*. If it occurs farther back, it is called *retrobulbar neuritis*. Papillitis is often difficult to distinguish from papilledema with an ophthalmoscope, as both have swollen and raised disc heads and indistinct disc margins. In contrast, retrobulbar neuritis produces no early visible signs in the eye. The clinical comment is, "The doctor sees nothing; the patient sees nothing."

Possible causes of optic neuritis include CNS tumors, multiple sclerosis, toxins (such as alcohol or lead), various drugs (chloramphenicol, for example), and viral infections. Early withdrawal of a toxin or drug usually results in complete recovery. In addition, if CNS problems are ruled out, chances are good that the neuritis will heal spontaneously, and that full vision will return, usually within a few weeks. Sometimes short-term systemic steroids are used to assist in the recovery process. Recurrences may occur with multiple sclerosis, however, with gradual visual deficit.

Optic Nerve Atrophy (Optic Nerve Degeneration)

The child with optic nerve atrophy has a white, gray, or pale disc that is normal in size and not elevated. If the atrophy is asymmetrical, a positive Marcus-Gunn pupillary sign may also be present. Remember that premature and full-term infants can also have paler discs in their early months, as may children of any age with moderate myopia.

The most common type of optic atrophy in children is the primary type, which is caused by optic nerve disease and results in a white disc. It may be due to demyelinization (multiple sclerosis, for example); a tumor; hereditary disease; or infection (for example, meningitis). A few young adult males have Leber's optic atrophy, which is caused by an X-linked recessive gene. Secondary optic nerve atrophy may follow inflammation or edema of the optic disc. It may also be caused by glaucoma, diabetes, or lead poisoning. The discs of these patients are grayish from a loss of the smaller vessels or nerve fibers.

Optic Nerve Hypoplasia

In contrast to those with optic nerve atrophy, children with optic nerve hypoplasia have a disc that is congenitally smaller in size than normal. In addition, they usually have a permanent significant loss of vision and variably decreased fields. If both discs are involved, the child may also have nystagmus; if one disc is involved, the child may have strabismus. Any child with optic nerve hypoplasia usually requires a complete CNS examination to rule out other possible CNS defects.

NYSTAGMUS

Nystagmus is a rhythmic involuntary back and forth movement of the eye(s) occurring independently of their regular movements. This movement can be described in many ways: monocular or binocular; symmetrical or asymmetrical; horizontal, vertical, or rotary; jerk or pendular; slow to fast; coarse to fine; and induced or spontaneous.

Most nystagmus occurs in the horizontal directions. Some drugs such as antihistamines, barbiturates, and anticonvulsants can cause either horizontal or vertical nystagmus. However, a child with any spontaneous nystagmus should be referred immediately to an ophthalmologist for a complete work-up to rule out any CNS lesions.

Jerk nystagmus involves a slow movement of the eyes toward one direction, followed by a quick rebound movement to the other. It is labeled according to the direction in which it moves faster. In contrast, patients with pendular nystagmus have the same speed of movement toward both directions. Most nystagmoid movements decrease when the patient is asleep.

The rate of nystagmus is considered slow when the beats are less than 40/min, medium when they range between 40 and 100, and fast if they are greater than 100. In addition, when the nystagmus deviates less than 5 degrees it is called a *fine* or *low amplitude,* as opposed to a coarse or high amplitude when the deviation is more than 15 degrees. In general, the greater the amplitude, the greater the loss of vision from the nystagmus.

Physiologic (Induced) Nystagmus

Physiologic nystagmus is a normal response of the eyes to various visual, auditory, or positional stimuli. Optokinetic or visually induced nystagmus (OKN) occurs when the subject views repetitive objects (Chapter 2). Likewise, stimulation of the vestibular system with rotation also induces nystagmus (Chapter 2). A third type of physiologic nystagmus is *end point* or *pseudonystagmus*. It consists of very fine back-and-forth eye movements when a subject is looking at the extreme ends of gaze.

Pathologic (Spontaneous) Nystagmus

Nystagmus present without the eliciting stimuli mentioned previously must be considered abnormal and may indicate poor vision or neurologic disease.

Congenital Nystagmus

Congenital nystagmus develops in the first year or two of life. It is conveniently subclassified into the primary motor and sensory types. The *primary motor type* occurs in a normal visual system in which there is instability in the brain centers controlling eye position; it can lead to decreased vision. In contrast, children with *sensory nystagmus* initially have a significant loss of vision; their nystagmus is due to their poor vision. Of interest is that the onset of blindness before the age of 2 years often results in nystagmus, although its onset after the age of 6 years does not. Children who become blind between the ages of 2 and 6 years may or may not develop nystagmus.

Children with primary motor nystagmus may have a neutral or null point, in which the nystagmus is diminished or even disappears in one position of gaze. As a result, many of these children develop head turns to maintain the position of minimal nystagmus, allowing maximal visual acuity. (Nystagmus normally causes visual acuity to decrease.) In addition, these children may see better at near than at distance because convergence of the eyes at near decreases the nystagmoid movements. As a result, one treatment for primary motor congenital nystagmus is to overcorrect the child's vision with minus lenses, as a means of promoting convergence. Prisms may be used for a similar purpose. Surgery may be indicated for some children, particularly if a child's neutral point is not in the primary position, causing the child to develop a head turn. By rotating the null point to the primary position through surgical intervention, the head turn can be alleviated. Finally, as some children grow older, the speed of their nystagmus may decrease.

Manifest motor nystagmus is observable with both eyes uncovered, whereas the latent variety does not become significantly noticeable until one eye is occluded.

Since many children do not have an eye covered before their first eye screening, you may be the first to notice a child's latent nystagmus. If this is the case, screen these children with both eyes only, as occlusion of one eye will stimulate the nystagmoid movements and result in poorer vision. Also significant is the tendency for these children to develop strabismus and resulting ambylopia. Refer children without a past history of latent nystagmus, or with positive findings of strabismus or amblyopia.

Acquired Nystagmus

The most common type of acquired nystagmus in children is *spasmus nutans*. Characteristically, it first appears between the ages of 2–12 months, although it may appear up to 3 years of age. These children have fine and rapid nystagmoid movements of one eye more than the other. In addition, they may develop head nodding, and to a lesser extent, head turning. Several years later (ranging from 4 months to 9 years, with an average of 3 years), the signs disappear. Usually the nystagmus disappears last.

The etiology of spasmus nutans has been attributed to a number of environmental causes. For example, home illumination, malnutrition, and maladaptive behavior have all been cited, but they have never been proved. If no associated CNS disease or stabismus is found, the child has a good probability of having no residual damage.

Monocular acquired nystagmus can also result from an optic nerve glioma, a third ventricle tumor, or amblyopia (particularly in adults). Thus, most ophthalmologists prefer to rule out any tumors before making the diagnosis of spasmus nutans.

VISUAL FIELDS

At the same time that a person uses the macula to focus straight ahead, the peripheral retina is transmitting information about the surrounding area (although not as sharply as the macula does). The term *visual fields* refers to the testing of this peripheral or nonmacular vision.

Figure 8-1 shows a set of normal visual fields. When each eye is tested separately, the field normally extends about 90 degrees to the lateral quadrant of each eye, 70 degrees down, 60 degrees to the medial quadrant, and about 40 degrees to the upper one. A person is considered legally blind if the visual field is less than 20 degrees in diameter in the better eye. Inside the normal field is a blind spot, or scotoma, that corresponds to the physiologic loss of vision from the optic disc. Pathologic blind spots can occur in any area of a visual field. A scotoma that equals the loss of vision in one-half of an eye is called a *hemianopsia*.

The type of field loss usually clearly indicates where in the visual system the cause is located. For example, when any loss occurs in one eye only, we know that its cause is located before the optic chiasm (Fig. 1-1). Etiologies posterior to the chiasm will result in decreased fields on the same side of each eye. Problems that occur on the right side of the brain result in field losses to the left of each eye and are called *left homonymous* ("same name"; here, "same side") field losses. Similarly, a lesion on the left side will result in a right homonymous field loss. Possible causes of any visual field loss include trauma, tumors, or cerebral vascular disorders.

Any child who has had head trauma or a history of bumping into objects on one side only is a candidate for visual field screening. Frequently the child will not be aware of the loss, having learned to compensate for it unconsciously by turning the head more (much as a child with an artificial eye does) or by scanning with increased eye movements.

Children below the age of 5 or 6 years can only have a gross estimate of their visual fields made, as they are too young to comply with more formal types of testing. For these younger children, the *confrontation method* is used. Cover one eye of the child and place the child at arm's length in front of you, with your eyes at the same level. With one hand hold an interesting near target, such as a finger puppet or animated wiggle picture, directly in front of the child's nose and have the child continue to focus on it. With your other hand, hold another stimulus and repeatedly bring this into the various quadrants of the nonoccluded eye from outside the child's line of vision. To assess the child's responses accurately, close your opposite eye so that your only vision will be on the same side as that of the child. For example, if the child's right eye is occluded, close your left eye. Then, assuming that you have normal visual fields, you can determine whether the child is fixating on the moving object at the correct distance. Remember to take the moving target out to a nonseeing area initially and then bring it into the child's visual field. Once you have tested the child's responses laterally, medially, up, and down, repeat the process with the other eye.

For preschool and kindergarten children, you can adapt the testing into a game. For instance, you can use your fingers as the peripheral target and have the children count how many they see or call out "now" when they see them. Or, you can briefly show one, two, or five fingers in an outer field area, then remove them, and ask children to show you with their fingers what they saw. This method is particularly helpful for children who have difficulty in keeping their head straight, or for children who do not yet know how to count.

If you have an older child in whom you suspect a field loss, you may wish to try one of the following, in addition to the confrontation method. Place before the child a wide book and ask the child to read it aloud without turning the head. If the child makes mistakes or leaves out some of the words on one side only, a visual field loss should be suspected, and a referral should be made. Or draw three horizontal lines of different sizes at various locations on a piece of notebook paper. Then ask the child to divide each line in half, without turning the head. The child fails if the divisions occur markedly off-center. (This last test may indicate either a visual field loss or a visual perception problem.)

Formal visual field testing usually includes the use of a perimeter or tangent screen (Fig. 8-2). Either method is safe and painless.

A *perimeter* is a bowl-shaped machine, in which the child is asked to fixate at a spot in its center. Then the examiner flashes or moves spots of light into the various areas, asking the child to press a button or call out upon seeing the light. Usually a small peep hole allows the examiner to watch the child continually and ensure that the child is maintaining central fixation. The *Goldmann perimeter* is the classic manually operated type, but in recent years computerized machines have been developed. From the child's responses a diagram of the visual fields can be constructed (as in Figure 8-1).

As the perimeter is used to test the child's peripheral fields, the *tangent screen* is designed to test the 30 degrees in the center of one's fields. (Do not confuse this with the testing of central visual acuity, however.) Tangent screens are usually made of felt, measure 1 meter in each direction, and have a dot located in the center at which the patient fixates. The other eye is occluded, and the patient is seated 1 meter from the screen. The examiner then picks up a stick with a target on one side and slowly moves the stick from the periphery into the patient's line of vision. Each location at which the patient views the target coming into the line of vision is marked with a pin on the screen. From the results, the examiner can then determine the child's central fields. Tangent screening is especially helpful for children or adults who may have glaucoma or CNS lesions.

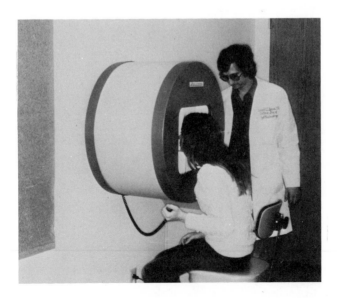

Fig. 8-2. A tangent screen on the left: an adolescent girl participating in computerized perimetry on the right.

The *Amsler Grid* is also used for patients who may have a central field loss or distortion, although it is not as refined as the tangent screen (Fig. 8-3). The patient is asked to look at the center of the grid with one eye covered. A normal response is that the patient can see the surrounding outline of the grid, as well as all of the squares inside of it. In addition, all of the lines should appear straight. Any reported differences should lead to a referral for a more complete work-up.

VISUALLY EVOKED POTENTIAL/RESPONSE

The visually evoked potential or response (VEP/VER) is actually an electro-encephalogram (EEG) of the patient's occipital area. Flashing single or repeated lights into a patient's eye allows small changes in the occipital EEG to be made and electrically recorded. The appearance of these changes assures the examiner that the visual pathway is intact. However, changes of low amplitude or no changes at all indicate that part of the visual pathway has been interrupted or blocked, preventing the light stimuli to reach the occipitus adequately. The source of inadequate transmission cannot be determined from a VEP but may result from prob-

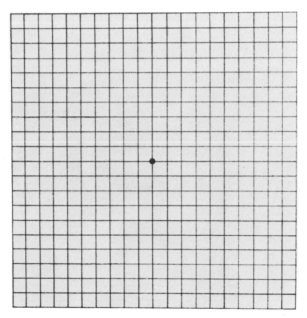

Fig. 8-3.   The Amsler Grid: the original grid is actually a black background with white lines. Printed courtesy of Hamblin (instruments) LTD., London.

lems in the retina, optic nerve, or anywhere else along the visual pathway to the visual cortex. A VEP is particularly useful in ruling out blindness of an unknown cause in infants, estimating amblyopia, and ruling out malingering. However, it is not used for a child with a known retinal or optic nerve problem because it supplies no new information.

Although the machine may be frightening to the child or parents, VEPs are actually quite painless. Three electrodes are placed on the child's scalp, and a black patch is placed over the eye that is not being tested (only one eye is tested at a time). Then the light flashes begin. Minimal cooperation is needed from the child, and thus sedation is rarely necessary. VEPs can be performed on a child of any age. In many cases, after adapting to the lights (preferably through play preparation) or being comforted by a parent and perhaps a bottle or favorite toy or blanket, the child settles down for the duration of the 30 minutes of testing.

VEPs have also lately proved to be an objective method of measuring an infant's visual acuity. However, the machines are quite expensive and require a certain amount of training for their proper use.

X-RAYS

Sometimes x-rays of the skull and cranial sutures, as well as special views of the orbits and optic foramen, are ordered to provide additional information.

SELECTED BIBLIOGRAPHY

Buncic JR, Lloyd LA: Pediatric neuroophthalmology, in Crawford JS, Morin JD, (eds): *The Eye in Childhood,* New York, Grune & Stratton, 1983

Gaston DC: Visual fields. J Ophthalmic Nurs Tech 3:24–31, 1984

Glaser JS: *Neuro-ophthalmology.* New York, Harper & Row, 1978

Johnson JH, Cryan M: Homonymous hemianopsia: Assessment and nursing management. Am J Nurs 79:2131–2135, 1979

Keltner JL: Neuro-ophthalmology for the pediatrician. Pediatr Ann 12:586–602, 1983

Norman S: The pupil check. Am J Nurs 82:588–591, 1982

Chapter Nine

Glaucoma

The definition of glaucoma is increased intraocular pressure (IOP). Although glaucoma is rare in children, its incidence increases with age. Hence, 10–15 percent of persons over 70 have it. Unfortunately, the increased pressure ultimately causes optic disc damage with visual field and acuity losses, making glaucoma the second cause of blindness in the United States. When glaucoma appears in children, early diagnosis and treatment may significantly lessen the risk for blindness.

Figure 9-1 shows the normal anatomy and flow of aqueous humor through the anterior portion of the eye. The aqueous humor is secreted by the ciliary body and then begins its journey through the posterior chamber between the iris and the lens. With normal pressure and flow, it then proceeds through the pupil into the anterior chamber, to the angle of the iris, through the trabecular meshwork, and into the canal of Schlemm. Here it becomes part of the scleral venous system and ultimately joins the body's general circulation.

Glaucoma occurs when one or more components of this freeway system becomes blocked or inoperable. Usually the cause is at the angle/trabecular area, where the flow is decreased or totally obstructed. This results in the build-up of aqueous humor pressure, eventually creating so much pressure within the eye that the cells of the optic disc become ischemic and necrosed. In addition, in children less than 2 years old the anterior portion of the eye is much more pliable than in older persons and can also be effected by increased pressure. Much less frequently, aqueous humor can build up within the eye because of its hypersecretion by the ciliary body. Contrary to popular belief, no relation exists between systemic hypertension and glaucoma; they are independent entities.

TYPES OF GLAUCOMA

Developmental Glaucoma

Developmental glaucoma is actually a broad term used to describe the several different types of glaucoma present in childhood. The most well-known is *congenital glaucoma*. About 75 percent of these cases have bilateral involvement,

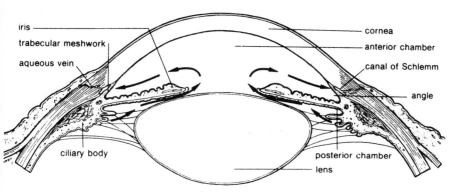

Fig. 9-1. Normal flow of aqueous humor.

and there is an increased incidence in males. It is speculated that congenital glaucoma is inherited through an autosomal recessive gene with a weak penetration. 80 percent of all cases are diagnosed by the first year of life. The later the development of the symptoms, the better the visual prognosis.

The classic triad of initial symptoms includes excessive tearing (epiphora), photophobia, and lid spasm (blepharospasm). As pressure increases, the cornea become edematous, develops a hazy appearance, and enlarges. Enlarged opaque corneas are called *buphthalmic* (''ox eyes''); hence *buphthalmos* is an older name for congenital glaucoma. Upon examination of the optic disc, significant cup enlargement may be noted. Finally, a child may exhibit pseudo-mental retardation, because the loss of vision, photophobia, and so on, cause atypical behavior. However, with proper treatment for the glaucoma the atypical behavior disappears.

Surgery is the usual treatment for congenital glaucoma, although medications may be used until the surgery is performed. The most common surgical procedures are goniotomy and trabeculectomy. Unfortunately, these procedures may have to be repeated several times for optimal success. Even if the intraocular pressure is kept within normal limits by surgical interventions, the child may have residual visual acuity or field losses from either optic disc damage or corneal opacifications. In addition, it is not uncommon for a child with congenital glaucoma to develop myopia and astigmatism. If a refractive amblyopia occurs, it is carefully treated with glasses and patching.

Juvenile glaucoma is defined as any glaucoma that develops between the ages of 3 and 30 years (some authorities say ages 4–21 or 6–35). Most of the children who develop juvenile glaucoma have myopia, and many of their families have a history of open-angle glaucoma. Males have a slightly increased incidence over females. Children with this type of glaucoma do not have pain or megalo-cornea but do have definite visual field and acuity losses. They also have

NURSING GOALS, OUTCOME STANDARDS, AND DIAGNOSES

Because glaucoma is rare in children, most pediatric nurses have minimal contact with it. Therefore, Chapter 9 has two primary nursing goals.

The first concerns the child with glaucoma: *each child with glaucoma has the best possible visual functioning*. Its outcomes are identical to those in Chapter 7, if one substitutes the word *glaucoma* for *retinal disorder* and replaces the list of children at risk with those found in the history section of this chapter. The nursing diagnoses are also quite similar to those in Chapter 7, with the following additions:

- *Anxiety:* Also regarding IOP procedures or results.
- *Potential for injury:* Coughing, lifting, and contact sports can also increase intraocular pressure.
- *Alterations in parenting:* Especially regarding children with congenital glaucoma.
- *Disturbance in body image:* May also occur secondary to corneal hazing.
- *Alteration in tissue perfusion:* In glaucoma, this can refer to the abnormal flow of aqueous humor or to the ischemia of the optic nerve and other cells due to increased IOP.
- *Noncompliance:* Particularly by children who are on a complex medication regimen or in respect to follow-up visits.
- *Sensory deficit:* Unfortunately, the effect on the optic nerve and vision cannot be predicted.

The second goal emphasizes the prevention of glaucoma: *all family members have minimal effects from glaucoma*. It is based on the premise that the larger role for pediatric nurses regarding glaucoma is to educate children and their families about it, as the chances of its occurring in older family members and neighbors are significant.

Outcome Standard 1

At least one member of each family can define glaucoma in simple terms, indicate whether it is present in first- and second-degree relatives, state that glaucoma can lead to blindness in many adults and that diagnosis through regular eye exams and compliance with treatment lead to the best prognosis.

Outcome Standard 2

Students in junior and senior high schools are given at least one health class on glaucoma.

Suggested Interventions:
- The nurse obtains copies of glaucoma literature for the general public

and distributes this literature in the office and school settings. The NSPB prints two basic pamphlets, *Glaucoma—Sneak Thief of Sight* (available in English, Chinese, and Spanish at $5.00/100 copies) and the *Glaucoma Alert Program Guide,* with forms, posters, and plans ($5.00/copy). In addition, they have a 25-minute movie, *Seeing,* available for a $10.00 rental fee. It tells the story of a 30-year-old-woman who develops glaucoma and includes a leader's discussion guide, poster, and take-home literature. (The nurse can use this to prepare a Parent-Teacher Association presentation for local schools.) The Patient Information Library also has a 16-page booklet on glaucoma and its treatments, with good illustrations.

• The nurse contacts local schools to see whether glaucoma is explained in the upper grades and assists in any way to ensure that such information is incorporated into the health education program.

marked cupping with possible atrophy of their optic discs, and their intraocular pressures range in the 30s and 40s. Unfortunately, this type of glaucoma is in general very difficult to treat, either medically or surgically.

Two other groups of children who develop glaucoma include those who have a hereditary or familial disorder that has an associated incidence of glaucoma, and children with other diseases that likewise have an increased risk for glaucoma (see the section on history).

Open-Angle (Simple, Chronic) Glaucoma

Although rare in infants, open-angle glaucoma comprises 80-90 percent of all glaucoma cases. It is characterized by a gradual, painless visual field loss, initially in the peripheral area (tunnel vision). As a result, simple glaucoma has been labeled the "sneak thief of the night" because patients have no symptoms and are usually not aware of their visual field loss until extensive irreversible damage has occured. The mechanism of simple glaucoma appears to be a malfunctioning of the trabecular meshwork. In children the type that most closely resembles chronic open-angle glaucoma is juvenile glaucoma.

Closed-Angle (Acute) Glaucoma

Closed-angle glaucoma occurs when the iris is pushed forward and blocks the trabecular angle. This causes an immediate elevation of ocular pressure. Within hours the patient develops headaches, nausea, vomiting, intense pain, a red eye, and a fixed and dilated pupil. Because of these rapidly appearing symptoms, such diagnoses as gastrointestinal viruses or appendicitis have been made, causing loss of valuable time. Surgery (peripheral iridectomy) or laser treatment must be

185

performed as soon as possible to prevent significant damage to the optic nerve by the greatly increased intraocular pressure. Prior to surgery, miotics, osmotics, or carbonic anhydrase inhibitors may be given to help lower the pressure. Although this variety is not common in children, it may occur with eye inflammation or infection or when the lens is pushed forward by a process such as RLF.

DIAGNOSTIC ASSESSMENTS

History

Glaucoma, whether in children or adults, can follow an autosomal recessive inheritance pattern. Therefore, always inquire about a history of glaucoma or blindness in immediate family members.

In addition, glaucoma in childhood can be associated with numerous syndromes and anomalies. Among these are Wilm's tumor, Sturge-Weber's syndrome, neurofibromatosis (von Rechlinghausen disease), rubella, Axenfeld's syndrome, Reiger's anomaly, Peter's anomaly, Marfan's syndrome, Pierre-Robin syndrome, homocystinuria, and Lowe's syndrome. Any child suspected of having one of these syndromes should be referred for a complete ophthalmic work-up as soon as possible, if one has not already been done. Conversely, any child with a history of glaucoma should have a complete physical examination to rule out any of the problems listed. Finally, a number of ophthalmic problems such as uveitis, retinoblastoma, retrolental fibroplasia, persistent hypoplastic primary vitreous, aniridia, ocular trauma, and the long-term use of tropical ophthalmic steroids are associated with glaucoma.

In terms of a history of ophthalmic complaints, be attuned to parental reports of young infants with excessive tearing, photophobia, a red eye, or lid spasms. For example, a parent may state that their infant always hides his head in the blankets; this could indicate photophobia. In addition, many parents begin to feel that something is abnormal when they notice their child's enlarged or hazy cornea. However, all of the signs of congenital glaucoma can be signs of other unassociated problems. For example, the excess tearing may represent a lacrimal obstruction, upper respiratory infection, or conjunctivitis. The use of forceps during delivery may have caused a unilateral corneal haziness. Nevertheless, if you have any suspicion that glaucoma may be indicated, refer the child immediately.

Visual Acuity And Fields

Examiners attempt to assess both the visual acuity and the visual fields of a child with suspected or documented glaucoma. With a young infant, however, such assessments may be next to impossible.

Corneal Measurements

Since children less than 2 years old have pliable corneas that can be affected by glaucoma, measurement of the corneas may provide additional diagnostic information. For the most accurate measurement, the ophthalmologist uses a caliper to measure the horizontal and vertical diameters of the cornea. Any measurements greater than 12mm are considered abnormal.

Tonometry (IOP Measurement)

Tonometry is the means of measuring intraocular pressure, (IOP), which normally ranges between 12 and 20 mm Hg. Higher pressures can damage the optic disc, although individuals vary in how much pressure is necessary to cause damage. The diagnosis of glaucoma is never based on one IOP recording alone, however. In addition, pressures can vary throughout the day for each individual (usually higher in the morning) and certain medications such as barbiturates can decrease it.

The Schiotz tonometer is the oldest method of determining IOP still in use today (Fig. 9-2). It is small, quick, safe, portable, easy to use, and relatively inexpensive ($165.00). It functions by having various weights indent a plunger against the cornea. The greater the pressure within the eye, the lower the reading will be on the scale at the top of the instrument because the increased pressure will not allow any further indentation. A chart, last revised in 1955, allows you to convert the scale recording to an intraocular pressure.

If you work in a setting where you may be taking IOPs with the Schiotz tonometer, follow this procedure. First, assure that the plunger (indentor, footplate) can move freely; for proper functioning it should be cleaned daily with alcohol, and its chamber routinely cleaned with a pipe cleaner. Some Schiotz tonometers have ultraviolet containers that sterilize the instrument after each use; however, the plunger still requires separate care. Then insert one drop of a topical anesthetic in each eye while the child is lying flat and wait 15–20 seconds for it to become effective. Infants and young children frequently become uncooperative at this point, and an *examination under anesthesia* (EUA) may have to be arranged by the ophthalmologist for more accurate results. (Crying and breath holding are notorious for increasing IOP). However, for screening purposes with a cooperative child, ask the child to focus on an item of interest that you have previously attached to the ceiling directly above the child's eyes. Then, being careful not to put any pressure on the eye (which would increase the IOP), gently place the plunger with the 5.5-weight attached against the center of the cornea; read the results to the closest half-unit (the indicator will continue to move slightly). So that you don't interfere with the child's focusing, approach each eye from its own side. If you need to reposition the tonometer, lift rather than slide it on the cornea. Slight corneal abrasions are not uncommon after the use of the Schiotz tonometer.

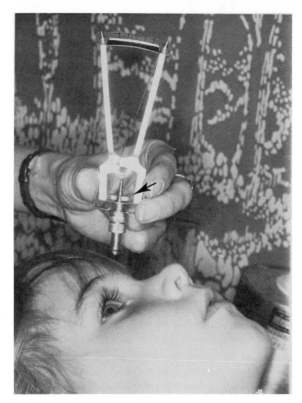

Fig. 9-2.   The Schiotz tonometer. Note the scale at the top and the
indentor (plunger) at the bottom. The interchangeable weight is indicated by the arrow.

You can record your results in several ways. For example, T_S 5.5 $^{\text{OD 6 u}}_{\text{OS 5.5 u}}$ means
that the tension (T) or IOP using the Schiotz (S) was 6 units (14.6 mm Hg ac-
cording to the chart) in the right eye, and 5.5 units (15.9 mm Hg) in the left
eye, using the 5.5 weight. On the tonometer this would show as 1.1 and 1.0,
respectively; that is, 1.1 times the 5.5 weight equals 6.0, for instance. If you
prefer, you can simply write out your findings, preceded by *IOP* = or *T* =.
However, do remember to note which eye is examined, which method is used,
the time of day, and any medications (especially barbiturates, cycloplegics, or
antiglaucoma medications) that the child has taken recently. Refer any child with
a pressure greater than 20 mm Hg.

Outside of a screening or general practice setting, the Schiotz tonometer has
been replaced by more sophisticated and accurate equipment. The *applanation*

tonometer is most commonly found in the professional eye examiner's office and is attached to a slit lamp. *Applanation* refers to flatness; the instrument works by having a small plastic arm flatten against the center of the cornea (Fig. 9-3). Fluress eyedrops (fluorescein with a topical anesthetic) are administered prior to the test, and the child is asked to look at the blue light on the slit lamp. After each use, the plastic arm should be cleaned with alcohol. The recording from an applanation tonometer may be written as $T_A = x$. Some patients have problems with the applanation method because their eyes begin to blink as the machine approaches, but many cooperative children can be taught to accept IOP measurement by this method.

The *Perkins* and *Draeger* portable applanation tonometers have been quite beneficial for patients who cannot sit or who are under anesthesia. As with all tonometers, the eyes must be centered for accurate measurement.

Tonographs are machines that record the IOP on graph paper. For instance, the *pneumotonograph* sends out a puff of air against the cornea at a steady rate, and the resulting IOPs are recorded. A tonofilm or sheath covers the part that touches the patient's eye (and can be easily lost when transporting the machine).

Finally, the *finger tension,* or *tactile method* is a way of approximating the IOP. In this method, you place two fingers over the patient's closed eyelids and compare the feel to your own, which is soft. However, its only benefit is in patients who have closed-angle glaucoma, since in order to manifest a difference, the IOP must be extremely high. Hence, it is not a useful procedure with children.

Optic Disc

The use of the ophthalmoscope for assessing the normal optic disc is discussed in Chapter 7. For children with known or suspected glaucoma, the assessment of the optic cup–disc ratio provides a key in determining the effect of increased IOP on the child's visual status.

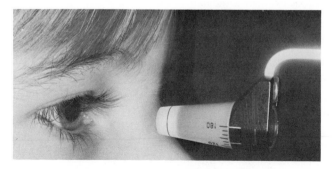

Fig. 9-3. Close-up of the applanation tonometer.

Gonioscopy

Gonioscopy is a procedure used in the office or operating room to get a well-rounded view of the anterior portion of the eye, not normally visible with the ophthalmoscope. This is accomplished with special contact lens instruments, such as the *Koeppe lens,* the *goniolens,* and the *gonioprism.* A solution of 2.5 percent methylcellulose may be first placed on the cornea to provide a firm contact for the lens, although the child's tears may provide a similar function.

TREATMENT

Medications

Various groups of medications are used to treat glaucoma. They are divided according to their method of action.

The Cholinergics (Miotics, Parasympathomimetics)

Pilocarpine hydrochloride (HCI) is one of the better known antiglaucoma medications. It comes in a multitude of strengths, from 0.25 percent to 10 percent, although normally up to 6 percent is used for children. Pilocarpine may be written on a report as P_x, with x equaling the strength. Its total effect lasts for up to 8 hours; hence, it is usually taken three or four times daily.

A shorter-acting cousin of pilocarpine is *carbachol.* Sometimes these two drugs are interchanged when a patient develops a tolerance to one of them. Both carbachol and pilocarpine cause miosis through contraction of the ciliary muscles. In this way, the angle of the iris is widened, and the outflow of aqueous humor is increased through the trabecular meshwork.

Pilocarpine and carbachol are not used as frequently in children as in adults in the initial stages of treatment because their miotic effect in children can cause increased ciliary spasms and fluctuating myopia. For a similar reason, another group of miotics known as the *anticholinesterases* (physostigmine, neostigmine, diisopropyl fluorophosphate, echothiophate iodine, and demecarium bromide) is rarely used in children with glaucoma.

Adrenergic Agents (Mydriatics, Sympathomimetics)

Topical *epinephrine* is used in glaucoma as an adjunct to the miotic drugs. It decreases the production of aqueous humor by reducing the volume of secreted aqueous humor and may be written as E_x. Topical epinephrine slightly dilates the pupils.

Timolol maleate is a beta-adrenergic blocker that has been specifically developed in the past decade for the treatment of glaucoma. It also is assumed to decrease the outflow of aqueous humor. It may be written as $T_{0.25}$ or $T_{0.5}$, depending on its concentration. Timolol has no effect on the pupil size or accommodation and hence does not cause ciliary spasms. It is given only once a day. Its side effects are similar to those of other beta-blockers. These include light-headedness, and an increased incidence of asthma and bradycardia.

Marijuana, although not an adrenergic agent, has been used on an experimental basis to decrease the flow of aqueous humor. However, to date it has not been as effective as the miotics and mydriatics.

Carbonic Anhydrase Inhibitors

Acetazolamide (Diamox; Lederle) is a potent carbonic anhydrase inhibitor that decreases the amount of aqueous humor being produced by the ciliary muscles. Acetazolamide is given orally, except in urgent cases when it can be given intramuscularly or intravenously. Since it is a sulfa derivative, it can cause rash or renal calculi in addition to its other side effects: gastrointestinal (GI) complaints, tingling in the hands and feet, and drowsiness. Its diuretic effect can deplete potassium, and a potassium supplement with increased intake of fluids may be advised.

Hyperosmotic Agents

A hyperosmotic agent may be used for temporary but rapid decrease of IOP when a child is in an inpatient setting. The osmotic agent helps transport the fluid from within the eye into the bloodstream and is most helpful for children with congenital glaucoma in the preoperative stages or for those who have glaucoma from a hyphema or penetrating wound.

Mannitol, glycerol, isosorbide, and urea are the commonly used hyperosmotic agents. They all cause extreme thirst and marked diuresis, but the child's intake must be well controlled or the purpose of the medication will be defeated. An indwelling catheter may be ordered to accommodate the marked diuresis. Strict intake and output records must be kept. The child may complain of headaches, possibly due to cerebral dehydration; try keeping the child lying flat to help decrease these headaches. Also watch for any signs of confusion or coma secondary to severe dehydration.

Surgical Treatment

Surgery is generally the preferred method of treatment for children with congenital glaucoma. Until the actual surgery, various medications may be used to help lower the IOP and prevent any subsequent damage to the optic disc. Surgery may also be indicated for children with other types of glaucoma if progressive optic disc changes occur.

Examination Under Anesthesia (EUA)

Small children are usually uncooperative during an eye examination and the assessment of their IOP. Hence, an examination under anesthesia (EUA) may be scheduled. Often the child is kept at home until the morning of the examination.

However, because general anesthesia is used, the child is allowed nothing orally after midnight except maybe clear liquids until 3:00 A.M. or so. Normally EUAs take 15–45 minutes, in addition to the time spent in the recovery room. After voiding and tolerating liquids, the child is sent home. Occasionally, the ophthalmologist may perform one of the following glaucoma procedures immediately after an EUA, depending on the findings and any plans made with the parents prior to the examination.

Goniotomy

A goniotomy is often the first choice among many ophthalmologists to correct congenital glaucoma, especially if corneal opacities are not sufficiently severe to prevent visualization of the angle. In this procedure, a special knife is used to cut the membrane at the trabecular meshwork that is interfering with the outflow of aqueous humor. About 30 percent of goniotomies are not always successful at first, but they can be safely repeated several times. A goniopuncture is a similar procedure, with slight modifications. Following surgery, some anti-inflammatory medications are usually ordered, and the eye is covered until the wound has healed.

Trabeculectomy and Other Filtering Procedures

A *trabeculectomy* is a procedure that alters the trabecular meshwork to allow aqueous humor to drain adequately into the canal of Schlemm. In a *peripheral iridectomy,* several minute holes are made into the iris to allow aqueous humor to drain directly from the posterior chamber into the anterior chamber. Other filtering procedures permit the aqueous to flow into the subconjunctival space and then into the general circulation. Some of these procedures are trephining, iridencleisis, cyclodialysis, cyclocryotherapy, and cyclodiathermy; they are named after the specific method used to open the "freeway" system. However, in children most of these procedures (except the trabeculectomies) are used as a last resort because they can cause cataracts, intraocular hemorrhage, vitreous loss, and subluxation of the lens. After some of these filtering procedures, a child may have a bleb visible under the upper lid, representing the new scleral–conjunctival area into which the aqueous humor is now flowing. Ambulation is quick (same or next day), but protection of the eye as well as administration of appropriate medications to the eye area will be necessary for a week or two. Of course, close follow-up to determine whether the IOP remains within normal limits is necessary.

Laser

The National Eye Institute is sponsoring a study on the effects of laser treatment for patients with open- and closed-angle glaucomas. The laser forms a new drainage area in the trabecular meshwork, and the results so far appear promising, particularly in respect to closed-angle glaucoma.

Enucleation

When a patient is blind because the optic nerve has been completely destroyed by glaucoma, the IOP can nevertheless remain elevated, causing intense pain. For example, a diabetic may continue to have vitreal hemorrhaging, thus increasing the IOP to painful limits. In such cases the eye is removed when medications can no longer make the patient comfortable (see Chapter 7 for a discussion on enucleations).

SELECTED BIBLIOGRAPHY

Boyd-Monk H: Screening for glaucoma. Nursing 79 9: 42–45, 1979

Kwitko ML: *Glaucoma in Infants and Children.* New York, Appleton-Century-Crofts, 1973

McPherson SD: The challenge and responsibilities of a community approach to glaucoma control. Sight Sav Rev 50:15–20, 1980

Penland LR, Penland WR: The school's role in preventing blindness from glaucoma. J Sch Health 50:125–127, 1980

Chapter Ten

Cataracts

A cataract is a loss of transparency of the crystalline lens. It results from physical or chemical alterations within the lens, although many persons still incorrectly believe that it is caused by a film or growth on the eye. In ancient times it was felt that a cataract represented water cascading within the eye, and hence its name originates from the Latin word for "waterfall." Cataracts are also known as *lens opacities* or *clouds*.

Despite new surgical treatments in technologically advanced countries, cataracts remain the leading cause of blindness in the world. In children they are the prime cause of deprivation amblyopia (Chapter 4).

ANATOMY

The crystalline lens, cornea, anterior chamber, and vitreous are all transparent media through which light rays are refracted and focused onto the retina (Figure 3-2). The lens maintains its transparency by being avascular. In the younger years, it consists of approximately two-thirds water and one-third protein. With age, however, the water content decreases. This results in a natural yellowing and hardening of the lens, which may affect color vision and be associated with the formation of senile cataracts. In addition, if certain other metabolic substances (electrolytes, minerals, and so on) build up within the lens, other types of cataracts can develop.

Each lens consists of a nucleus (center) and a cortex (periphery,) surrounded by a capsule. The capsule is divided into anterior and posterior portions. In young children the nucleus is normally not very large or solid, as it is partially formed by lens fibers that continually arise in the cortex. With time, these fibers slowly work their way toward the center as newer fibers are formed in the periphery. As a result, the nucleus is quite solid in the elderly. This difference becomes important in the selection of the surgical procedure to use when removing a cataract.

NURSING GOALS, OUTCOME STANDARDS AND DIAGNOSES

As in several previous chapters, the primary nursing goal is that *each child with a cataract has maximal visual functioning*. This is not an easy goal, however, because unless a young child with a cataract that is blocking the visual axis receives proper treatment as early as possible, the potential for maximizing visual acuity can be markedly reduced.

Outcome Standard 1

Each child under 9 years of age with a suspected or documented cataract is seen for an initial visit by an ophthalmologist within 10 days of the cataract's being suspected or identified.

Outcome Standard 2

Each child with a documented cataract receives the recommended treatment for the cataract, in a timely fashion.

Outcome Standard 3

Examinations and treatment procedures are performed with minimal risk to the child's psychosocial and physical well-being.

Suggested Interventions:
- The nurse helps to identify children at risk for having or developing a cataract. For example, children with a history of eye trauma or certain syndromes or physical findings that have a significant association with cataracts should be examined at frequent intervals, especially in their early years, in case a cataract develops. In addition, all newborn infants should have an ophthalmoscopic examination by their pediatrician, the neonatal nurse practitioner, or by the house staff, within 3 days of birth. Any child with an obvious white spot in an eye must be immediately referred for an ophthalmic consultation.
- The nurse follows all children with suspected or known cataracts to ensure that all have been seen by an ophthalmologist and have received appropriate treatment. This follow-up can be done by phone, mail, or personal contact with the child's parents, ophthalmologist, or primary care provider, or through a visiting nurse referral.
- The nurse assists in decreasing any financial, psychosocial, or other barriers that may prevent a child from being seen by an ophthalmologist or receiving proper treatment.
- If the child needs surgery, see Outcome Standards 5 and 6 in Chapter 5 for preparation of the child, family, and staff.
- If the child has amblyopia secondary to cataracts, see Outcome Standards 3, 4, and 5 in Chapter 4.

- If the child is now aphakic and needs contact lenses or glasses, see Outcome Standards 2, 3, 4, and 5 in Chapter 3. Also advise the child's family to have a spare pair of glasses or contact lenses available, in case the original becomes lost or damaged.
- If the child is postoperative, follow up on the home administration of medications and return visits for intraocular pressure, visual acuity, and refraction checks.

Outcome Standard 4

Older patients and the parents of all children with cataracts or aphakia define *aphakia, cataract,* and *lens* and verbalize the implications and recommendations for their child's cataract.

Suggested Intervention:
- The nurse clarifies and offers repeated explanations as necessary about the diagnosis and treatment plan, using written information whenever possible to supplement the teaching program. Unfortunately, current educational materials on cataracts rarely can be applied to cataracts in children, so read carefully any literature before distributing it. In addition, remember to include significant others in these sessions whenever possible (decrease *knowledge deficit*).

Outcome Standard 5

Older patients and the parents of all children with cataracts or aphakia verbalize the impact of the cataract or aphakia on their daily lives.

Suggested Interventions:
- The nurse identifies any *sensory deficits* secondary to the cataract and reviews with the family any recommended ways to diminish them. These deficits may include decreased vision secondary to amblyopia, aphakia, or the cataract itself; altered peripheral vision, magnification, or aneisikonia due to aphakic glasses; decreased fusion from amblyopia; photophobia secondary to aphakia; or altered color vision.
- The nurse provides the child and family several opportunities to discuss the impact of the cataract and treatment on their lives. For example, if the child was born with a cataract, *alterations in parenting or dysfunctional grieving* may occur. Or if the cataract developed from trauma or illness, *alterations in family processes* may result. Some parents may become overprotective, and others may subtly reject the child. *Coping* abilities of various family members may become *ineffective,* particularly in view of a tedious visual rehabilitative program. Some parents feel quite alone and can benefit from meeting other parents who have coped with a similar problem. At these times they can also discuss their *anxieties or fears* about the possibility of decreased vision, any associated anomalies, surgery or its possible complication, hospitalization, and so on.

196

The child may experience a *disturbance in self-concept* related to the cataract, glasses, or any associated strabismus. Any decreased vision will increase the child's *potential for injury*. In addition, the family should take proper precautions in protecting the child's remaining vision. If the child has recently had surgery, *physical mobility* will be *impaired* as a result of restrictions on bending, straining, and contact sports.

• The nurse makes referrals as needed to outside agencies and health professionals, such as special educators, public health nurses, parent groups, appropriate role models, counselors, and vocational rehabilitation services.

DIAGNOSIS

Cataracts are identified in children in one of three ways. An opacity can be directly noted (causing a "white pupil"), the child can have other ocular or physical problems that warrant further ophthalmologic examination, or the child has reduced visual acuity.

Ophthalmoscopy is one of the main tools used in the assessment of cataracts. If one can't see a red reflex (Chapter 7), or if it is partially obstructed, then an opacity exists in the cornea, lens, or vitreous. To help identify the affected area, the examiner notes the color of the opacity and then moves the ophthalmoscope slightly in any direction. If the opacity moves in the opposite direction and is white, it is most likely on the cornea. If it does not move at all, then the opacity is usually on the anterior of the lens. If it moves in the same direction as the ophthalmoscope, it is probably in the vitreous or the posterior of the lens. Vitreal opacities tend to move with wavy motions. Remember, however, that the more posterior the opacity, the harder it is to see with direct illumination. Usually posterior opacities are dark because they have blocked the red reflex on its return from the retina. Hence, it is only their shadow that can be seen (retroillumination).

Often parents believe that any white spot in the eye is a cataract. As explained, this belief is incorrect. In fact, one ophthalmologist listed 26 possible diagnoses that must be considered when a white pupil *(leukokoria)* is present.[1] These include advanced RLF, retinoblastoma, and persistent hypoplastic primary vitreous (PHPV). Usually, however, the findings from the ophthalmoscope and slit lamp can rapidly establish the diagnosis of a cataract.

The *slit lamp* is a binocular microscope with various light capabilities. It is especially helpful for seeing opacities in the anterior of the lens.

Also of primary importance is the estimation of the child's *visual acuity* through age-appropriate methods, since cataracts are not removed unless they interfere with vision (Fig. 10-1). For example, an opacity that does not reduce vision and can only be seen with a slit lamp requires no treatment except regular vision checks. Older children or adults with decreased vision secondary to cataracts may be especially aware of their decreased vision at night or in bright lights.

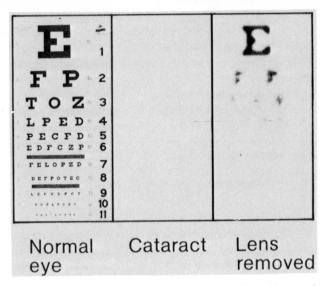

Fig. 10-1.   Snellen chart illustrating visual acuities with normal, cateractous (complete), and aphakic eyes (Courtesy of IOLAB Corporation).

CLASSIFICATION OF CATARACTS

Although no clear-cut classification system exists for cataracts, the following considerations may be helpful.

Is the cataract congenital or acquired? *Congenital* cataracts can be due to any viral, metabolic, hereditary, or unknown process that occurs before birth and results in abnormal development of the lens. It may be difficult to distinguish a congenital cataract from an acquired one, however, because a number of congenital cataracts are not recognized until the infant is several months old. *Acquired* cataracts tend to have a better visual prognosis than congenital cataracts because they don't interfere with vision during the critical period of a child's vision, that is, the first several months of life. Some acquired cataracts develop from trauma, especially from blunt blows to the anterior portion of the eye or a penetrating metal foreign body; these cataracts may not appear until some time after the injury. Children can also develop acquired cataracts from radiation, long-term use of steroids, total parenteral nutrition, enzyme deficiencies, and diabetes. As already discussed, senile cataracts develop from the aging process of the lens and account for 95 percent of all cataracts.

To classify the cataract further, next determine whether it is stationary or progressive. Most congenital cataracts are of the *stationary* type and do not enlarge. On the other hand, toxic, traumatic, and senile cataracts tend to be *progressive*.

Finally, if the cataract is not complete you may wish to know which part of the lens is involved. In children nuclear cataracts may occur from damage during the embryonic or fetal stages. A lamellar or zonular cataract can also result from damage at specific stages of lens development and involves one layer of the cortex. Such cataracts may advance in puberty but often do not interfere with vision until that time. Childhood cataracts can also be labeled as *axial, polar, cortical,* or *sutural (Y-shaped),* and by such descriptive terms as *floriform, dustlike, spokelike, stellar,* and *snowflake.*

ASSOCIATED OCULAR AND PHYSICAL ABNORMALITIES

When a cataract is noted, complete ocular and physical examinations are necessary, since numerous problems coincide with their presence. Similarly, a child diagnosed with a physical problem that has a high incidence of cataracts should be referred immediately for a complete ophthalmic work-up.

It has been estimated that 60 percent of children with congenital cataracts have other ocular problems.[2] Most common are *nystagmus, strabismus,* and *microophthalmia.*

Recent studies indicate that the onset of nystagmus in children with cataracts may herald the onset of irreversible damage to the visual system.[3] In children with congenital cataracts, nystagmus is almost always present by the age of 6 months and often sooner.

Associated with the nystagmus is the development of deprivation amblyopia. Following early surgical removal of a cataract, a vigorous program of patching with simultaneous correction of refractive errors is necessary to treat this amblyopia.

Children with *PHPV* (Chapter 7) have unilateral dense posterior cataracts. Although these cataracts can be removed, their presence with PHPV usually indicates a poor visual prognosis for that eye.

The physical problems that have a high incidence of cataracts include some genetic, metabolic, and chromosomal abnormalities, as well as certain prenatal infections, postnatal complications, or long-term medications. For example, three-fourths of children with *galactosemia* can develop *oil droplet cataracts* if their diagnosis is not made early. Hence, in many pediatric centers a urine screening for reducing substances is automatically done when an infant has symptoms of cataracts, hepatomegaly, or septicemia. With early dietary treatment for the galactosemia, the cataracts will often disappear or at least will not interfere with the child's vision.

Children with *Down syndrome* may have congenital or acquired cataracts. However, the incidence of cataracts in these children increases remarkably during their pubertal years. Children with *trisomy 13* also have a high incidence of cataracts.

Congenital rubella is well known for having characteristic cataracts as one of its classic triad of symptoms (deafness and cardiac problems are the other two). Fortunately, it is quite rare nowadays. When it does occur, the cataracts can be dense and can significantly interfere with vision. If surgical removal is performed, remember that the rubella virus can be quite active in the eye and nose for up to 2-1/2 years after birth. Hence, special isolation procedures are usually required during the hospitalization, as well as special handling procedures when removing the lens. Contact your local public health department to see what specific techniques are necessary. Also remember that these children's pupils may not dilate well and that the children may have prolonged post operative inflammation. Following surgery, the children can have significant hyperopia, usually because their eyes are small. Generally, their visual prognosis is guarded.

Children with *Lowe syndrome* (oculocerebrorenal syndrome) have an 85 percent incidence of cataracts. Some babies who had *hypoglycemia* following birth or who developed tetany from *hypocalcemia* may develop lamellar cataracts. Moderate doses of *oral steroids* (in adults, at least 15 mg/day for longer than a year) can cause posterior subcapsular cataracts, which appear as lacy shadows on ophthalmoscopy. They may not interfere with vision for years and occasionally disappear after the steroids are discontinued. Children who receive local radiation to the ocular area because of retinoblastoma (RB) or other tumors can also develop cataracts.

TREATMENT

The determination of when a cataract interferes with vision is different for everyone. One elderly person with cataracts may be quite satisfied with 20/70 vision, although another is not happy at all. With children, however, attempts are almost universally made to maximize visual acuity, provided that the family consents to the visual rehabilitation program required postoperatively and that the ophthalmologist feels that a gain in the child's visual acuity is possible.

Unfortunately, there are no medications or nonsurgical methods that can prevent cataracts or make them disappear. On occasion, dilating drops may be used to allow more light to pass around a partial cataract through the pupil. If vision improves by this method, surgery can be delayed.

Contrary to popular belief, cataracts do not have to "ripen" or "mature" before they can be removed. This is particularly true for children under the age of 9, whose cataracts may be blocking some retinal cells and lead to the formation of amblyopia.

The current preferred treatment for congenital cataracts that interfere with vision is surgical removal as soon as possible after birth; if they are not removed by 3-6 months of age, the visual prognosis is considered to be poor. This immediacy is even greater for a child with a *monocular congenital cataract* because the visual pathway from the eye with the cataract does not receive the same input as that in the better eye. Hence, deprivation amblyopia quickly sets in. Previously, children with monocular cataracts were felt to have no chance for any visual rehabilitation, but now immediate surgical removal followed by an intense program with a contact lens and patching has proved quite beneficial. In one study, eight babies with congenital monocular cataracts not related to any known disorder or syndrome all developed vision of at least 20/80 in the eye that had the cataract.[4] Surgery was performed within days or weeks after birth. Following surgery, both eyes were totally patched to prevent uneven retinal stimulation. Four days later, the first contact lens was fitted, and unilateral patching of the better eye occurred for 4–8 hours/day, as needed. During the first year the average number of contact lenses needed by each child was nine. Unfortunately, none of these children developed binocularity (fusion) after surgery, and all developed an esotropia that was eventually corrected surgically.

Children with *bilateral congenital cataracts* have likewise benefited from early surgical intervention. One ophthalmologist has often obtained visual acuities of 20/60 or better when these children were treated before 8 weeks of age.[5] To avoid uneven retinal stimulation after one cataract has been removed, the other cataract is preferably removed within 48 hours. In between, the child is patched bilaterally. Shortly after both surgeries, the child is fitted with glasses or contact lenses, and a patching regimen is begun if needed. Progress is monitored by frequent assessment of visual evoked potentials and retinoscopy, to help determine whether amblyopia or any change in the child's refraction has occurred. Like children with monocular congenital cataracts, most of these children later developed strabismus.

The treatment plan for children under 9 years of age with *acquired cataracts* that interfere with vision is basically the same as that for children with congenital cataracts. Children who develop cataracts after visual maturity (6–9 years of age) do not develop amblyopia; hence, the timing of their surgery is dependent upon their personal needs and preferences.

Surgical Treatment

Preoperative Care

Prior to surgery, a regimen of mydriatic drops to keep the eyes widely dilated during surgery is instituted. Although to a medication nurse on a pediatric surgical floor, drops administered every 5 minutes times 3 seem a great nuisance, viewing a surgery for which you prepare patients or administer medications first-hand can make a difference in your perspective afterward. With adults, local anesthesia is frequently used. However, in children general anesthesia is a must. Naturally, parents will be concerned about their child's response to anesthesia and the outcome of the surgery.

Surgical Procedures

Civilizations as old as that of the Hindus practiced a form of cataract surgery termed *couching,* a technique still used in some countries today. This refers to introducing a sharp instrument into the eye to dislodge the lens and let it fall into the vitreous cavity, away from the pupillary axis. The more common practice in Western countries today is either to remove the lens entirely through an incision in the cornea *(intracapsular extraction),* or to remove all but the posterior surface of the lens capsule *(extracapsular cataract extraction,* or *ECCE).*

In children, the former technique, total lens removal, cannot be performed because of the strong adherence of the lens to zonular fibers and the vitreous face. An attempt to remove a lens in toto would pull part of the ocular contents with it. To avoid this problem, a needle-and-aspiration technique has been devised, using instruments to control pressure within the eye with fluid infusion, while exerting a controlled small amount of suction to aspirate the lens material.

Generally, one or two small incisions are made at the edge of the cornea (the *limbus* area). The anterior surface of the lens is pierced with a sharp instrument to expose the lens substance. The lens fibers are then aspirated carefully until they are gone. If a dense area is encountered, some instruments such as the Ocutome are capable of also cutting the lens material. When the lens has been removed, a posterior lens surface, or *capsule,* is usually still intact. It is well known that in children, this membrane will almost always become fibrous and white within a year or two, creating another barrier to good vision. Whether to open it at the time of the initial surgery or wait until it opacifies and perform another operation is still being debated. When the surgery has been completed, the small corneal wounds are sewn closed with fine suture material. A small opening in the iris, termed an *iridectomy,* may be made.

Postoperative care

Only a generation ago patients were required to stay in bed for many days after cataract surgery, with sandbags on the sides of their head to help them keep still. This was a difficult task for both pediatric patients and nurses. Now some children can go home the day of surgery or on the next day. Usually the child is kept indoors for a few days, playing as tolerated. Afterward the child can resume normal activities, minus contact sports for several weeks. Children who are old enough to understand are instructed to refrain from stooping and straining, for example, putting on their shoes, during the first few weeks. In addition, they should be prevented from rubbing their eyes. By 6–8 weeks postoperatively, the eye should be fully healed. To prevent infection and promote healing, however, the child will need medications administered daily over several weeks. Ophthalmic antibiotics and steroids will be given, as well as 1 percent atropine to keep the eye dilated and prevent the formation of adhesions *(synechiae)* and ciliary spasms. As a dressing, a pressure patch is placed after surgery and removed by the surgeon in 1 or 2 days. Then a plastic bubble or shield is placed over the eye to provide protection for a month or so. Small children may need to wear mitts until they have accepted the cover or their wound has healed. Finally, the intraocular pressure must be kept within normal limits. Hence, in the first few days after surgery, infants should not be allowed to cry for more than a few minutes, since crying increases this pressure. Nurses and parents should be aware that pain-induced behavior, along with nausea, vomiting, and a bubble in the eye, could indicate pupillary block (closed-angle glaucoma), especially within a few days after surgery. The child's position should be changed, and the surgeon should be notified immediately if such symptoms appear. In addition, the child's intraocular pressure must be checked every 1–2 months, since the anterior chamber has been altered with the surgery, and the flow of aqueous humor may be impeded, possibly causing glaucoma.

Visual Rehabilitation After Cataract Surgery

After a cataract has been removed, the child is said to be *aphakic,* or without a lens. Because of this, the child can no longer accommodate or focus clearly at close range with the involved eye. In addition, children below the age of 9 can develop amblyopia unless a visual rehabilitation program is started immediately after surgery.

Glasses

Glasses are currently recommended for children who have had bilateral cataracts removed and cannot use contact lenses for one reason or another. Unfortunately, a number of problems accompany the use of aphakic glasses. For example, to correct a child's aphakia and refractive error adequately, the glasses must contain 15–40 D of power, in a bifocal style. This causes the glasses to be quite thick, particularly in their center. In turn, this increased thickness causes 25–30 percent magnification of all objects, with associated depth perception changes. For example, if a child is reaching for a toy, but it appears 30 percent larger than it really is, the toy will appear closer and the child may misjudge how far to reach for it. Obviously, time will be needed for the child to adjust. Similarly, because the center of the glasses is thicker than the periphery, the child will have decreased and distorted peripheral vision. Long vertical lines such as trees may appear wavy, and the child may initially lose balance because of these peripheral distortions. Children learn with time, however, to turn their heads and look through the center of their glasses to view peripheral items, rather than merely moving their eyes and looking out of the periphery.

Cataract glasses can likewise magnify the appearance of the eyes, giving the child a "bull's eye" appearance. Some parents (and children, depending on their age) find this unattractive, and problems may result from such feelings.

In addition, parents may have difficulty in keeping the glasses on their child (see Chapter 3). Or, if the child is very young, glasses may be difficult to fit because the child's nasal bridge has not yet completely grown. Finally, aphakic glasses can be quite heavy, unless plastic (which is preferred for children anyway) is used in place of tempered glass lenses.

Contact Lenses

Contact lenses are currently the preferred method of visual rehabilitation for children who have had a monocular cataract removed and are often used for children with bilateral cataracts because they magnify objects by only 7 percent, rather than the 25 percent magnification of aphakic glasses. Since the other eye of children with monocular cataracts usually views objects in their normal size, any magnification by the treated eye will result in *aneisikonia,* or difference in the size of images as they focus on the retina. The greater this difference, the greater the chances for amblyopia to develop secondary to the confusion caused by the aneisikonia. Contact lenses also provide more normal peripheral vision. However, since the majority of children's work (play) is at near range, they are either given glasses for this close work, or their contact lenses are overplussed by 1–3 D.

Ophthalmologists differ in their selection of contact lenses for children with aphakia. Some prefer the gas permeable hard lenses, which must be removed daily. Others like the extended-wear silicone or soft lenses, which require insertion and cleaning only once every month or so.

Eventually, an infant or toddler gets around to exploring a contact lens. Perhaps it accidentally falls out, is loosened by crying, or is rubbed out. In this exploration process some children have even eaten the lens! The repeated loss of lenses can be costly, so many families obtain contact lens insurance to assist them in keeping up with their child's natural explorations and activities. (See Chapter 3 for further details about contact lenses.)

Intraocular Lenses (IOLs, or Lens Implants)

IOLs are permanent plastic lenses placed into the eye at the time of cataract extraction or in another surgical procedure after extraction. They are usually made of the plastic PMMA and have attachments called *haptics* that are made of various materials and hold the lens in place (Fig. 10-2). Although these lenses have been in existence for several decades and have been successful in many patients, there is much controversy surrounding their use in children and young adults.

The benefits of IOLs include little, if any, magnification of objects; normal depth perception; and no need for insertion or cleaning. Most patients require additional glasses for near vision.

Reported possible complications from IOL insertion include increased risks of intraocular infection and vitreous loss during surgery, as well as postoperative inflammation, secondary glaucoma, macular changes, retinal detachment, and corneal edema. In addition, IOLs are not uniformly recommended for patients with glaucoma, extreme myopia, or a history of iritis or retinal detachment.

For children, a number of additional complications exist. Since IOLs are

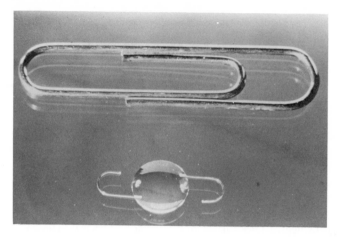

Fig. 10-2. Example of an intraocular lens (Courtesy of IOLAB Corporation).

considered foreign bodies in the eye, and since most IOL patients have been over 65 years of age, their long-term tolerance remains unknown. How will the body's immune system react over 30, 40, or 50 years to this foreign body? Will there be a considerable increase in the already known complications over long periods of time? Will the plastic lenses or haptics eventually change and produce irritants? Will the haptics themselves remain in place for long periods or require numerous reattachment surgeries?

On the other hand, the possibility of using IOLs for children is being pursued with much interest, especially for children who have cataracts secondary to trauma. As stated, the visual rehabilitation of a child using glasses or contact lenses after a cataract removal can be quite tedious. The possibilities for developing amblyopia, aneisikonia, and the decreased opportunities for developing fusion are high. As a result, the number of children attaining adequate visual acuity after their cataract surgery is markedly lower than the number of adults who have such surgery and use glasses or contact lenses afterward.

In summary, some ophthalmologists are looking at the IOL to help improve a child's vision, and others are directing their efforts towards the newer types of contact lenses. Only time and careful studies can tell which will prove better.

DISLOCATED LENSES

Dislocated lenses are not related to cataracts. The medical term for a dislocated lens is *ectopia lentis*. When a lens is only partially dislocated, it is said to be *subluxated*. A lens may become dislocated when the zonules (which usually keep the lens in place) become weakened or disrupted. Ectopia lentis is almost always inherited and hence bilateral; sometimes, however, children develop a dislocated lens secondary to trauma.

You may be able to notice a dislocated lens by shining a light from the side into the anterior of the eye and noting whether the edge of the lens is visible in the pupillary area (normally, it is not). If the lens stays behind the iris but still in view, the child will have varying (and often significant) amounts of astigmatism because the lens will be only partially refracting light. If the lens is totally invisible, the patient is considered to be aphakic. If the lens moves into the anterior chamber, acute glaucoma will result from the blockage of the aqueous humor's flow.

Dislocated lenses can also be associated with several syndromes. The one most commonly associated with it is *Marfan's syndrome*. Eighty percent of these patients eventually develop dislocated lenses, more than half of them by the age of 5. The dislocated lens will often be upward and nasal. These children can also develop other ocular problems, such as myopia, retinal detachment and heterochromia.

Children with homocystinuria also frequently have dislocated lenses. However, their lenses usually dislocate downward and nasally.

REFERENCES

1. Catalano JD: Leukokoria—the differential diagnosis of a white pupil. Pediatr Ann 12: 499, 1983
2. O'Neill JF: Cataracts in infants and children. Pediatr Ann 9:27, 1980
3. Parks MM: Visual results in aphakic children. Am J Ophthalmol 94:448, 1982
4. Beller R, Hoyt CS, Marg E, et al: Good visual function after neonatal surgery for congenital monocular cataracts. Am J Ophthalmol 91:559, 1981
5. Gelbart SS, Hoyt CS, Jastrebski G, et al: Long-term visual results in bilateral congenital cataracts. Am J Ophthalmol 93:615, 1982

SELECTED BIBLIOGRAPHY

Boyd-Monk H: Cataract surgery. Nurs 77 7:56–61, 1977
Crawford JS, Morin JD; The lens, in Crawford JS, Morin JD (eds): *The Eye in Childhood*, New York, Grune and Stratton, 1983
Hiles DA (ed): *Intraocular Lens Implants in Children*. New York, Grune and Stratton, 1980
Hiles DA: Infantile cataracts. Pediatr Ann 12:556–572, 1983
Raab EL: Cataracts and glaucoma in the infant and preschool child: Detection, systemic aspects, and treatment. Sight Sav Rev 50:5–14, 1980

Chapter Eleven

The External Eye

External eye problems involve the eyelids, tear duct apparatus, the conjunctiva, and the cornea. In addition, the sclera, iris, and pupil are often examined at the same time because these structures are so amenable to external examination; however, technically they are internal structures of the eye. External problems can be congenital or caused by allergy, disease, infection, or injury. The more common ones that nurses encounter in their pediatric patients are discussed in this chapter and the next.

BEGINNING THE ASSESSMENT

Equipment

You should have the following equipment available to help in making assessments: age-appropriate visual acuity screening equipment (see Tables 1-3 and 1-4), a penlight, a lens that can magnify at least four times, cotton tip applicators, tape, sterile eye or gauze pads, a ruler calibrated in millimeters, sterile ophthalmic irrigating solution, and a plastic or metal eyeguard. In addition, identify how and where you can quickly flush a child's eye in case of emergency. Nurses who work in conjunction with a physician may also have access to topical ophthalmic anesthetics, fluorescein strips, and culture and smear equipment.

History

What is the child's chief complaint, and when was it first noticed? How rapidly did it appear? Has the child had this problem before? Do other family members or peers have a similar problem? Has the child had a recent episode of trauma? Does the child have a history of allergies, or has the child received any topical ophthalmic medications recently? Does the child wear glasses or contact lenses? What is the child's general health? The answers to these questions will provide you with a firm basis to begin your physical assessment of the eye(s).

NURSING GOALS, OUTCOME STANDARDS, AND DIAGNOSES

Although external eye problems are varied, the primary nursing goal for all is that *each child with an external eye problem ultimately has optimal visual and psychosocial functioning*. For children with a transient or acute type of external eye problem, such as viral conjunctivitis or styes, optimal functioning is often reestablished once the problem has abated or disappeared. In contrast, for children with a long-standing external eye problem (for example, ptosis or dry eyes) optimal functioning must be pursued as soon as the eye problem is identified.

Outcome Standard 1

Any child with a suspected or documented external eye problem is seen by a primary care provider or ophthalmologist and receives any recommended treatment and follow-up.

Suggested Interventions:

• The nurse identifies children with suspected or documented external eye problems and refers these children appropriately. Individual problems are discussed in this chapter, and Table 11-1 summarizes many of the common abnormal findings of external eye problems. In general, children with possible involvement of their cornea, iris, sclera, or pupil should be referred to an ophthalmologist, as should children with long-standing problems of their lids, lacrimal system, or conjunctiva. Children with other external eye problems can be referred to a physician or nurse practitioner. Keep a list of ophthalmologists and primary care providers available, in case the family does not currently have access to one.

• The nurse educates parents, teachers, other health staff, and significant others about the signs and symptoms of possible eye trouble in children, as listed in Table 1-1.

• The nurse ensures that each child with an external eye problem receives proper treatment and identifies and assists with any problems that might prevent such treatment (counteracts *impaired home maintenance management, noncompliance, knowledge deficit*).

• The nurse assists the family and child in carrying out home-care instructions. For example, parents may not be aware of proper handwashing and waste disposal precautions or the importance and proper technique of administering antibiotic drops (decrease *knowledge deficit, noncompliance*).

Outcome Standard 2

The visual acuity of a child with an external eye problem either remains unaffected by the external eye problem or, if affected, improves with early treatment and follow-up.

Suggested Interventions:

Some children experience a *sensory deficit* because their vision is impaired secondary to either the disease or the treatment. For example, bacterial keratitis can blind a child's eye, ophthalmic ointments can blur vision, and patching can also interfere with vision. Unfortunately, the outcome of a child's vision may not be known for several weeks or even months after some ocular diseases. If bilateral low vision or blindness is present, ensure that appropriate recommendations in Chapter 13 are pursued.

Outcome Standard 3

Family members and peers of a child with a contagious external eye problem do not develop a similar problem. (See interventions listed for the first and next Outcome Standards.)

Outcome Standard 4

Older patients and the parents of all children with an external eye problem define the specific external eye problem, how and why treatment is recommended, frequency and importance of follow-up visits, and possible consequences if such treatment and follow-up is not carried out.

Outcome Standard 5

Older patients and the parents of all children with an external eye problem verbalize the impact of the external eye problem on their daily lives.

Suggested Interventions:
- The nurse clarifies and offers repeated explanations about the diagnosis and treatment plan (decrease *knowledge deficit*).
- The nurse provides the patient and family the opportunity to discuss the impact of the external eye problem on their daily lives. For younger children, such an opportunity may involve the use of puppets, dolls, pictures or story books.

Since external eye problems are visible, the child may have a *disturbance of body-image* or may experience *social isolation* by becoming withdrawn or being rejected by peers. If the problem is contagious, social isolation will also be created by the child's need to remain at home. Explain that the problem will eventually disappear and assist the child in developing *diversional activities* in the meantime.

A child may also develop *fears,* such as fear of blindness, fear of temporary or permanent disfigurement, or regarding diagnostic or therapeutic procedures and equipment. Explores these fears with the child through age-appropriate measures. Even young children are aware that an injury to the eye can cause blindness, and they may become quite *anxious* about it. If a significant loss of vision does occur, *dysfunctional grieving* or *ineffective coping* by the child or family may also develop.

Many children with external eye problems also have an increased *potential for injury,* as the problem can extend to the other eye, other ocular structures, or other family members or peers. A few external eye problems, such as orbital cellulitis, can actually spread beyond the child's eye to other body parts, including the brain.

Finally, external eye problems may cause *alterations in comfort,* and measures to decrease any pain complaints should be offered when possible.

Visual Acuity

Another important but often forgotten step is the determination of the child's visual acuity before any other assessments or treatments are done. The only exceptions concern children with chemical burns of the eye (in which case immediate flushing is required) and those having problems that are life-threatening. A quick, rough estimate is adequate (preferably with correction, if possible, or using the pinhole technique) and will provide you and follow-up providers with important baseline information and documentation. Remember to screen only one eye at a time, however. If any sudden change has occurred, refer the child immediately to an ophthalmologist, since a corneal or internal problem is probably occurring.

Pain

Children may describe ocular pain in many ways. They may complain of photophobia, burning, headaches, a foreign body sensation, itching, or local or generalized pain. Younger children may be irritable or rub their eyes or hide their faces. Your early assessment of the type of pain complaint can often help you quickly complete your assessment and determine the proper sources of referral. However, remember that some children with serious internal eye problems or injuries may have no complaints or minor complaints of pain.

Any complaints or behaviors related to *photophobia* usually indicate that the cornea or iris is involved. Young infants, especially premature ones, tend to have small to moderate amounts of photophobia, and their eyes should be protected from bright lights until they are older. Nevertheless, ensure that these children do not have other signs of glaucoma (Chapter 9). Older infants and toddlers who hide their faces in lighted rooms, or prefer to play in darker rooms should be referred to an ophthalmologist immediately, as permanent damage to their vision may be occurring from an underlying problem. Besides glaucoma, photophobia can also accompany iritis or keratitis.

Itching indicates an allergic response of the eyelids or conjunctiva and does not usually present any potential for permanent damage. Therefore, referrals can be made according to the severity of the child's complaints.

A *gritty sensation* ("something in my eye") may represent a foreign body on the conjunctiva or cornea or may allude to a corneal abrasion, viral conjunctivitis, dry eyes, or, quite rarely, exophthalmos. Again, because the cornea may be involved, immediate referral is necessary if the sensation does not decrease over a brief period of time.

210

Burning can represent a local reaction to such irritants as smoke or smog, or it can result from the toxic products of a bacterial infection of the lids or conjunctiva.

Headaches are frequently considered to be associated with eye problems yet infrequently are. Instead, they usually have nonocular origins. A child who complains of headaches of sudden onset or who has had chronic headaches with normal vision (with or without the pinhole test) should be referred to the primary care provider for a general evaluation. However, if a child's vision improves with the pinhole test, refer the child to an ophthalmologist or optometrist, since this result may indicate a refractive error.

In contrast, severe *local pain* located within the eye can indicate iritis, glaucoma (rare in children), a foreign body or other injury, or corneal inflammation (abrasion or keratitis). These children should be referred immediately to an ophthalmologist.

Referrals

You can refer children with suspected or documented problems of their lids or conjunctiva or those who have initial problems with their tear ducts to either their primary care provider or ophthalmologist. Children with suspected or documented problems of the cornea, iris, or other internal structures, however, should be referred to an ophthalmologist only. Have on hand the names of several primary care providers and ophthalmologists to whom you can refer children if families need such information and remember to send along your visual acuity results and other pertinent findings.

COMMON DISORDERS OF THE EXTERNAL EYE

After the history and visual acuity screening, most examiners proceed in a systematic fashion in assessing the external eye area. For example, some go from top to bottom, medial to lateral, and outside to inside. With experience, you will probably develop your own style.

THE EYELIDS

Anatomy and Assessment

The purpose of the eyelids is to protect the eyes, physically, through a barrier in front of the eyes, and chemically, through the tears that are produced in and around the eyelids.

For our purposes the eyelids have five main layers. Outermost is the loosely connected skin covering, which is one of the thinnest skin coverings of the body. Beneath this is the *orbicularis oculi muscle,* which closes the eyelid when activated by the seventh cranial nerve. In the middle of the eyelids are the *tarsal plates*. These are the connective tissue of the eyelids that give the lids their form and shape. Next the *meibomian or tarsal glands* appear as numerous vertical yellow streaks on the inside of the lids, assisting in tear production and flow. Finally, the *palpebral conjunctiva* comprises the innermost layer of the lids.

The *levator palpebrae muscle* starts approximately at the lid fold and extends up to the brow area. This muscle is responsible for opening the lids and is innervated by the third cranial nerve. When a child looks straight ahead, the eyelids should be open to such a degree that they cover the top portion of the iris but do not interfere with the pupil.

The *palpebral fissures* (rima palpebrarum) are those spaces where the eyelids open (Fig. 11-1). The *outer (lateral) canthus* is the area where the upper and lower lids connect at the temporal side of the head, and the *inner (medial) canthus* connects the lids at the nasal side.

To examine the lids, instruct the child to look straight ahead, then up, and then down. If you are doing a more thorough assessment, evert the lids to examine them for signs of inflammation or lesions. To evert the lower lid, have the patient look up while you place your thumb or finger about 1/2 in below the eye. Then gently pull down until you can adequately inspect the area. To evert the upper lid you will need a cotton applicator. Place it against the outside of the upper lid about 1/2 in above the lid margin. Then have the patient look down (and keep looking down) to relax the levator palpebrae muscle. Also tell the child to relax the other muscles in the eye area as much as possible. Then gently pull the upper lid down and forward by holding on to the eyelashes. Quickly turn the eyelid inside out by pressing the applicator into the lids, being careful not to press on the eye itself. After you inspect the area, gently pull the eyelids forward and let the patient look up and blink to return the eyelid to its normal position. A pocket flashlight and magnifying lens may help in your assessment.

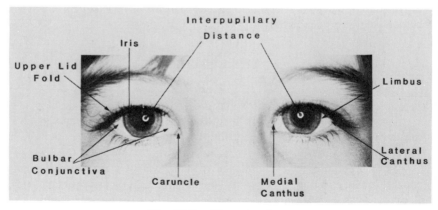

Fig. 11-1.   The external eye.

Table 11-1

Common areas of external eye assessment in children, normal findings, and possible abnormal findings (list not all inclusive)

Area of Assessment	Normal Findings	Possible Abnormal Findings
Visual acuity	Normal, with correction if necessary	Refractive errors Infection, inflammation, or trauma to cornea, intraocular network (including the iris), or orbital bones
Pain		
Itching	None	Allergic or marginal blepharitis Allergic conjunctivitis Lice on eyelashes Dry eyes
Burning	None	Blepharitis Conjunctivitis Irritants (smog, for example) Dry eyes
Gritty sensation	None	Viral or allergic conjunctivitis Foreign body Corneal abrasion or ultraviolet burns Keratitis Dry eyes Trauma Blepharitis Exophthalmos
Headaches	None	If no change in visual acuity, often nonocular in origin If vision improves with pinhole test, refractive error Iritis, glaucoma or other internal source

(continued)

Table 11-1 *(continued)*

Area of Assessment	Normal Findings	Possible Abnormal Findings
Pain (continued)		
Photophobia	None, except in bright lights or going from dark to light, or in young infants who do not have other signs of glaucoma	Iritis Glaucoma Keratitis Corneal abrasion or ultraviolet burns Viral conjunctivitis or keratoconjunctivitis Foreign body Dry eyes Hyphema
Local, superficial	None	Herpes keratitis Corneal abrasions or ultraviolet burns Foreign body Hordeolum (stye) Dacryocystitis Trauma
Deep, diffuse	None	Iritis Glaucoma Sinus problems Trauma (orbital fracture, for example) Referred pain from other areas
With eye movements	None	Orbital cellulitis Optic neuritis
Eyelids Shape	Semicircular, with or without epicanthal folds	Lid coloboma Lid laceration or scar

Color	Similar to child's skin tone	Marginal blepharitis: red at edges Hemangioma: red Blow to the eye: ecchymotic Other inflammation (chalazion, style): red Orbital cellulitis: violet Dermatomyositis: violet
Turgor	No swelling	Recent, prolonged crying Systemic or local allergies Marginal blepharitis Conjunctivitis Foreign body: usually one eye only Dacryocystitis: nasal side Local or orbital cellulitis Orbital fracture Systemic fluid retention (for example, nephrosis)
	No nodules present	Chalazion or hordeolum Dacryocele: nasal side of eye
	No crusts or scales on lids or lashes	Marginal blepharitis secondary to: *Staphylococcus* infection: hard, yellow scales Seborrhea: gray, greasy scales Allergy Lice Bacterial conjunctivitis Nasolacrimal duct obstruction
Function	Lids open completely (pupils totally visible if child looks straight ahead)	Ptosis secondary to: Congenital or hereditary defect

(continued)

Table 11-1 (*continued*)

Area of Assessment	Normal Findings	Possible Abnormal Findings
		Myasthenia gravis
		Cranial nerve III or other CNS problem
		Lid swelling (trauma, allergies, and so on)
	Sclera not visible above or below iris if child looks straight ahead	Thyroid disease
		Proptosis secondary to:
		Orbital cellulitis
		Orbital tumor
		Infection
		Lid retraction
		CNS disease
	Stay open	Gradually close when fatigued in myasthenia gravis
	Close completely, except in some persons of Asian background	Cranial nerve VII dysfunction
	Blink about every 4 seconds	CNS problem
		Dry eyes
	No twitching	Myasthenia gravis
Tears		
Amount	Keep eyes moist without excess	Crying: excess
		Allergy: excess
		Common cold: excess
		Foreign body and corneal abrasions: excess
		Dacryocystitis: excess
		Nasolacrimal duct obstruction: excess, without runny nose

	Normal	Deviations
		Congenital glaucoma: excess with runny nose, photophobia, or corneal haze
		Other inflammation (blepharitis, keratitis, iritis): excess
		Dry eye syndrome: decrease
		Sjogren's syndrome: decrease, possibly with dry mouth
		Stevens Johnson syndrome: decrease

Conjunctiva

Color:

	Normal	Deviations

Bulbar conjunctiva	Transparent, with some small blood vessels apparent	Focal bright redness
		  Subconjunctival hemorrhage
		  Conjunctival foreign body
		  Orbital fracture
		Diffuse pattern of redness
		  Any conjunctivitis
		  Keratitis, including ultraviolet burns
		  Systemic illness (Kawasaki's, for example)
		  Orbital cellulitis
		Circumcorneal flush
		  Iritis
		  Keratitis
		  Uveitis
		White triangular piece onto cornea: pterygium
		Yellowish-white nodule, not on cornea: pingueculum

Palpebral conjunctiva	Reddish pink and smooth	Anemia: pale Chronic illness: pale Inflammation: bright red Vernal conjunctivitis: cobblestone texture

(continued)

Table 11-1 (*continued*)

Area of Assessment	Normal Findings	Possible Abnormal Findings
Sclera	White, except in persons with darker skin colors, then has yellowish hue	Newborns: light blue Osteogenesis imperfecta: blue Marfan's syndrome: blue Jaundice: yellow

Discharge	None	Watery
		  Viral conjunctivitis
		  Herpes keratitis
		Stringy
		  Allergic conjunctivitis
		  Inclusion blennorrhea
		Purulent or mucopurulent
		  Bacterial conjunctivitis
		  Bacterial keratitis
		  Dacryocystitis (near puncta)

Cornea		

Color	Transparent, clear	Congenital glaucoma: corneal haze
		Corneal opacities secondary to:
		  Congenital anomalies
		  Infection
		  Burns
		  Use of forceps during delivery
		  Other trauma
		Cataracts (may appear as corneal opacity)

Surface	Smooth, with sharp light reflex	Corneal abrasion: irregular reflex Strabismus: uneven reflex (Chapter 4)

	No bright green areas with fluorescein staining	Corneal abrasions: small pools Herpes keratitis: branchlike Scars on cornea
Size	10–12 mm	Congenital megalocornea: large Congenital glaucoma: large Microcornea: small
Shape	Round when viewed from side	Keratoconus: cone-shaped appearance
Reflex	Brisk blinking response with cotton wisp	Herpes simplex keratitis: decreased CNS disorder: decreased
Iris		
Shape	Round	Coloboma of iris (''tear drop pupil'') Trauma
Color	Equal between both eyes, or slight, long-standing variation	If sudden change in one eye, rule out trauma or malignancy Red or black hue: hyphema White or gray appearance: hypopyon
	Some markings are normal	

(continued)

Table 11-1 (*continued*)

Area of Assessment	Normal Findings	Possible Abnormal Findings
Pupil		
Size	3–5 mm, depending on lighting; 25 percent of normal population has 1-mm difference between pupils	Dilated secondary to: Recent administration of mydriatics Blunt trauma Glaucoma (usually in adults) Constricted secondary to: Iritis Miotic drugs CNS disease (for example, Horner's syndrome)
Shape	Round	Trauma Iritis Adhesions
Extraocular Muscles		
Movements	Normal and complete	Orbital cellulitis: decreased Strabismus: abnormal Orbital fracture: decreased Cranial nerve palsy: abnormal CNS lesion: abnormal

Some Common Eyelid Problems

The prefix *blephar-* is often used in describing a problem of the eyelids, such as *blepharitis*. Table 11-1 includes the common areas of assessment of the eyelids and lists possible problems that may be present when a particular finding is abnormal.

Colobomas

Colobomas are congenital structural defects of any part of the eye. Fortunately, skillful plastic surgery can often satisfactorily correct all but the most dramatic of these defects when they occur on the lids. Lid colobomas are often associated with syndromes.

Epicanthal Folds

Some children, especially infants and those of Asian descent, may have epicanthal folds. These are half-moon shaped folds of skin at the inner canthus that may give the incorrect impression that the child has strabismus (see pseudo-strabismus in Chapter 5 and Fig. 5-1).

Marginal Blepharitis

Marginal blepharitis is a common lid inflammation characterized by scaling, redness, swelling, and sometimes itching and a discharge. As its name implies, such signs occur at the edge of the lid, near the lashes. Unless the infection or inflammation spreads to other ocular structures, there is usually no danger of its permanently damaging a child's vision.

A *staphylococcal infection* is the most common cause of marginal blepharitis. It is manifested by hard, yellow scales that cling to the lash edges, sometimes with small ulcerated areas and pus. Treatment includes soaking the lids gently with baby shampoo or warm compresses for a few minutes, several times a day, then gently removing the crusts with a cotton applicator and administering an antibiotic such as bacitracin. Patients and their families should be advised about good handwashing and dressing disposal techniques and cautioned against rubbing their eyes. Unfortunately, this type of blepharitis tends to recur and can involve other ocular structures, such as the cornea.

Seborrhea can also cause marginal blepharitis. Unlike those in a staph infection, the scales of seborrhea are gray and greasy and can be easily removed with a cotton applicator. These patients often have an associated seborrhea of the scalp, and about 30 percent have a combination of seborrhea and infection (usually staph). Treatment, following a culture to rule out infection, is with ammoniated mercury ointment.

Lice can also cause blepharitis and are identified by the presence of white nits (eggs), small moving spots, and the patient's complaint of associated itching. Treatment involves frequent washing of the lids with a mild baby shampoo or special ointment and manual removal of the lice and nits.

Finally, blepharitis can also be caused by an allergy that produces *contact dermatitis*. Soaps and makeup are frequent precursors. The patient should try to determine what the causative agent may be and to eliminate its use. Topical steroids are occasionally used to treat contact dermatitis.

Chalazions and Hordeolums (Styes)

A *chalazion* is a granulomatous cyst of a meibomian gland. It feels hard and may appear on either the outside or inside lid. Unlike a hordeolum, however, it may not be tender, can be present for months, and is usually located in the center of the lids, away from the margins. Treatment consists of warm soaks several times a day and the use of antibiotics if an infection is present. Infrequently a chalazion may cause astigmatism or create discomfort by abrading the cornea. Hence, incision or surgical excision may be necessary, preferably from the inner surface of the lid. However, since chalazions can disappear spontaneously, a waiting period of several months may be beneficial. Unfortunately, they may recur and can be multiple.

In contrast, *hordeolums* are infections of a sebaceous gland or hair follicle near the eyelashes. They are differentiated from chalazions by their short duration; their tendency to be acutely painful, swollen, and inflamed; and presence of pus in their boillike structure. Hordeolums require treatment with antibiotics, as *Staphylococcus aureus* is a common cause. In addition, patients should be reminded of good handwashing techniques and must be cautioned against squeezing them because cellulitis can rapidly develop. Gentle, warm compresses may also promote healing. Like chalazions, hordeolums can spontaneously heal by rupturing and draining.

Ptosis (Blepharoptosis)

Ptosis is an inability of one or both eyelids to open completely. Although it usually occurs in children as an idiopathic congenital problem of the levator palpebrae muscle, it can also result from a third cranial nerve palsy, trauma, or myasthenia gravis. It can also be inherited.

Several problems can occur secondary to ptosis. First, decreased vision from deprivation amblyopia can occur if the eyelids cover the pupil. However, most children with severe ptosis tilt their heads back so that they can see adequately. Another problem concerns the child's self-image, as the drooping eyelid(s) tends to give the child a dull and indifferent appearance.

The diagnostic work-up includes visual acuity testing and refraction to rule out amblyopia, assessment of the extraocular muscles (especially the superior rectus muscle) to help rule out myasthenia gravis and third cranial nerve palsy, and evaluation of the levator function. For example, a child with ptosis of the left eye may open the left eyelid only 3 mm although the child may be able to open the right eyelid a full 13 mm.

In acquired cases, the evaluation may include a Tensilon (Roche) (edrophonium chloride) or neostigmine test to help rule out myasthenia gravis. In children, ocular signs and symptoms are often the first evidence of this neurologic disease and may include complaints of diplopia, strabismus, or lid twitching, as well as ptosis. The ptosis may be variable and asymmetric and may develop at the end of the day when the levator muscle becomes fatigued or when the patient is looking in the up gaze for some time. Blinking or temporarily closing the eyes may cause it to decrease or disappear.

If you should assist with the Tensilon procedure, prepare the child accordingly. Depending on the child's age, you may wish to use a doll for demonstration. Try to plan the preparation so that there is minimal time between it and the actual procedure.

After the IV is in place, a small test dose is given to determine whether the child has any idiosyncratic reactions. Then atropine may be given; otherwise, it is kept available in case the child has a strong anticholinesterase response (for example, sweating, nausea, vomiting, tearing). Following this, the rest of the Tensilon is given. If a child has ptosis secondary to myasthenia gravis, the lid(s) will assume a normal position about 30–60 seconds after the administration of the Tensilon, continuing until the Tensilon begins to wear off a few minutes later. A child with ptosis secondary to other causes will have no eyelid response to the Tensilon but may have increased complaints of its side effects. Monitor the child's pulse at intervals throughout the procedure.

Tensilon tests can also be performed while a tonograph is attached to the child's eyes. As the lid(s) assumes the normal position, a spike will be noticed on the tonograph recording.

Surgery is the only treatment for cases of ptosis not caused by myasthenia gravis. However, surgery is sometimes delayed several years to give the child time to develop the use of the frontalis muscle at the forehead, which also assists in opening the lids. One common surgical procedure is the *levator resection,* in which the levator and tarsus muscles are shortened. For more severe cases, a sling may be made to connect the levator muscle with the frontalis muscle, sometimes using fascia lata from the patient's thigh. In these cases, the child will have stitches on both the eye and leg areas, and the eye will look worse (swollen, ecchymotic, observable stitches) before it looks better in several weeks. The child may be double-patched for a few days after surgery to protect the cornea against exposure, so prepare the child for this and orient the child to the environment prior to surgery. Usually children can be as active as tolerated postoperatively, although in this day of television and other visual stimuli, they may quickly become bored and frustrated secondary to the patching. If possible, obtain some of the story tapes now available to help them pass the time and encourage their parents to stay with them as much as possible. Usually surgery is successful on the first attempt, but repeat procedures may be necessary for a few children.

Edema

Edema often occurs around the eyelids because the skin of the lids is so loosely connected to the layers beneath it. The most common cause of lid edema is a local or systemic allergy, such as an allergy to makeup. Other causes have more serious implications and include preseptal or orbital cellulitis and some renal diseases. When only one eye is involved, a foreign body or infection should be suspected. Palliative relief to help decrease the edema consists of applying cold compresses for 5 minutes, several times a day. Edema may be more noticeable when a child wakes up in the morning.

Orbital Cellulitis

Orbital cellulitis is a most serious ocular problem characterized by swollen red lids that sometimes have a violet hue. In addition, the child may have proptosis, pain on movement of the eyes, decreased eye movements, injected conjunctiva (if visible through the lid edema), blurred vision, fever, and malaise. Its onset is sudden and usually involves one eye only. Sinus films may help the physician identify a paranasal sinus infection (especially of the ethmoid sinus), which often precedes orbital cellulitis. In younger children *Haemophilus influenzae* is a most common causative agent; in older children and adults it is *Staphylococcus*.

Orbital cellulitis requires rapid diagnosis, culture, and treatment with intravenous antibiotics to prevent the inflammation from spreading into the central nervous system (CNS) pathway or causing a cavernous sinus thrombosis. Interventions by an ear, nose, and throat specialist may also be necessary.

Lid Hemangiomas

Lid hemangiomas are benign, highly vascular nodules that frequently appear during the first weeks after birth and continue to enlarge during the child's first year. They eventually reach a plateau and usually regress markedly. Besides being quite noticeable in their rapid growth phase, their increased bulk can press on the cornea, causing astigmatism. This in turn may cause anisometropic amblyopia. Infrequently, ptosis or strabismus may develop. Various treatments have been tried (for example, steroids, sclerosing agents), but none has proved totally satisfactory.

Proptosis (Exophthalmos)

Proptosis, or forward displacement of the eye with widening of the lids, is uncommon in children. When it does occur, it may be due to an orbital tumor, infection (orbital cellulitis), thyroid disease, or trauma. In true cases of proptosis you can see the white of the sclera between the iris and upper and lower lids. Hence, it is different from lid retraction, in which the eye does not protrude but the upper lid remains more open than usual.

Proptosis can progress rapidly or gradually. To measure it, the ophthalmologist may use a Luedde or Hertel instrument. The first is a transparent ruler and the latter is a metal bar connecting two rulers with attached mirrors, which can measure both eyes simultaneously.

Patients with proptosis may complain of a gritty sensation in their eyes secondary to increased exposure of the cornea, especially in the morning. To decrease these complaints, they can use artificial tears as necessary. In addition, they may need to cover their eyes at night to prevent corneal damage. Patients with proptosis are at increased risk for developing other ocular problems, such as optic nerve damage.

Entropion and Ectropion

Entropion refers to the lids' (and lashes') turning inward. Infrequently the turned-in lashes can cause irritation to the cornea. In contrast, *ectropion* describes lids that turn outward. Patients with this disorder may have conjunctival irritation from dryness or exposure, since the protective barrier of the lid has slipped away. Both disorders are most common in older people.

THE LACRIMAL SYSTEM

Anatomy

Tears have many functions. They wash away foreign particles, thereby protecting the cornea and conjunctiva. They lubricate the eye so that the lid can open and close freely. They maximize the optics of the cornea by keeping it clear and they deliver oxygen to the cornea. They help prevent infection secondary to their lysozyme content, and they also keep the eye cool. In addition, there is some recent evidence that tears may wash away chemicals that build up during emotional swings.

Unbelievable as it may seem, only about 1 cc of tear fluid is made every day under normal circumstances. This is called the *basic secretion,* and it is necessary for proper functioning. In addition, intense light, certain chemicals or irritants, and strong emotions can cause increased tearing through *reflex lacrimation.* Opinions still vary whether newborns have tears at birth or develop them 2–3 weeks later.

The tears themselves are isotonic. The tear fluid actually consists of three layers, with the middle layer being the thickest and composed mostly of salts and water.

The lacrimal, or tearing, system is another freeway of the eye that depends on free flowing traffic for its many functions. For example, basic secretion originates from glands in the palpebral conjunctiva. Blinking then propels the tear fluid down and medially across the eyes into the *puncta lacrimale* (Fig. 11-2). These are small openings on the medial aspects of the upper and lower lids that begin the drainage of the small amount of basic secretion that has not evaporated while on the eye. As suspected, the lower puncta carries away the majority of leftover fluid. From the puncta the fluid enters the upper and lower lacrimal canaliculi, which in turn flow into the lacrimal sac. Here muscles contract and relax, causing the fluid to be further propelled into the nasolacrimal duct, where under normal conditions it evaporates completely.

Reflex tears originate in the lacrimal gland, located in the outer third of the

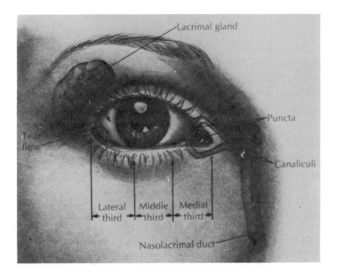

Fig. 11-2.   The lacrimal system.

orbital area between the upper lid and brow. Normally this gland is not palpable. From here the tear fluid travels through the dozen or so lacrimal ducts underneath the upper lid and joins with the basic secretion.

Common Disorders of the Lacrimal System

Nasolacrimal Duct Obstruction (Congenital Stenosis)

Obstruction of the nasolacrimal duct (NLD) is the most common lacrimal problem of early childhood. It is characterized by epiphora (excessive tearing) and some residual mucus on the edge of the lashes. These symptoms usually appear several weeks or months after birth and can be unilateral or bilateral. However, unlike congenital glaucoma (which also involves epiphora), there is no associated photophobia or runny nose.

Quite frequently the obstruction clears spontaneously, as it is secondary to a natural anatomic change that has been delayed. As a result, the first treatment usually recommended is to gently massage the lacrimal sac area three or four times a day to help clear the area of debris and plugs. Before leaving the office, parents should give a return demonstration of this massage, starting at the lower inner orbital rim (not at the side of the nose or over the eye) and pressing toward the corner of the eye. If no infection is present, massaging downward will help open the duct. However, if there is a current infection, massaging upward will help push the debris out of the puncta, where it can be manually removed. In addition, both systemic and local antibiotics are prescribed for children with concurrent infections or as prophylaxis against the development of such.

Usually the duct will open in 2–4 months. However, if a child reaches the age of 6–12 months and the massaging has not resulted in any improvement, the duct may have to be probed. Probing can be done under general or local anesthesia, in the operating room or office, or as an outpatient surgical procedure. It is not a sterile procedure. It involves the insertion of fine probes into the puncta lacrimale, which are then threaded along the canaliculi and lacrimal sac into the nasolacrimal duct. When the probing is completed, fluorescein dye is inserted into the puncta. When it can be withdrawn in the nasal cavity with a syringe, the duct is open.

Sometimes an NLD probing has to be repeated. If this should still fail, silicone tubing may be inserted, or a dacryocystorhinostomy (DCR) may be done. In this latter procedure, a piece of the nasal bone is permanently removed, and the mucous membranes of the lacrimal sac and nasal pharyngeal areas are connected. General anesthesia is required. Occasionally the surgeon may place polyethylene tubes in the nose for several months (they are not readily visible), or the nasal area may be packed for a few days. Children having these more involved procedures will often have a small incision on the side of their nose, and may spend several days in the hospital before their discharge.

Dacryocystocele (Mucocele)

A *dacryocystocele* is a less common type of NLD obstruction, characterized by accumulation of mucous in the lacrimal sac of newborns secondary to obstruction. It appears as a bluish lump on the nasal aspect of the involved eye and requires probing within a few days to prevent infection and discomfort.

Dacryocystitis

Dacryocystitis is an inflammation of the lacrimal sac or nasolacrimal duct. Patients with acute cases have excessive tearing, redness, swelling, pain, fevers, and a purulent discharge from the puncta that increases when pressure is applied to the lacrimal sac area. Treatment is with oral antibiotics, following a culture. In some cases, incision and drainage of the area may also be necessary.

Dry Eyes and the Schirmer's Test

Although sometimes loosely used, the diagnosis of *dry eyes* or *decreased tearing* technically implies some damage to the cornea or conjunctiva. It can be secondary to an idiopathic or physiologic cause or result from a fifth or seventh cranial nerve lesion.

The combination of dry eyes and dry mouth or decreased vaginal secretions is called *Sjogren's syndrome* and is a frequent complaint of patients with autoimmune diseases. It occurs predominantly in females.

Patients with dry eyes may complain of photophobia or a burning or itching sensation or report that something seems to be in their eye(s). Or they may complain that they don't form tears, even when they are crying. On examination, the conjunctiva may be inflamed, secondary to irritation of the dry mucosa.

A simple semiquantitative way of measuring tear production is by the *Schirmer's test*. This consists of placing one small strip of filter paper over the lower lid of each eye and measuring the tear production at the end of a specified time (usually 5 minutes). The strips are prepackaged and standardized with complete instructions. With this test normal basic secretion is 15 mm or more over a 5-minute period. Less than 10 mm is considered abnormal. One way of writing the results is *Schirmer's R: 8/5 min; L: 17/5 min,* implying in this case that the right eye may have decreased tear production. Some examiners prefer to administer a topical eye anesthetic prior to the test so that the insertion of the filter paper does not irritate the conjunctiva or cornea, thereby increasing tear flow. When a chemical irritant is given with the Schirmer's to promote reflex lacrimation, it is called a *Schirmer's II test*.

Another test for detecting dry conjunctiva or corneal mucosa is the *Rose-Bengal dye test,* whereby one drop of Rose-bengal dye is placed onto the eye and immediately washed away with sterile normal saline. A slit lamp examination follows, looking for any area that becomes stained and hence indicative of dryness.

The treatment for dry eyes is palliative, with the frequent insertion of artificial tears (usually every 2 hours, if not more often). Students with dry eyes should keep a spare bottle of these tears at school. Infrequently the lacrimal puncta may be temporarily or permanently occluded with small silicone plugs or cautery, respectively, to allow for the build-up of tears.

THE CONJUNCTIVA

Anatomy

The *conjunctiva* is a thin mucous membrane that separates the orbit from the environment. Its *palpebral* part lines the inside of the lids, and the *bulbar* conjunctiva covers most of the front of the eyeball up to the cornea. The invisible histologic connection of the conjunctiva and cornea is called the *limbus* (Fig. 11-1); the palpebral and bulbar conjunctiva are connected by pocketlike areas called the *fornices* (singular, *fornix*). Finally, the small triangular shaped area near each medial canthus is called a *caruncle*.

Although the bulbar conjunctiva is transparent, it has some small blood vessels. When inflamed, these vessels can become quite noticeable. Otherwise, the bulbar conjunctiva takes on the color of the sclera that lies beneath it, although the palpebral conjunctiva normally has a reddish hue. The sclera is the thick, tough shell that surrounds the entire eye and gives the eye its shape (Fig. 3-2).

Assessment Techniques

When taking a history of a child with a suspected conjunctival problem, be sure to inquire about the following. Does the child have any allergies, or has this complaint occurred before (common in allergic conjunctivitis)? Has the child had a recent episode of trauma, or sun exposure (ultraviolet burns can cause symptoms of conjunctivitis)? Has the child been near other children with a "pink eye" (viral or bacterial conjunctivitis can be quite contagious)?

Also consider the child's age. Infants less than 1 months are at risk for developing bacterial, chlamydial, or viral infections, some quite serious, secondary to their passage through the birth canal. These infections usually occur within a few days after birth and require immediate attention. Furthermore, newborns frequently develop chemical conjunctivitis a day or two after birth secondary to silver nitrate prophylaxis. Recurrent bacterial conjunctivitis in infants between the ages of 1 and 8 months may indicate an obstructed nasolacrimal duct. Older children can develop any type of conjunctivitis, although the viral type is most common in school-aged children.

The techniques for assessing the conjunctiva are similar to those for the lids. Have the child look up, down, and to the sides to view the bulbar conjunctiva, and evert both lids if you wish to inspect the palpebral portions.

Redness, or *hyperemia,* of the conjunctiva is the characteristic sign of conjunctivitis. However, it is not the degree of the hyperemia that is so significant, but its pattern and distribution. In cases of pure conjunctivitis—whatever its cause— the inflamed vessels originate in the periphery of the conjunctiva and travel toward the cornea. The vessels themselves may be tortuous and have a diffuse distribution. This pattern is also seen in some systemic diseases that have ocular manifestations, such as Stevens-Johnson syndrome or Kawasaki's disease. In contrast, when the inflammation involves the cornea or iris, the inflamed vessels may lead from the cornea toward the periphery and are radial in design. This distribution is known by many terms, such as *circumcorneal inflammation or redness, perilimbal injection, limbal flush, pericorneal halo,* and *ciliary flush.* The distribution is often 2–3 mm in radius and occurs because the anterior chamber and ciliary vessels are supplied by the same system of vessels that supplies the circumcorneal conjunctiva. Hence, inflammation in the anterior chamber is evidenced in the bulbar conjunctiva. Any circumcorneal redness requires immediate referral to an ophthalmologist.

If you are having difficulty in determining a patient's hyperemic pattern, try the following. Gently press the patient's lower lid against the conjunctiva while the patient looks up and slowly pull the lid downward while maintaining this gentle pressure. If the hyperemia is secondary to conjunctivitis, there will be a noticeable period of nonredness, as you are decreasing the conjunctival blood supply by applying continued pressure on the periphery. In contrast, hyperemia secondary to a circumcorneal inflammation will cause only momentary nonredness; since its supply comes from the anterior chamber system, pressure over peripheral blood vessels will not decrease its blood supply.

However, corneal trauma or infection can also cause a diffuse conjunctival pattern. Therefore, you must consider some other aspects in your assessment. For example, children with pure conjunctivitis will have no complaints of pain and no change in their visual acuity, whereas children with involvement of the cornea or iris may have such changes. Furthermore, if only one area of the conjunctiva is bright red, the child may have a subconjunctival hemorrhage, or foreign body.

Discharge is another characteristic feature of conjunctivitis. To assess its presence and type, evert the lower lids, as discharge tends to collect in the lower fornices. If cultures are necessary, obtain them from this area. Pay special attention to the amount and consistency of the discharge. Does it overflow the lower lids or increase in the morning? These features often indicate bacterial infection. In addition, bacterial infections usually cause a purulent (puslike) or mucopurulent discharge; viral infections cause a watery type, and allergies and chlamydial inflammations cause a stringy kind.

Excessive tearing (epiphora) occurs in many ocular inflammations and hence is not necessarily indicative of conjunctivitis. However, infants may have tearing and recurrent bacterial conjunctivitis secondary to an obstructed nasolacrimal duct.

Swelling of the lids may occur secondary to a bacterial, viral, chlamydial, or allergic inflammatory process of the conjunctiva. Occasionally the conjunctiva itself will become so edematous that it puffs out over the lower eyelid. This is known as *chemosis*.

Pupillary or intraocular pressure changes never occur in conjunctivitis. Patients with such changes should be immediately referred, as they may have iritis, glaucoma, intraocular trauma, or CNS problems.

Finally, children with conjunctivitis will occasionally have associated *systemic symptoms,* such as enlarged lymph nodes (especially the preauricular nodes), fever, or upper respiratory infection. These usually occur with viral types of conjunctivitis, although they may accompany the bacterial types, as well.

Cultures and Smears

Cultures of the conjunctiva should be taken from the lower fornix, where exudates accumulate. Some examiners use the commercially available culture collectors, others use more specific media for transport and growth. In either case, a topical anesthetic should not be applied before culturing, as it can inhibit bacterial growth. And, of course, all cultures should be taken to the laboratory for proper plating and incubation as quickly as possible.

Conjunctival smears are obtained from a conjunctival scraping, which is similar in nature to the cervical Papanicolaou's (Pap) smear. The smears are done after any necessary cultures have been obtained, so that a topical anesthetic can then be applied. Most examiners use the Kimura type of platinum spatula, as it has a blunt edge, can be quickly sterilized with an alcohol lamp, and cools within 30 seconds after removal from the flame. However, other sterile blunt metal instruments can also suffice. A child who is old enough to cooperate should look up as the examiner scraps the palpebral portion of the lower lid. Then the smear should be rapidly transferred onto premarked glass slides and immersed in a glass jar with 95 percent ethanol as a preservative. For best results, this entire process should occur within 10 seconds. Then send the slides to the lab for Gram and Giemsa staining.

The Gram stain will help identify any bacteria that may be present, and the Giemsa stain will allow examination of cell infiltrates to the area. For example, the presence of any neutrophils indicates an acute inflammatory process such as a bacterial infection, whereas the presence of many monocytes represents a chronic or viral inflammation, and the presence of many eosinophils shows an allergic response. In addition, inclusion bodies indicating a chlamydial infection may be identified on a Giemsa stain. Finally, although rare in children, precancerous or malignant cells may also be identified from a conjunctival smear.

Types of Conjunctivitis

Bacterial Conjunctivitis

Bacterial conjunctivitis can sometimes be difficult to distinguish from viral conjunctivitis, as both types cause varying degrees of diffuse hyperemia and both may have associated lymphadenopathy. Furthermore, both commonly start in one eye and spread to the other by the child's hands, and both can be highly contagious. However, bacterial conjunctivitis tends to cause a mucopurulent or purulent discharge. This is especially true in the morning, when the child may have difficulty opening the eyes and may develop crusts on the lids as the discharge dries. In addition, bacterial conjunctivitis usually yields positive culture results.

A wide variety of bacteria can cause conjunctivitis in children. The most common type is *Staphylococcus aureus* (gram-positive), which may be acute or chronic. Its discharge tends to be yellowish and quite thick, and the child may also have small ulcerated areas on the lid margins. Some other types of bacteria that can cause conjunctivitis are *H. influenzae* (gram-positive), *Pseudomonas* species (gram-negative), and *Streptococcus* species (gram-positive). Conjunctivitis from *Neisseria gonorrhoeae* (gram-negative) in newborns is now uncommon secondary to the use of silver nitrate or prophylactic antibiotics.

Fortunately, most cases of bacterial conjunctivitis are self-limiting, spontaneously disappearing within 1–2 weeks without leaving any residual damage. However, newborns and a very small percentage of other children are at risk for developing complications. In addition, bacterial conjunctivitis is highly contagious. Hence, treatment with antibiotics is preferred.

Many examiners treat suspected cases with a broad spectrum antibiotic such as Sulamyd (Schering) or Neosporin (Burroughs Wellcome). If cultures are taken (usually only on neonates or when a quite purulent discharge is present), more specific antibiotics may be prescribed. For example, sulfonamides, erythromycin, bacitracin, and tetracycline are often used for gram-positive bacteria, and gentamicin and polymyxin B are frequently prescribed for gram-negative bacteria. In addition, many examiners concurrently prescribe systemic antibiotics for children infected with *Streptococcus pneumoniae, beta-Streptococccus,* or *Neisseria gonorrhoeae.*

Ophthalmic antibiotic solutions may be given quite frequently, for example, every 2 hours, but ophthalmic ointments need only be inserted three or four times daily. However, since the ointment often blurs vision, its use may be restricted, especially in older children, to hours of sleep.

Any prescribed ophthalmic antibiotics should be continued for at least 72 hours after the disappearance of all symptoms. All oral antibiotics should be taken for their entire prescribed course. Children and their parents will often need repeated instruction about this, as the tendency is for them to stop taking the antibiotics as soon as symptoms have disappeared. Any child with a nonallergic conjunctivitis, should be kept out of school until all symptoms subside. If no improvement occurs within 2–3 days, the parents should be instructed to call their examiner immediately; sometimes a child may be having an allergic reaction to an antibiotic, or the bacteria is not sensitive to it. Recurrent bacterial conjunctivitis in older infants should cause one to suspect an obstruction of the nasolacrimal duct, especially if excessive tearing without photophobia is also present.

Additional treatment recommendations include saline washes to remove the discharge and crusts (these should occur just before the next administration of any topical antibiotics), the promotion of good handwashing and waste disposal techniques (no sharing of wash cloths or towels), and reminding the child to refrain from rubbing the eyes. Warm soaks or compresses should not be used, since they can promote bacterial growth. Likewise, occlusion of the eye can also promote bacterial flourishing.

Gonococcal Ophthalmia Neonatorum: Prophylaxis

Ophthalmia neonatorum refers to any bilateral conjunctivitis that appears in infants less than 1 month of age. The most infamous type of ophthalmia neonatorum is gonococcal, although chemical conjunctivitis secondary to the use of silver nitrate is the most common type seen.

The use of silver nitrate ($AgNO_3$) as a prophylactic measure against gonococcal ophthalmia neonatorum was first employed by Credé in 1881. Since that time it has become a widespread practice, mandated by most states and territories of the United States, as well as by numerous other countries.

The current recommended method of administration is one drop of 1 percent silver nitrate in the conjunctival sac of each eye, inserted within 1 hour of birth. Each drop should coat the entire conjunctival sac, and the eyes should not be rinsed afterward. Several studies have shown that rinsing does not decrease the chemical conjunctivitis that commonly follows administration of silver nitrate but may possibly decrease its prophylactic benefits. Furthermore, the use of normal saline as an irrigant can actually increase the severity of some cases of conjunctivitis.

Individual ampules of the 1 percent solution, manufactured in beeswax, are preferred. This not only decreases the possibility of cross contamination but also eliminates the possibility of the solution's evaporating and becoming greater than 1 percent in strength (which could cause permanent corneal damage).

Silver nitrate is considered to be a prophylactic measure only against *Neiserria gonorrhoeae*. It works by binding with surface protein of the *N. gonorrhoeae* organism, ultimately interfering with the bacterium's metabolism. In addition, the associated mild chemical conjunctivitis brings a host of neutrophils to the area, which further helps to destroy the bacteria. However, when a woman has premature rupturing of her membranes, the bacteria may gain early access and hence not be adequately destroyed by the silver nitrate prophylaxis.

In addition to the mild bulbar and palpebral conjunctivitis caused by silver nitrate prophylaxis, some lid edema and the appearance of a purulent discharge 1–2 days after birth can also occur. Chemical conjunctivitis can be differentiated from other causes of conjunctivitis in the newborn period by its rapid onset (3–24 hours after birth), its negative cultures (although culturing is rarely necessary), and its spontaneous disappearance within 3–5 days after onset. Rarely does it cause any permanent damage. Treatment consists of gently wiping away the discharge with sterile gauze or cotton.

Some states allow the option of administering tetracycline ophthalmic ointment or erythromycin ophthalmic ointment in place of silver nitrate. This recommendation has been approved by the American Academy of Pediatrics, the Center for Disease Control, and the NSPB.

A few parents are opposed to having their baby develop the chemical conjunctivitis and possibly some permanent damage from the 1 percent silver nitrate when they are certain that the mother is not infected with the *N. gonorrhoeae* bacterium. In addition, others feel that the chemical conjunctivitis from the silver nitrate interferes with the bonding process immediately after birth because the baby's vision may be altered, the baby may be irritable from the discomfort, or because of the time spent, although quite brief, in administering the drops. To assist staff in handling these situations, some hospitals have developed written waivers of liability for mothers to sign if they elect not to have the drops administered to their child. Other hospitals offer the option of antibiotics for these cases or delay the administration of the silver nitrate for up to an hour, so that the bonding experience can begin uninterrupted. Furthermore, many physicians now obtain routine cervical cultures for *N. gonorrhoeae* from all expectant women throughout their pregnancies, to identify who is at greater risk for infecting the child. Whatever the alternatives, delivery room and nursery staff must remain sensitive to parental preferences, while promoting the child's right to optimum vision.

Gonococccal Ophthalmia Neonatorum—The Infection

The major sign of an ocular infection from *N. gonorrhoeae* is a bilateral purulent ocular discharge that appears about 2–5 days after birth and becomes copious 1–2 days later. Marked hyperemia and chemosis are also evident. Whenever any infant less than 6 weeks of age exhibits such history and findings, a smear and culture should be immediately taken. If the gram stain is negative, the infant should be isolated and quickly started on topical sulfacetamide or tetracycline and parenteral aqueous penicillin. Prompt treatment is necessary to prevent corneal damage with subsequent permanent loss of vision and possible loss of the eye itself, as well as cross contamination within the nursery or unit. Culture results within 24–48 hours will confirm or negate the presence of *N. gonorrhoeae* infection.

The discharge should be cleaned several times a day, using meticulous technique and proper handwashing and waste disposal. In addition, an ophthalmologist should examine the child's corneas on a regular basis, to determine whether any corneal damage is occurring. Once a case has been positively identified from culture results, it must be reported to the local or state health department. Finally, these children need close follow-up after their hospital discharge to ensure that antibiotic treatment is continuing as necessary. A referral to a community health nurse is recommended.

Older children and adults can also develop a gonococcal ocular infection. Hence, parents of neonates with such an infection should likewise be treated on an ambulatory basis. *N. gonorrhoeae* must be considered a possible causative agent whenever any patient has a copious purulent eye discharge.

Viral Conjunctivitis

A number of authorities have estimated that adenoviruses are the most common cause of acute conjunctivitis in the school-aged population; however, many of these cases may be so mild that the child or family does not seek professional consultation. Yet viral conjunctivitis is highly contagious; when it is suspected, the child should be confined to the home until the symptoms disappear, usually in 10–14 days.

The symptoms of viral conjunctivitis can be quite similar to those of the bacterial type; therefore, the two may be difficult to distinguish. The bulbar conjunctiva is often entirely pink secondary to the inflamed blood vessels (hence the term *pink-eye*) with more intense discoloration near the periphery. The child may complain of a scratchy sensation in the eye and have a rather noticeable watery discharge, swelling of the lower lids, photophobia, and enlarged but nontender preauricular nodes. Some children also have associated fevers and upper respiratory symptoms, and a few may have viral conjunctivitis secondary to rubella, varicella, measles, mumps, or flu. However, there should be no change in the child's visual acuity during the conjunctivitis; otherwise, the cornea is most likely also involved, as in epidemic keratoconjunctivitis (EKC) or herpes simplex. Of course, if bacterial cultures are taken they will be negative (many examiners do not culture such an acute type of conjunctivitis unless the discharge is purulent), but a conjunctival scraping may show increased mononuclear cells.

Treatment is palliative, with cold compresses to the eyes several times a day to alleviate discomfort and to help remove secretions. All family members should be instructed about good handwashing and waste-disposal techniques. Since topical steroids can augment the problems of herpes simplex keratoconjunctivitis, they are used only by an ophthalmologist to treat viral conjunctivitis, and then with great care.

Inclusion Conjunctivitis (Blennorhea, TRIC)

Inclusion conjunctivitis is caused by a chlamydial agent (the TRIC agent). *Chlamydia* are microbes that are closely related to viruses and bacteria (they have been reclassified from one group to the other several times) and are transmitted between sexually active persons. In adults, the genitourinary symptoms are mild.

Inclusion conjunctivitis comprises different types. Newborns between 5 and 15 days of age are at risk for developing a chlamydial infection secondary to their passage through the birth canal. Initial symptoms include swollen eyelids and injected conjunctiva, especially near the lower fornices. A few days later the child develops a bilateral copious mucopurulent discharge similar to that seen in gonococcal infections but has a later onset. Fortunately, the implications of a chlamydial infection in the neonate are usually benign. Although recurrence is common, the child often has no damage to the eyes or vision. Diagnosis may be assisted by Wright's or Giemsa staining of scrapings from the lower palpebral conjunctiva, and culture. The stain will identify the cytoplasmic inclusion bodies of the chlamydia and will have an increased number of polymorphic nuclear cells. Cultures will be negative. Treatment is with 10 percent ophthalmic sodium sulfacetamide or tetracycline ointment four times a day, for 10 days to 3 weeks. If a chlamydial pneumonitis is also present, it should be treated with systemic antibiotics. Untreated chlamydial infections can last up to 1 year.

"Swimming pool" conjunctivitis is the second type of chlamydial infection and is so named because persons become infected with it after swimming in contaminated water. These children may have enlarged nodes, and the discharge appears within 3–4 days. In addition, follicles are more noticeable, especially in the lower palpebral conjunctiva. Treatment is with ophthalmic sulfonamide or tetracycline.

The third type of chlamydial infection is trachoma, evidenced by a slow, progressive conjunctivitis that causes the lids to thicken. The infection ultimately invades the cornea. Trachoma is a leading cause of blindness in the world but is rare in the United States. When it does occur, it is more commonly seen in the southwest. Treatment is with ophthalmic sulfa or tetracycline ointments.

Finally, the most common form of chlamydial conjunctivitis seen in the United States is the sexually transmitted form. Although it is more commonly seen in adults, its incidence is increasing among adolescents. Treatment is with systemic erythromycin or tetracycline.

Allergic Conjunctivitis

Allergic conjunctivitis is fairly common in children and adolescents, with a higher incidence in boys. Usually the hyperemia of the conjunctiva is mild. The lids may be edematous, with the upper lids having ptosis. The discharge is characteristically stringy and milky, and excessive tearing may also be present. Itching is a common complaint, especially in the vernal variety. Conjunctival scrapings show an increased number of eosinophils, and of course, cultures are negative. Frequently these children have signs and symptoms of allergies elsewhere, such as rhinitis, eczema, or asthma.

The etiology of allergic conjunctivitis may be a local irritant (for example, hair spray, cosmetics, laundry detergent or softeners, or ophthalmic medications) or systemic. The ideal treatment is to remove the source of allergy. When the source is unknown, cold compresses several times a day may be beneficial, especially for complaints of itching. When nonocular symptoms are also present, oral antihistamines may be prescribed. However, older children may only want to take these at bedtime, since antihistamines can cause drowsiness. If ocular symptoms become severe, topical steroids may be used cautiously. Remember that children using topical steroids need to have their intraocular pressure (IOP) checked regularly, so ensure that they return for their follow-up visits. Infrequently systemic steroids are used for even more serious cases, and the child may need an allergy work-up with a possible desensitization program.

Vernal Conjunctivitis

Vernal conjunctivitis, or *spring catarrh,* is a bilateral recurrent seasonal type of allergic conjunctivitis. It is most common in the spring and summer months and occurs predominantly in children and adolescents who live in warm climates.

It can be distinguished from other types of allergic conjunctivitis by the presence of cobblestonelike papillae on the palpebral conjunctiva of both the upper and lower lids. In addition, these children may have complaints of photophobia, as well as the usual signs and symptoms of allergic conjunctivitis and a history of spring allergies in their family.

Vernal conjunctivitis can last for 4–10 years. As a result, topical steroids can only be used for brief intervals, perhaps several weeks a year when symptoms are worse. Furthermore, herpes simplex must always be ruled out before steroid treatment is instituted. Ophthalmic vasoconstrictors such as naphazoline may also be helpful, but desensitization programs have not been as successful as initially desired. Despite the chronicity of vernal conjunctivitis, the prognosis is usually quite good. Infrequently some children develop corneal irritation secondary to the raised papillae on the lids, but otherwise vision remains within normal limits and other ocular structures are not involved.

Pterygium

A *pterygium* is a superficial triangular piece of bulbar conjunctiva that usually starts growing at the inner conjunctiva and grows toward the cornea. It is much more common in adults, especially persons who live in desert areas or who work outdoors. A pterygium is not a significant ocular problem unless the excess tissue encroaches on the cornea, ultimately obstructing the pupil and decreasing the patient's vision. If corneal obstruction does occur, surgery is necessary to remove the excess tissue. Unfortunately, pterygiums frequently recur.

Pingueculum

A *pingueculum* is a small and slightly raised nodule, usually located on the nasal side of the bulbar conjunctiva. It is yellowish-white in color. Like that of the pterygium, its incidence increases with age. It is usually of no ocular significance unless it becomes inflamed or enlarged.

THE CORNEA

Anatomy and Assessment

The cornea is the transparent covering over the iris. Its primary function is to refract light rays (see Chapter 3). To do this effectively it must stay transparent, with a smooth and rounded surface. Because the cornea plays such a major role in a persons' vision, any child with a suspected or verified corneal problem should be referred immediately to an ophthalmologist for a thorough evaluation, treatment, and follow-up.

In the newborn the cornea ranges from 6 to 10 mm in diameter, but by the age of 1 year it reaches its adult size of 12 mm. *Megalocornea* (greater than 12 mm in diameter) can occur in children with congenital glaucoma,

Marfan's syndrome, or as an idiopathic or familial problem. *Microcornea* (less than 10 mm in diameter) is often associated with other ocular structures that are small.

The cornea has five layers. The outermost is the *epithelium,* which is quite resistent to infection. It is at this layer that corneal abrasions normally occur (see Chapter 12). The next layer is *Bowman's layer,* and the middle one is the *stroma,* which comprises 90 percent of the cornea and is made of connective tissue. The other two layers are *Descemet's membrane* and the thin *endothelium.*

Patient complaints indicating possible corneal involvement include photophobia, decreased vision, and pain (either a gritty sensation or severe superficial pain). Assessment includes taking the child's visual acuity and examining the cornea for a smooth and rounded surface and transparency.

One way of checking for these properties is with a flashlight, held about 4–6 inches from the eye. When directed from in front of the patient, the light reflex on the cornea should be distinct and sharp; an abrasion may cause an irregular reflex. When the flashlight is directed from the temporal side the cornea can be tested for a round, curved surface. A slight bulging is normal, but a cone-shaped appearance indicates *keratoconus.* Not visible to this gross assessment is the irregularity of the surface that causes astigmatism. From this flashlight technique you can also note the depth and clarity of the anterior chamber. In addition, a white or gray discoloration indicates a *hypopyon,* or pus, in the anterior chamber, and a red or black hue indicates a *hyphema.* The iris should be flat.

Another method of assessing the surface of the cornea in children with suspected problems is by placing a drop of irrigating solution or normal saline onto a prepackaged fluorescein strip, so that it drips into the lower fornix area. Fluorescein strips are preferred over fluorescein ophthalmic solution because once opened, some fluorescein solutions can become contaminated with *Pseudomonas.* Irrigating solutions can likewise become contaminated, so it is best to purchase small containers and to use only freshly opened solutions (less than 12 hours old). Once inserted, the child should gently blink the eyes to promote dispersion of the fluorescein over the cornea; excess fluorescein can be washed away with normal saline or irrigating solution. (Remember, however, that fluorescein is considered a drug, and nurses need standing or direct orders from a physician to administer it.) The examiner then uses a blue light (from the slit lamp or by placing a blue filter over a regular pocket flashlight) and examines the surface of the cornea. Any abrasions or other breaks in the cornea's normally smooth surface will appear as green dots or lines. For example, herpes simplex keratitis causes branchlike jagged lines to appear on the cornea's surface. The fluorescein will turn to yellow as it washes out of the eye over a period of 15–30 minutes.

Opacities can be noticed by direct observation, by illumination with a flashlight and hand-held magnifying lens, or by an ophthalmoscope. In general, any opacity that moves in the opposite direction from the ophthalmoscope is located on the cornea (see Chapter 7). Corneal opacities may be congenital or caused by chemical burns or keratitis. In addition, congenital glaucoma may cause a steamy appearance to the cornea, as can injury to the cornea by forceps; this latter type usually clears after a few months. Finally, corneal opacities may infrequently be caused by inborn errors of metabolism.

To remain transparent, the cornea must be kept moist at all times. This is accomplished by the lacrimal system and blinking. If a patient has dry eyes or inadequate blinking or cannot close the eyes completely, use of artificial tears at frequent intervals (every 1–2 hours) is necessary. Patients who are unconscious should have their lids taped shut if they can not adequately close or have artificial tears inserted.

The examiner may use a drop of topical anesthetic in the assessment to decrease the pain from corneal problems immediately. Patients may request more of this anesthetic and should be told that repeated administration of topical eye anesthetics can lead to permanent corneal damage and therefore cannot be prescribed, regardless of the amount of relief that they offer.

Finally, the cornea is innervated by the fifth cranial nerve. To test this reflex, take a cotton wisp and gently touch it to the center of the cornea, being careful not to touch the lashes. Patients with a normal response will quickly blink their eyes. (In some areas, a physician's order is necessary to test the corneal reflex.) Use the patient's other eye for comparison. Although this test is not commonly performed except in neuroophthalmologic examinations, the corneal reflex may also be decreased in persons with herpes simplex keratitis.

COMMON DISORDERS OF THE CORNEA

Keratitis

Keratitis, inflammation of the cornea, can be caused by bacterial, viral, or fungal infections or by dry eyes, burns, or trauma. It occurs infrequently; when it occurs, it require immediate attention by an ophthalmologist, as it can lead to corneal opacities, ulcers, or perforation with corresponding permanent loss of vision. Children strongly suspected of having keratitis are those who have a painful red eye with tearing, photophobia, and decreased vision.

Bacterial Keratitis

Bacterial keratitis is commonly caused by *Staphylococcus aureus, Streptococcus pneumoniae,* and *Pseudomonas.* The first two types may be associated with a bacterial infection of the lid, conjunctiva, or lacrimal sac, or with a corneal abrasion; the last type can result from contaminated ophthalmic irrigating or fluorescein solutions. Patients may have significantly decreased visual acuity, as well as a purulent discharge and perhaps a *hypopyon* (pus in the anterior chamber). Only one eye may be involved.

Because bacterial keratitis can lead to corneal ulcers or complete loss of the eye, patients require immediate hospitalization for the insertion of topical antibiotic and cycloplegic drops, as well as the intravenous infusion of systemic antibiotics. (Remember, however, that the cornea is avascular, so the topical drops actually play a much more important role than do the systemic antibiotics.) Patients may also receive antibiotics injected into the subconjunctival space. Until culture results are known, broad spectrum antibiotics may be used. Debridement of the epithelium with a sterile spatula may also be done.

Despite early identification of bacterial keratitis, much permanent damage may have already occurred to the cornea. Therefore, some patients may benefit at a later date from a corneal transplant *(keratoplasty)*.

Viral Keratitis

The most common type of viral keratitis is caused by the *Herpes simplex* virus. It is estimated that this virus is present in at least 60 percent of 5-year-olds, and 90 percent of all adults in the United States, usually lying dormant in the fifth cranial nerve ganglion. The type I virus is well-known for causing canker sores or fever blisters, but on rare occasions it can cause epithelial keratitis. Usually there is no relationship between the mouth and ocular manifestations. Type II *Herpes simplex* infection is more commonly associated with genital signs and symptoms but may cause ocular problems.

Children with ocular involvement may complain of blurred vision, tearing, and a gritty painful sensation. Upon examination the child displays circumcorneal injection and perhaps a watery discharge and some yellow crusts on the lids. Administration of fluorescein and the use of a slit-lamp or blue filter show the characteristic green dendritic shape, similar to tree branches or coral, with a little knob at the end of each branch. In addition, the fifth cranial nerve may have decreased sensation, evidenced by lightly touching the cornea with a wisp of cotton and receiving a decreased blink response. Remember to dispose properly of waste products and to cleanse all equipment thoroughly after each assessment.

A cardinal rule governing the treatment of *Herpes simplex* keratitis is that steroids are rarely used, and then only under the close observation of an ophthalmologist. Otherwise, the virus can flourish in the presence of steroids. If only the epithelium is involved (as in most cases) an antiviral medication such as idoxuridine (IDU; Stoxil), vidarabine (VIRA-A; Parke-Davis), adenine arabinoside, or trifluridine (Viroptic; Burroughs Wellcome) may be prescribed on a round-the-clock basis. (Herpes is one of the few viral diseases that have a specific therapy.) If no improvement occurs within 7–14 days, however, these medications are often discontinued because of the increased risk of their side effects (for example, closure of the lacrimal puncta, pain, or hypersensitivity). Ophthalmologists may also choose to debride the cornea by scraping away the involved epithelial cells with a sterile platinum spatula, and frequently cycloplegic drops are ordered. Without treatment, most cases of herpes simplex keratitis heal spontaneously in 2 weeks or so but may involve deeper corneal layers.

Generally, the prognosis is good for cases in which only the epithelium has been involved. However, if deeper corneal layers such as the stroma have been involved, the prognosis is worse, and permanent decreased vision can result from corneal scarring or intraocular infection. Unfortunately, herpes simplex keratitis can recur with or without previous proper treatment.

Similar to *Herpes simplex,* the *varicella virus* can also lay dormant along the trigeminal nerve and surface years later to cause the hemifacial rash of *Herpes zoster.* If the rash involves the tip of the nose, the patient often will develop ocular manifestations. *Herpes zoster* keratitis can be chronic, requires treatment on a long-term basis, and frequently recurs. Unlike the treatment of *Herpes simplex* keratitis, however, topical steroids are the preferred treatment for these patients. Remember that careful handwashing and waste disposal techniques are most important for patients who have skin vesicles or pustules, since they contain active varicella virus. In addition, do not allow such patients in school or in waiting areas and preferably arrange for them to be seen in an isolated area until their vesicles have healed. Finally, thoroughly cleanse all equipment immediately after the examination of the patient.

Active varicella (not the dormant type) can infrequently cause vesicles on the conjunctiva. However, they usually heal spontaneously and do not cause any permanent damage. Adenoviruses can also cause keratitis, and their treatment consists of careful use of topical steroids (once keratitis by *Herpes simplex* has been ruled out), as well as mydriatic drops.

Keratoconus

The term *keratoconus* refers to a cornea that has changed from a rounded to a cone shape. It results from a noninflammatory degenerative process and is usually bilateral. Although it is rare in young children, those at risk for developing it include teenagers who have a history of keratoconus or high astigmatism in their families and children with Down syndrome.

The patient may initially complain of blurred vision secondary to a resulting myopic astigmatism. Upon examination, the cone-shaped appearance may be noticed by shining a flashlight from the side across the front of the eye.

Initial treatment uses contact lenses to help neutralize the corneal astigmatism. If adequate improvement does not result, a keratoplasty may be tried. Eventually the central cornea can become so thin that it perforates and scars.

Corneal Transplants (Keratoplasty)

Corneal transplants have been performed for many years and have significantly benefitted many persons who have had decreased vision because of corneal opacities or ulcers. As a group, however, children have had poorer overall results than adults. Contributing success factors include the child's age and diagnosis, with children 10 years of age or older and those with isolated keratoconus or acquired corneal opacities having better results. Younger children tend to have flaccid corneas (with associated increased risk of surgical complications) and a higher incidence of graft rejection. Children with opacities secondary to congenital anomalies tend to have amblyopia, which can decrease any gains in vision that the keratoplasty might have effected. Some recent variations on the lamellar keratoplasty method have been developed, however, and may become useful in children's eye problems.

Usually families have only 12–48 hours between notification that a cornea has been found and the actual surgery. No tissue typing is required, and no pediatric donor is necessary for a pediatric patient. After admission and necessary laboratory work, the child may receive medication to lower the IOP. Although the IOP is normal in corneal transplant patients, decreased pressure provides better operative conditions.

Once in the operating room, general anesthesia is administered, although local anesthesia may be used with adult or teen-aged patients. Then a 5- to 8-mm circle is cut out of the central portions of the patient's and donor's corneas. In the lamellar method the top layers of the corneas are involved, whereas in the penetrating method the entire cornea is transplanted. The new cornea is normally attached with a continuous stellarlike suture.

Postoperatively, the child is ambulatory within 24 hours, wearing a fox shield for protection; younger children may need to wear elbow restraints. Air bubbles may be visible near the operative site for several days. Because numerous medications will be necessary, some of them for months, parents will need to learn how to administer these properly. In addition, they need to learn the signs of graft rejection (redness, increased discomfort, corneal opacification) and must be instructed to call the ophthalmologist immediately should any of these signs appear. When possible, the child should sleep on the noninvolved side and avoid straining, bending, crying, or any other activities that can cause a sudden increase in eye pressure. The eye shield is necessary until the area has healed and the sutures are removed, usually in 6–8 weeks. (In adults, the sutures are often kept in place until 1–2 years later!) Parents will obviously be anxious about the results of the transplant and may need to be reminded that determining the maximal benefits of the surgery may require 6–12 months. Finally, in addition to graft rejection, patients with a corneal transplant can develop a high degree of astigmatism or a cataractous lens; in younger patients amblyopia may also develop. Hence, frequent postoperative visits are recommended.

A more difficult aspect of corneal transplantation concerns the child as the donor, rather than as the recipient. The corneas taken from children 5 years or older who have died from an accident or acute illness tend to be quite successful as transplants, and the eyes from all donors can be used for some surgical, educational, or research purpose. For some parents, the donation of their child's corneas may provide a small but important consolation after their child's death. Therefore, approach parents in a matter-of-fact way about the possibility of donating their child's eyes (or about an *eye transplant,* the popular but mislead-ing term for a corneal transplant). If you receive a positive response quickly con-tact your nearest Eye Bank, Lion's Club, or university medical center. The Eye Bank Association of America can also provide you with additional information (see Appendix C). In general, all eyes are kept closed in comatose patients. When a possible donor dies, ice should be placed over the eyes immediately, and the Eye Bank should be quickly notified if the parents consent to donating the corneas. The eyes are then enucleated within 4 hours (this does not cause disfigurement), and transplantation should occur within 1–3 days.

THE IRIS

Anatomy and Assessment

The iris is the visible colored part of the eye and rests between the anterior and posterior chambers (Fig. 3-2). Its main purpose is to regulate the amount of light entering the pupil through muscles attached to it (see Chapters 3 and 8). The iris, along with the ciliary body and choroid, forms the uveal tract.

The color of the iris is established in 50 percent of infants by the age of 6 months and in 90 percent by their first birthday. In contrast to popular belief, blue eyes contain little pigment, whereas dark eyes have a lot. A difference in the color of the irides of a child, called *heterochromia,* is usually a normal variant. However, a sudden change of iris color may signify trauma, or in adults, a tumor or glaucoma. Following trauma, a child may have a red or black color before the iris, which represents a hyphema. Inflammation or infection can cause a white appearance, signifying a hypopyon.

Various markings on the iris may also be normal. For example, children with Down syndrome frequently have Brushfield spots. As their name indicates, these spots appear as brushlike strokes and do not interfere with the child's vision. Any sudden change in the size or color of a marking, however, should be care-fully examined by an ophthalmologist, since it may indicate a malignant mela-noma (rare in children).

Some Disorders of the Iris
Coloboma

Normally the iris is round. When this is not the case, the child may have a *coloboma* or *congenital structural defect.* An iris coloboma is usually located in the inferonasal (6 o'clock) area of the iris and is shaped like a tear drop. It may occasionally be associated with other congenital defects, or infrequently, it may extend to other ocular structures or result from an iridectomy. Occasionally iris colobomas run in families.

Iritis

Technically, the term *iritis* refers to inflammation of the iris only. However, the term is also frequently (but incorrectly) used to describe *iridocyclitis,* or inflammation of the iris and ciliary body (also known as *anterior uveitis).*

Although iritis is an internal disorder, it is usually manifested by external complaints. Its most common symptoms are localized pain, blurred vision, tearing, and photophobia secondary to ciliary spasms. Upon examination the pupil may be irregularly shaped, and there may be circumcorneal redness. Some patients may complain of aching of the brow. With a slit lamp, the ophthalmologist may see cells (evidenced as spots of light) floating in the aqueous or settled at the bottom. In addition, the inflammation can cause adhesions to form between the iris and the lens or cornea. When present in the anterior chamber, these adhesions are called *synechiae* and prevent the pupil from dilating. Finally, patients can develop secondary glaucoma from these adhesions, as well as cataracts or band keratopathy from the inflammatory process.

Iritis can be acute or chronic. Children with juvenile rheumatoid arthritis—especially those who have the pauciarticular type with a positive antinuclear antibody (ANA) test—are particularly at risk for developing a slow and insidious type of iritis that rarely causes pain, photophobia, or redness in its early stages; some of these patients develop iritis before or after their arthritic problems are manifested. Therefore, children with juvenile rheumatoid arthritis need slit-lamp examinations every 3–12 months, depending on their type of disease onset and their ANA test results. Some ophthalmologists also request that these patients dilate their pupils every week to determine whether the pupils remain round and actually dilate; if they cannot, synechiae may have formed. When iritis does develop in these children, it may be difficult to treat and may infrequently result in glaucoma, either from the iritis itself, from steroid treatment, or from a combination of both.

Other children at risk for developing iritis include those with ankylosing spondylitis, sarcoidosis, Reiter's syndrome, retinal detachment, or a corneal problem such as herpes. In addition, iritis can also develop in a child who has recently had mumps, chicken pox, or measles.

The treatment for iritis centers on keeping the pupil dilated with mydriatics/cycloplegics to prevent the formation of adhesions and frequent administration of topical steroids to provide anti-inflammatory effects. Infrequently, systemic steroids may also be given. Finally, these children must return for all recommended follow-up appointments to assure that the iritis is responding adequately to the treatment regimen.

Albinism

Albinism is a genetic defect (either hereditary or the result of a mutation) that causes a decrease in the pigment of a person's iris and choroid *(ocular albinism)* and sometimes of the hair and skin *(oculocutaneous* or *generalized albinism)*. No relationship exists between the color of a child's iris and the occurrence of albinism.

A key diagnostic tool centers on the use of an ophthalmoscope. Normally only a red reflex occurs through the pupil. However, if the iris also transilluminates, that is, if a red or pink reflex is reflected back through the pupil and iris, then the child has albinism. Other associated symptoms and signs include a variable decrease in the child's visual acuity, nystagmus, photophobia, and an increased incidence of strabismus and refractive errors.

Children with albinism are unable to metabolize normally the amino acid tyrosine. Those children who totally lack tyrosinase, the enzyme responsible for metabolizing tyrosine, tend to have a poorer visual prognosis than those who have some enzyme activity. Ocular albinism cannot be identified at birth but usually becomes apparent when the child is prepubescent, and the enzyme deficiency becomes more noticeable. In contrast, oculocutaneous albinism is readily identifiable at birth or shortly thereafter.

Treatment for albinism is palliative, employing opaque scleral contact lenses. These limit the amount of light entering the eye and correct the child's refractive error.

Aniridia

Aniridia is a congenital defect of the iris in which the iris does not develop completely and properly. Total aniridia is rare. Instead, a child usually has some development of the irides *(hypoplasia)*. Most cases of aniridia are bilateral and are frequently dominantly inherited.

In addition to the photophobia, nystagmus, and significant visual loss that these children have, they are also at risk for developing cataracts and early glaucoma. Furthermore, some children with aniridia may develop renal abnormalities or a Wilm's tumor. Other associated anomalies include CNS and skeletal defects and macular hypoplasia. Therefore, most children with aniridia need close ocular and medical follow-up, at least for the first 2–3 years of their lives.

The treatment of aniridia is with a special tinted or painted contact lens, which limits the amount of light entering the eye and hence decreases photophobia and increases the child's refractive abilities. Surgery is not indicated unless glaucoma or cataracts develop. Don't forget to refer these children to appropriate stimulation and educational settings at an early age.

THE PUPILS

The pupils should be examined for their shape, size (both individually and compared to the other), and responses to light and accommodation. These assessments are discussed in detail in Chapter 8.

NEONATES

Although neonates have many external eye findings similar to those of older children, several exceptions and specific problems do exist. (See also the discussion of chemical and bacterial conjunctivitis in the newborn.)

The eyes begin to develop in the third week of gestation. By birth they are almost fully developed, except for the macula and optic nerve, which histologically develop within the first year. Because the orbits of the eyes are so large at birth (almost adult size) the eyes appear prominent on the newborn's face. Children with widely spaced eyes have *hypertelorism* and may have other physical anomalies.

Many infants blink in response to loud noises or bright lights. Some infants are photophobic (especially premature babies) but outgrow this condition in a month or two. (Remember to look for the other signs of congenital glaucoma in these children, however; see Chapter 9). In addition, any nurse who has tried to instill eyedrops in a neonate knows that a baby can keep the eyes shut quite tightly in response to touch *(blepharospasm)*. However, true protective blinking (versus reflexive) does not develop until the age of 6 months or so. Tears form somewhere between birth and 3 months of age.

A newborn's irides may have a grayish hue and may not develop their own natural color until 6–12 months of age. Often the sclera has a bluish tint, as it is still thin. However, this normal tint is less blue than that seen in infants with osteogenesis imperfecta. Some infants have reddish or pinkish stork's beak marks on their upper eyelids at birth *(telangiectasia);* these also disappear, usually within the first year.

Many newborns have pseudoptosis and pseudostrabismus due to epicanthal folds. This appearance of strabismus diminishes as the nasal bridge develops in the first 1–2 years of life. In addition, a few newborns have actual strabismus. If the eye position is variable, it may be caused by decreased coordination skills of the newborn's eyes, and the strabismus may disappear in a month or two as these skills improve. If one eye is always misaligned, however, or if after several months one eye continues to be misaligned for varying intervals, the parents should seek the assistance of an ophthalmologist (Chapter 5).

Subconjunctival hemorrhages are relatively common in newborns and disappear within 10 days after their appearance. Retinal hemorrhages, although not an external eye problem, are considered to be the most common ocular birth injury, estimated to occur in 25–50 percent of all newborns. However, these hemorrhages frequently go unnoticed because most normal newborns do not receive a detailed ophthalmoscopic examination of their eyes in their early newborn period. As with subconjunctival hemorrhages, the vast majority of newborn retinal hemorrhages are spontaneously absorbed.

Phototherapy for treatment of high bilirubin levels can cause a superficial keratitis if proper precautions are not taken to protect a baby's eyes. Many innovative methods of covering the eyes have been designed and are now commercially available. At least once every 4 hours, each baby receiving phototherapy should have the eyes uncovered for at least 15 minutes while awake and should be examined for the presence of any redness, unusual discharge, or marked photophobia (after allowing time for the baby's eyes to adjust to room light).

Forceps used in delivery can lead to swelling around one or both eyes and infrequently to haziness of the cornea(s). Although these problems usually disappear within a few weeks or months, some refractive errors may develop secondary to them.

The appearance of a "setting sun" sign is usually transient and benign, but it may indicate neurologic damage along the brain stem, as in hydrocephalus or kernicterus. To elicit it, quickly lower an infant (with proper neck support) from a sitting position to supine. A sign is positive when the irides go out toward the periphery of the eyes and appear to "set" below the lower eyelids.

Finally, numerous congenital, genetic, and metabolic syndromes can cause ocular problems and abnormalities to develop and are beyond the scope of this book. However, two environmental causes of ocular problems deserve mention. Radiation to a woman's uterus carrying a baby in the third to tenth week of gestation can result in microophthalmia, cataracts, or retinal problems for the fetus. Also now well-known is the effect on the fetus of a mother's chronic excess alcohol intake, causing such ocular abnormalities as short horizontal palpebral fissures, and less often, ptosis, strabismus, and microophthalmia.

BIBLIOGRAPHY

Beauchamp GR: Corneal transplantation in children. Clin Proc Child Nat Med Cent 35:212–215, 1979

Boyd-Monk H: Examining the external eye, p I. Nursing 80 10:58–63, May 1980

Boyd-Monk H: Examining the external eye, p II. Nursing 80 10:58–63, June 1980

Frey T: External diseases of the eye. Pediatr Ann 6:49–87, January 1977

Gallagher MA: Corneal transplantation. Am J Nurs 81:1845, 1981

Levenson L, Levenson J: Corneal transplantation. Am J Nurs 77:1160–1163, 1977

Lum B, Batzel RL, Barnett E: Reappraising newborn eye care. Am J Nurs 80:1602–1603, 1980

Mead Johnson and Company: *The Eyes: Number Three of a Series on Variations and Minor Departures in Normal Infants,* Evansville, Ind., 1972

Mechner F: Patient assessment: Examination of the eye, p 1. Am J Nurs 74:P1 1–24, November 1974

Moore RA, Schmitt BD: Conjunctivitis in children. Clin Pediatr 18:26–30, January 1979

National Society to Prevent Blindness: Control of ophthalmia neonatorum, publication #700, 1973

Pernoud FG: The red eye—a practical approach. Pediatr Ann 12:517–526, 1983

Rodney WM, Louie J, Puffer JC: Schirmer's test of lacrimation. Am Fam Physician 24:161–164, November 1981

Chapter Twelve

Ocular First Aid and Preventative Safety Measures

NURSING GOALS, OUTCOME STANDARDS, AND DIAGNOSES

The primary nursing goal for this chapter is that *the current incidence of ocular injuries in children and adults drastically declines.* This goal is not so unrealistic when one considers that the NSPB estimates that over 90 percent of all ocular injuries can be prevented. However, even with an overwhelming decline, some ocular injuries will still occur. Therefore, a second goal states that *children who experience ocular injuries have no change in their normal visual acuity;* or *if such a change occurs, it is only temporary.* This goal may be more difficult to attain, since not even the best first aid and subsequent treatment given in a prompt fashion can always prevent permanent visual changes from occurring. It is nevertheless, a standard to strive for while we simultaneously educate the public and fellow health professionals in the prevention of any additional ocular injuries.

Outcome Standard 1

The incidence of ocular injuries in children decreases by at least 10 percent each year.

Suggested Interventions:
- The nurse keeps statistics about all ocular injuries that are seen or treated in each nurse's unique job setting and evaluates these statistics at least once a year.
- On the basis of these figures and evaluations, the nurse communicates with key personnel to alter factors that may promote ocular injuries. For example, the nurse consults with coaches if a specific sports activity has resulted in injuries, or with an instructor or school principal regarding injuries in the lab or shop setting.
- The nurse encourages the formation of safety councils to help explore and evaluate potential or actual sources of ocular or other injuries. Preferably the

council would consist of various professional and consumer representatives, including one or two children.

- The nurse educates parents and other significant family members about potential ocular injuries in the home, school, and neighborhood environments. The nurse may use such methods as distributing appropriate pamphlets in the waiting room, giving 5-minute educational sessions to individuals or groups on a specific topic in the office or clinic setting, sponsoring a home mailing, speaking at a PTA meeting, and so on.
- The nurse educates teachers and health professionals about potential ocular injuries by participating in faculty meetings or in-service sessions, by distributing pertinent literature and articles, and by one-to-one meetings about a particular child or circumstance.
- The nurse educates children about potential ocular injuries with age-appropriate activities in the office, clinic, hospital, school, or home settings. Various resources are discussed throughout the chapter.
- The nurse educates the general public, community groups, and legislators about potential ocular injuries in children through letters, data collection, speeches, and articles for personal communication, newspapers, television, and radio. Sponsoring or participating in an "Eye Safety" week could also highlight various topics.

The primary nursing diagnoses for the above outcome are *knowledge deficit* and *potential for injury*.

Outcome Standard 2

Each child who has an ocular injury receives prompt and appropriate first aid.

Suggested Interventions:
- The nurse ensures that proper equipment to provide ocular first aid is available in the office, clinic, or school.
- The nurse educates parents, older children, other significant family members and child care providers about ocular first aid measures and provides written instructions (preferably with illustrations), in case such first aid is needed.
- The nurse ensures that educational, sports, and health staffs who work with children are properly trained in ocular first aid and have access to posters or pamphlets that briefly review the proper steps in providing such aid.

Related nursing diagnoses for the second outcome include *alterations in tissue perfusion, impaired skin integrity* (actual or potential), *knowledge deficit, sensory deficit* (altered vision), *alterations in comfort-pain, ineffective coping, anxiety,* and *impaired home or school maintenance management*.

Outcome Standard 3

Each child with an eye injury receives appropriate treatment and follow-up as necessary by a primary care or emergency room physician, or ophthalmologist.

Suggested Interventions:
- The nurse refers children to appropriate medical services as necessary. (The appropriate services are listed under each specific problem.)
- The nurse ensures that a list of nearby emergency rooms, trauma centers, ambulances, and ophthalmologists is kept easily available and includes accurate phone numbers, addresses, and directions.
- The nurse provides follow-up on children with ocular injuries that required medical follow-up and ensures that each child receives proper home care management and any necessary follow-up. If any financial, psychosocial, or other barriers prevent such home care or follow-up, the nurse helps to remove them.
- The nurse provides follow-up on all children with minor ocular injuries that did not receive medical follow-up, to ensure that the child has no change in visual acuity and no complaints of pain, photophobia, and so on.

These interventions primarily help decrease *noncompliance, knowledge deficit,* and *impaired home maintenance management,* which in turn decrease a host of other nursing diagnoses related to the actual injury or its effects.

Outcome Standards 4 and 5 are similar to the same outcome standards in Chapter 11 and refer to the child's and family's knowledge of the specific injury and its effect on their daily lives.

OCULAR FIRST AID

Proper first aid for ocular injuries can make the difference between a child's sight or blindness. But remember that first aid means just that: the *first* aid that a child receives until more appropriate care is available. Although a few children, such as those with a piece of dust in the eye, will not require any additional care, many cases cause us to wonder whether any permanent damage can result from a particular injury. Therefore, the slightest suspicion should result in an immediate referral of a child for medical care, preferably provided by an ophthalmologist.

Equipment

The amount and type of equipment that you keep on hand in anticipating an ocular injury depends on your role and setting. However, all nurses should have access to the equipment listed in Chapter 11. In addition, a lid retractor can be helpful for separating eyelids during flushing of chemical burns of the eye. (You may need a standing order or special instruction to use this.)

Visual Acuity

Unfortunately, in today's legal-minded society nurses must first ensure that they are not held liable for any damage that may occur from the injury itself. Therefore, except in cases of chemical burns or life-threatening problems, always obtain an estimate of the child's visual acuity before rendering any care. Such an estimate does not have to be an elaborate reiteration of a standard screening. Instead, depending on the circumstances, a rough estimate with a pocket near-vision card is adequate. Be careful not to apply any pressure on the eye while taking the estimate and remember to screen each eye separately. Also note whether the child has double or blurred vision and whether your estimate shows a decrease from the last recorded visual acuity. Any changes or complaints in a child's vision require immediate referral.

History

After the visual acuity estimate and depending on the nature and extent of the injury, you can complete the history and further assessment while providing urgent care. In general, the history should include the time and circumstances of the injury, what the child has done since the injury, and what, if any, first aid or treatment has already been administered and by whom. What symptoms and behaviors does the child now have? Any pain? Where? Is it localized or diffuse? Are any symptoms progressive? What is the child's past ocular and medical history? Was the child wearing glasses, contact lenses, or sports or industrial eyewear at the time of the injury? If so, what is the condition of this eyewear now? If you feel that the injury may require surgery, do not allow the child to eat or drink anything and note the time of the child's last intake. Also check any available records for the date of the last tetanus booster.

Beginning Your Assessment

During the assessment of an ocular injury, the nature of the injury will naturally draw your attention to specific locations of the eye. Descriptions of the more common eye injuries are described next. Don't forget to assess other areas of the eye, however. For example, you may wish to quickly determine extraocular muscle movements (Chapter 5), shine a penlight obliquely onto the cornea and anterior chamber (Chapter 11), evaluate the pupils' shape and light responses (Chapter 8), and gently palpate the bones of the orbital rim.

OCULAR INJURIES SEEN IN CHILDREN

Chemical Burns

Of all ocular injuries seen in children, chemical burns to the eye are by far the most urgent. In these cases, seconds count. The child's eye(s) should be immediately flushed with water or normal saline for 10–30 minutes; do not wait until the substance has been identified as an acid or alkali and do not concern yourself with how to neutralize it. Only after adequate irrigation has been completed should the child be brought to a medical or emergency facility.

The flushing should be gentle but thorough and continuous. A minimum of 2000 cc is necessary and may be administered with a plastic bottle, pitcher, bulb syringe, IV bag and tubing or by placing the child's head under a water faucet or over an eye fountain (usually found in laboratories and industrial settings). Direct the stream from the nose to the side of the head so that the caustic substance does not enter the other eye. Also have the patient roll the eyes around and look in different directions to help irrigate the entire eye and direct the fluid under the lids and into the corners of the eye.

Because of the natural tendency of the eyes to close when any outside substance comes near them, either the patient, you, or an assistant will need to help hold the lids apart. If you have access to any topical ophthalmic anesthetics or lid retractors, use them after starting irrigation to keep the lids open. Be careful, however, that you do not apply any pressure to the eye itself while keeping the lids open; apply pressure to the orbital bones.

While irrigation is being initiated, you can ask what substance is in the eye. Acids (bleach, hair lotions, and so on) penetrate the cornea and anterior chamber quickly. Their immediate action also causes tissue protein to coagulate, which helps to protect the rest of the eye, however. Hence, as a group, acid burns tend to heal better because they are nonprogressive. They require 10–20 minutes of initial irrigation.

In contrast, alkali burns (for example, lye, toilet bowl and oven cleaners, ammonia detergents, and substances containing fresh lime) are progressive: their damage can continue for days. They require 30 minutes of initial continuous irrigation, and many patients will require hospitalization for several days after the injury for observation, further lavage, and treatment with antibiotics, steroids, cycloplegics, or anticollagenase medications. Unfortunately, if corneal damage does occur, corneal transplants are not as successful with these patients as with others. In addition, patients with alkali burns may develop severe iritis and cataracts.

Finally, do not apply any bandages or patches while transporting a child with a chemical ocular burn to an emergency facility. Keeping the eyes uncovered allows additional chemicals to be washed out. If an alkali burn has occurred, continue irrigation enroute to the emergency facility, after 30 minutes of initial irrigation has been completed.

Ultraviolet Burns

A fair number of ultraviolet burns to the cornea occur secondary to the use of sunlamps, from the sun's reflection off snow, or from welding. Symptoms tend to occur 6–12 hours after exposure and are similar to those seen in corneal abrasions. That is, the patient complains of sudden, intense pain; blurred vision; a sandy or gritty feeling in the eye; and photophobia. Treatment is likewise similar to that for abrasions, consisting of patching of the eyes and referral to medical care. If the patient's skin is also burned, use a gauze wrap instead of tape to hold the bandages in place. Cold compresses to the area and aspirin may also help decrease the patient's discomfort. Usually the cornea heals in 24–36 hours without any residual damage.

Thermal Burns

Because of the lid reflex and the eyes' natural tendency to rotate up into the globe when near danger *(Bell's phenomenon),* thermal burns do not usually damage the eye itself beyond a superficial keratitis. When the lids are burned, they should be covered with saline moistened dressings, and these dressings should be changed at frequent intervals. Antibiotics are often prescribed. If the lids cannot close because of edema or tissue necrosis, the cornea must be protected by the administration of artificial tears. In severe cases, a *tarsorrhaphy* (temporary suturing of the eyelids together) may be necessary.

Corneal Abrasions

When the cornea has been scratched by a fingernail, dust particle, contact lens, or other matter, its top epithelial layer may become abraded, resulting in sudden pain, increased tearing, possible photophobia, and decreased visual acuity. Prolonged use of nonextended-wear contact lenses can also cause similar symptoms.

To verify the diagnosis, the examiner will administer a topical anesthetic and fluorescein; the fluorescein can be seen as a green pool in the abraded area with a slit lamp or direct ophthalmoscope with blue filter held at an oblique angle. In addition, the corneal light reflex may be irregular, and a shadow from the abrasion may be seen on the iris if a penlight is held at an angle.

Treatment consists of patching the eyelid closed for 1–2 days to allow the corneal epithelium time to heal without the constant irritation of blinking. To apply the patch, have the child close both eyes and place one or two eye pads or gauze over the involved eye. Then place several pieces of tape at an angle from the center of the forehead to the cheekbone. When properly done, the procedure will not allow the child to open the lid of the involved eye, although the eye is not shut so tightly that it causes impairment of the retinal circulation. In some cases, slightly warmed adhesive tape may be necessary for an adequate seal, and better results may also be obtained if you apply tincture of benzoin to the area and allow it to dry before applying the tape. Remember, however, that patching in infants, even for only 24 hours, may result in amblyopia. Hence, some examiners recommend that the patch be removed in infants for variable lengths of time during the day(s) of patching.

Additional treatment measures may include the administration of prophylactic antibiotics, cold compresses, or acetaminophen to decrease discomfort; sometimes cycloplegics or mydriatics can be used to decrease ciliary spasms. Steroids or the repeated use of topical ophthalmic anesthetics are never prescribed. If pain or other symptoms continue after 24 hours of patching, the patient should return to the examiner. The vast majority of corneal abrasions heal with no permanent effect on vision.

Subconjunctival Hemorrhage

When one quadrant of the conjunctiva suddenly becomes bright red, with little or no visibility of the white sclera beneath it, the child most likely has a subconjunctival hemorrhage. Subconjuncctival hemorrhages commonly occur in newborns, upon awakening in the morning and after such Valsalva maneuvers as sneezing or intense coughing. These hemorrhages are usually painless and do not themselves cause any decrease in vision or other ocular problems. Yet their rapid and dramatic appearance often frightens both parents and children.

If there is no history of recent trauma or bleeding disorder, cold compresses may promote absorption, which occurs in 1–2 weeks. If there is a history of recent or suspected trauma, a thorough examination by an ophthalmologist is in order to rule out other ocular damage. This is also true for subconjunctival hemorrhages that cover most or all of the visible sclera, or hemorrhages that do not clear in 1–2 weeks. (In fact, some ophthalmologists prefer to see all patients with a subconjunctival hemorrhage.)

Foreign Bodies

Specks

When a child complains of pain of sudden onset, possibly associated with tearing and light sensitivity, an eyelash or piece of dirt or dust may be on the conjunctiva. The child may not have any changes in the corneal epithelium, however. Do not let the child rub the eye, as the speck may then abrade the cornea or become embedded. Instead, have the child blink rapidly, look around in different directions while keeping the head still, or pull the upper lid out and over the lower one. Any of these measures frequently allows the excess tears to wash away the speck. If these do not result in improvement (for example, there may be more than one speck present), wash your hands and inspect the area yourself. If the speck is on the conjunctiva, use a moistened cotton applicator or corner of a clean hankie to remove the dirt or lash. Or in some settings, the eye may be irrigated with normal saline or balanced eye solution. Another method, depending on your setting and role, is to evert the upper eyelid (see Chapter 11). If the speck is on the cornea or cannot be easily removed from the conjunctiva, or if the pain continues or the child develops a decrease in visual acuity, patch the eye and refer the child for medical care.

At this time, the examiner will often apply a topical anesthetic and fluorescein to determine whether an abrasion has occurred and may use a special sterile instrument such as a spatula or spud to remove the foreign body. Antibiotics may be prescribed for several days, and other treatment measures similar to those for abrasions may be instituted.

Other Foreign Bodies and Penetrating Injuries

When another object has settled on or entered the eye (for example, glass, metal, or wood), do not make any attempts to remove it or wash it out. (Otherwise, you may be removing intraocular contents in the process.) Instead, assure that no rubbing, wiping, or pressure is applied to the eye (even if it is bleeding), to prevent further damage. You can, however, lightly patch the eye after quickly estimating the child's visual acuity. If possible, use a plastic or metal shield or a dry sterile pad to cover the eye and help keep it clean and protected. Then quickly send the child to a physician or emergency room.

If the object has penetrated the cornea completely, the child may have decreased vision, as well as an irregular pupil or extravasation of vitreal fluid. Again, do not remove the object or allow any pressure on it or the eye. Cover both eyes loosely to decrease eye movements after taking the child's visual acuity estimate and transfer the child to an emergency facility as quickly as possible with the head at a 30-degree angle.

When possible, send along a sample of the matter that caused the injury. For example, an object with magnetic properties can be removed much easier than one without. X-rays (by Sweet technique), a computerized axial tomography (CAT) scan, or an ultrasound assessment of the area may also be taken to help determine the extent of the penetration.

If the removal of the object and any necessary repair or suturing of the area cannot be done in the ambulatory setting, the child will be taken to the operating room. If you suspect this possibility, do not allow the child to eat or drink. After the surgery, dilating drops may be used to help prevent adhesions, and topical or systemic antibiotics and steroids may also be ordered. In addition, the child may need a tetanus booster, preferably given shortly after the injury.

The visual outcome for each injury varies, depending on the nature and extent of the injury. Some cases will take weeks for normal vision to return, and in a few instances the vision may actually become worse with time. If the lens is involved, a cataract often develops. If the foreign body contains iron or steel particles, a rust ring may develop on the cornea shortly after the injury and may also interfere with vision until it is removed.

Cuts (Lacerations)

When an area near the eye has been cut, care to prevent application of pressure to the eye is essential, in case the ocular contents have likewise been injured. Hence, if bleeding occurs, a dry, sterile dressing should be lightly applied over the area after quickly estimating the child's visual acuity. If the area continues to bleed freely, gently apply cold compresses, while transporting the child to the nearest emergency facility. The repair of any lid lacerations should preferably be done by a plastic surgeon or an ophthalmologist for best functioning and appearance of the lid. In addition, children with lid lacerations need a complete eye examination to determine whether there has been any other damage to their eyes. Antibiotics are usually prescribed after the repair of a lid laceration, and tetanus boosters are appropriate for those children with outdated immunizations.

Blows to the Eye Area (Contusions)

Periorbital ecchymosis, more commonly known as a *black eye,* is often disregarded as a source of intraocular injury. However, all patients with this problem should be referred to an ophthalmologist at once, especially if there are any complaints of double, blurred, or decreased vision, or pain that increases over time. Remember to estimate the child's visual acuity and record the type and size of the object that caused the injury before sending the child for medical care.

Children with no evidence of more serious damage will be directed to apply ice to the area for 5–15 minutes every hour for the first day after injury to decrease the bleeding and edema. Then the application of heat can help promote the absorption of extracellular fluids. Frequently the areas around both eyes become discolored after a period of time, even if only one side is injured. This discoloration is caused by the effects of gravity, with fluids crossing the nasal bridge during hours of sleep and settling into the lower lid and cheek areas during hours of waking.

Orbital Fractures

Seven bones protect the eye in its orbital area, with the weakest component lying directly beneath the eye. Therefore, when extensive pressure is applied to the orbit, this bone may break and produce what is commonly called a *blow out* fracture. A frequent complaint of patients with this problem is diplopia, and upon examination the child may not be able to look in the up gaze or do so without great pain. So check the child's extraocular muscle movements carefully (Chapter 5) after estimating vision. Professional eye examiners may do a *forced duction test,* which is a mechanical attempt under topical anesthesia to rotate the eye upward; if this is not possible, the diagnosis of an orbital fracture is confirmed, as the inferior rectus muscle has become entrapped by the fractured bone. Edema, lid ecchymosis, or subconjunctival hemorrhage may also be present. A special x-ray of the orbit (a Caldwell's or Water's view) or a CAT scan may also be done.

Treatment may be medically oriented, with a wait-and-see approach to determine whether any diplopia spontaneously resolves or enophthalmos develops. Antibiotics, oral decongestants, and applications of cold, then in a day or two of heat, are frequently instituted. In addition, the extraocular muscles may take time to return to their normal functioning. If surgical repair of the bone is necessary, it is usually performed within a few days to a few weeks after injury.

Fractures of other orbital bones can also occur, but they are less common. Their signs and symptoms vary, depending on what structures, if any, they have entrapped or damaged. As a rule, if an orbital fracture is suspected, do not allow the child to blow his nose in case the sinuses are damaged from the fracture.

Hyphemas

A *hyphema* is a hemorrhage into the anterior chamber. It traditionally has been most common in boys between the ages of 4 and 12 years, and usually results from some foreign body hitting against the eye. Rocks, BB gun pellets, darts, and sticks are common causes, as is child abuse. However, hyphemas can also infrequently result from tumors, vascular abnormalities, coagulation deficiencies, and other inherent problems; these are called *spontaneous hyphemas*.

The diagnosis of a hyphema is usually straightforward, compiled from a slit-lamp examination showing blood in the anterior chamber, a history of recent activities, and the complaints of pain, photophobia, and decreased visual acuity. Some children may also have nausea and vomiting and be restless, lethargic, or disoriented.

Hyphemas are graded according to the amount of blood in the anterior chamber. A common grading system uses four grades, with each having an additional one-quarter involvement. A grade 4, or total, hyphema is also called an *eightball* hyphema because it contains a large black clot. The incidence of complications increases with the severity of the hyphema. Fortunately, most hyphemas are grades 1 or 2.

If you suspect a hyphema, lightly cover the eye with a metal shield or the bottom half of a styrofoam cup and transport the child to the nearest medical facility. Children with all but the mildest hyphemas are hospitalized and confined to bedrest for about 5 days. In the past, bilateral patching was immediately instituted. However, this procedure often frightens the child and causes sensory deprivation. Its purpose of immobilizing the eyes was often defeated by increased agitation and anxiety. Hence, many examiners now choose to use a plastic or metal "fox" shield over the affected eye only and perhaps a sedative to help relax the child. Needless to say, children who have hyphemas are frequently very active; 5 days of bedrest in a hospital may seem like a prison sentence, and may make them even more restless.

In the hospital the head of the bed is usually elevated about 30 degrees to help the bleeding settle. Coagulation studies may be drawn, as well as a sickle cell test in black children, to help determine any underlying pathology. Intraocular pressures are evaluated at least daily and, should they become abnormal, are immediately treated with appropriate medications. Slit-lamp examinations are likewise performed daily to help note the absorption or recurrence of bleeding.

Physicians differ in their selection of medications used to treat hyphemas. Some choose mydriatics to help prevent synechiae and hyperemia; others choose miotics to promote absorption of blood. Some prefer neither, or may use steroids instead.

In most children the hyphema heals within 7–10 days, although decreased activity is in order for several weeks. The lower the grade, the better the prognosis for visual acuity in that eye.

The most common complication is rebleeding, which usually occurs between the second and fifth day posttrauma. Recently the use of oral steroids or aminocaproic acid has proved beneficial in decreasing the occurrence of rebleeding. Other complications include synechiae, persistent glaucoma, corneal staining, endophthalmitis, and phthisis bulbi. In addition, other ocular problems may develop secondary to trauma to adjacent structures.

Children with recurrent hemorrhages, persistent glaucoma, or corneal staining may require surgical intervention. Sometimes an anterior chamber irrigation (paracentesis) is performed to remove some of the fluid. Other procedures may be the infusion of fibrinolysin to dissolve clots, diathermy to the site of rebleeding, or phacoemulsification or cryoextraction of the clots.

PREVENTATIVE SAFETY MEASURES

Introduction

According to the NSPB, 90 percent of all eye injuries can be prevented! The Society also speculates that about 40 percent of all eye injuries occur in the home, and many others are sports-related. Boys are still the most frequent victims, and unfortunately, children in general receive a significantly higher proportion of eye injuries than do persons of other ages. Any resultant damage from an eye injury has a greater long-term effect when it occurs in a child than when it occurs in older people.

The NSPB has long been an authority on injuries and an arch supporter of eye safety. You will notice that many of the recommended teaching materials in this section are produced by the NSPB. These materials are quite inexpensive, and the prevention of even one eye injury through their use is well worth the cost.

Preventing injuries, any injuries, is somewhat like being a detective. For example, do the schools in your area (public and private) provide protective eyewear for students during competitive sports or certain at-risk physical education classes? Are parents, teachers, and others aware of the signs of eye trouble (Table 1-1), so that they can quickly detect postinjury problems? With some data collection and an increased sense of awareness, you will be able to identify many ways to prevent or decrease eye injuries.

Also become involved in promoting legislation that encourages eye safety.

Some of you may be interested in the safety of toys, and others may be troubled by the current tendency toward liberalizing firework laws. In the past, groups such as nurses have greatly influenced legislation on specific issues (for example, car seats for infants).

Finally, consider participating in "Save Your Vision Week," usually held during September. Depending on your own schedule and the needs of your patients, however, you can pick your own week or month. The topics discussed next will give you many ideas. The prevention of even one injury will be well worth your time and effort.

Toys

All parents should be counseled about selecting appropriate toys for their children, keeping in mind the age of each child and general safety and construction features of the toy. Nowadays many toys are marked with suggested age ranges. Some well-meaning relatives and friends, however, may still purchase toys that are beyond a child's cognitive or motor skills. Such mismatching can lead to misuse of the toy and can ultimately lead to injury. Other toys simply are not constructed well and may break easily, leaving sharp edges, or have inherently pointed or projectile properties. These toys should not be purchased at all (for example, the infamous BB gun).

Children should also be taught at young ages the dangers of pointed and sharp objects, such as scissors, broken glass, pencils, TV and radio antennas, and so on. Adequate supervision should be provided when they are using these items; the NSPB estimates that more than half of associated injuries from these objects occur when children are not supervised in their use. In addition, never allow a child to run or jump while holding a sharp or pointed object and keep these objects to a minimum in the child's environment. As children get older (6–10 years of age) they are more likely to be injured by projectile toys. Again, adequate supervision must be provided when darts, arrows, or rocks are being thrown.

The NSPB has put together an excellent eye safety education program called *The Eyes Have It* for children aged 5 to 8. It consists of an instructor's activity packet stressing safety principles during play ($3.00/packet). It can be used with an 8-minute 16mm color film of similar title (rental fee, $10.00). A pamphlet, *Play It Safe* ($4.00/100), supplements the program and is designed to reinforce these safety principles to the child's parents. You may wish to purchase the film for your office, clinic, or school ($100.00) or to use the activity packet for children in the waiting area.

In addition, the American Optometric Association has developed the cartoon character "Seymour Safety," who appears in a number of their safety pamphlets and related materials. For example, Seymour Safety bag puppets are an entertaining way of helping to reinforce vision safety principles. (See the end of this chapter for other listings of Seymour's resources.)

Television

Another area for promoting eye safety among children is by one's example and guidelines for watching television. For example, one should sit far enough away to view the screen comfortably; this will decrease the amount of eye movements necessary and hence minimize the occurrence of fatigue, or "television headache." However, the earlier concerns of sitting too close to color sets for fear that they would emit dangerous amounts of radiation does not apply to those sets made during 1969 and later, since federal regulations have restricted the amount of radiation that can be released by a color television over a 1-hour period to 0.5 milliroentgens (mR). Color sets made before 1969 should be evaluated individually, but all black-and-white sets are safe.

Another important parameter regarding television and one's eyes (the effect of television on one's brain is beyond the scope of this book) is the amount of lighting in the room. Ample lighting is preferable, to avoid a large amount of contrast between the TV screen and the rest of the room. In addition, a set that can be clearly focused, a screen that has a size relative to the size of the room, and a comfortable viewing angle between the viewer and the set are all-important. These and other points are discussed in the NSPB pamphlet *Television and Your Eyes* and in *To View or Not to View* by the American Optometric Association.

Lighting

Good lighting should be encouraged for all activities that require close visual skills; otherwise, the eyes may become fatigued. However, most ophthalmologists agree that excessive near work in poor light, or too much near work for prolonged period of time, does not lead to decreased vision.

Sports

One authority on sports eye injuries (Vinger) has estimated that more than 100,000 eye injuries occur to school-aged children every year as a result of sport activities. The NSPB has therefore taken a great interest in sport safety. We, as nurses and parents, should likewise be concerned and do everything within our power to help lower this incidence.

One of the NSPB's largest current efforts is directed toward players of racquet sports, as the incidence of eye injuries resulting from these sports has increased significantly in the last 10 years or so. To help promote eye safety in racquet sports, the American Society for Testing and Materials has recently released its F803 Standard. This standard states that players of racquet sports should wear industrial quality safety glasses (preferably with lenses and frames made of polycarbonate), or, if the player has a refractive error, to wear a sports eye protector with polycarbonate prescriptive lenses. All glasses should have temple curving and headband, but eyewear with adjustable nosepads is not acceptable. Remind players that contact lenses provide no resistance against impact.

The National Collegiate Athletic Association has already adopted these standards, and we hope that the general public will respond in a similar fashion. In the meantime, we can serve as role models and educators by wearing such eyewear ourselves during any racquet sports that we play and by encouraging our children and friends to do likewise. If your family belongs to a racquet sport club, consider purchasing one or more copies of the NSPB poster "Give your eyes a sporting chance. Use eyewear (for racquet sports): at $1.00 each for your club. With everyone's effort, the incidence of injuries to the head and eye from racquet sports can decrease dramatically. Such was the case with hockey, when the standards for facial protection were issued and followed on a widespread basis.

As for other sports, encourage players to wear the prescribed equipment (for example, helmet with faceguard in baseball and football), even when they are not in a formal practice session or game. The NSPB also suggests that you encourage schools to supply protective eyewear for students while they participate in competitive sports and selected physical education classes. The American Optometric Association encourages safety in biking in their 24-page activity pamphlet *Reflections of Bike Basics*. In addition, don't forget to keep records of any injuries caused by sports activities and to report them to appropriate persons at least yearly, along with any suggestions for decreasing these injuries.

Finally, children who are at risk for developing retinal detachment should not be allowed to participate in any contact sports, and children with vision in one eye only should be mandated to wear impact-resistant eyewear during all sports activities.

Chemicals in the Home

Many parents are keenly aware of keeping poisonous cleansers, medications, and so on, out of the reach of children. Yet too often an imaginary line is drawn between those items that can be ingested by mouth and those with sprays or nozzles that make ingestion much more difficult: parents may remember to keep the former under lock and key, but may forget that the latter can also damage a child's eyes if they are left around indiscreetly. Therefore, encourage parents to keep items with sprays and nozzles out of the reach of children.

In addition, when parents are using chemicals, cleansers, or sprays, they should set a good example and wear appropriate eyewear. (How many of us even own a pair of safety goggles?) Also remind parents to be consistent in using this eyewear: not just when cleaning the house, but also in the garage, in the garden (lawn mowing and pruning are two big sources of injury), and while participating in any hobbies or sports that have the potential for an eye injury. Otherwise, the effect of role modeling will be diluted. It is also important to remember that observers of such activities in the near vicinity can also be injured. Finally, remind children with contact lenses not to wear them when using chemicals or near fumes or fine particles in the air, even with safety eyewear. The fumes or particles can become trapped between the contact lens and the eye, causing irritation and possible damage to either. To help reinforce all of these principles, consider using the NSPB pamphlet *Eye Safety Is No Accident.*

Jumping Batteries

A fair number of eye injuries occur from persons incorrectly attempting to jump start a car battery. Therefore, remind instructors of driver education classes to reinforce this point in their curriculum and perhaps distribute to each student a sticker produced by the NSPB on how to jump start a battery correctly ($10.00 for 100 stickers). In addition, instructors should caution students not to use matches when looking under a car hood, especially to see whether there is enough water in the battery. The battery acid fumes can explode, causing acid burns and a hyphema.

Driving

Many states require that a person pass a vision screening prior to the issuance of a driver's permit or license. Frequently, 20/40 vision is required when both eyes are tested together. Some states also require that a person have a certain amount of fusion (depth perception). Adolescents who do not have adequate fusion may need to demonstrate that they can use other cues to determine distance correctly. Similarly, adolescents with certain types of color deficiency may need to demonstrate their ability to recognize traffic signals and car lights, and some persons with the more severe types of color deficiency may not be given a license to drive at all.

The American Optometric Association offers two pamphlets, *Driving Takes Seeing* and *Open Your Eyes to Vision in Driving Safety,* to assist instructors in reinforcing the importance of adequate vision and mental skills when driving.

Shops and Labs

Currently, 36 states have requirements about the use of protective eyewear in laboratory and shop classes in their respective schools (Table 12-1). Students in all schools, whether their state has requirements or not, should be required to wear proper industrial level safety eyewear during the following circumstances:[1]

A.   Vocational, technical, industrial arts, chemical, or chemical-physics courses of instruction involving exposure to:

---

[1]From the National Society to Prevent Blindness, *An Option To See,* page 3.

Table 12-1

States having legislation or regulations regarding the use of approved safety eyewear in selected educational and vocational programs*

Alabama	Louisiana	Oklahoma
Arkansas	Maine	Pennsylvania
Arizona	Maryland	Rhode Island
California	Massachusetts	South Carolina
Colorado	Michigan	South Dakota
Connecticut	Minnesota	Tennessee
Delaware	Mississippi	Texas
Florida	Missouri	Utah
Georgia	New Jersey	Virginia
Illinois	New Mexico	Washington
Indiana	New York	Wisconsin
Iowa	North Carolina	Wyoming
Kansas	Ohio	

*Modified from *An Option To See* by the National Society to Prevent Blindness, page 2

1. Hot molten metal or other molten materials
2. Milling, sawing, turning, shaping, cutting, grinding, or stamping of any solid materials
3. Heat treatment, tempering, or kiln firing of any metal or other materials
4. Gas or electric arc welding, or other forms of welding processes
5. Repair or servicing of any vehicle
6. Caustic or explosive materials

B. Chemical, physical, or combined chemical-physical laboratories involving caustic or explosive materials, hot liquids or solids, injurious radiations, or other hazards not enumerated

States and schools vary in whether this eyewear is provided free of charge to the students or whether the students must pay a small fee for them. In addition, students who normally wear contact lenses should be advised not to wear them near fumes, vapors, splashes, intensive heat, molten metals, or highly particulate matter, since some of these may become trapped between the contact lens and eye. Or they may damage the lens, leading to irritation and possible injury to the eye.

To assist instructors in enforcing the use of safety eyewear in these situations, the NSPB has developed the program *An Option to See* for students in grades 7 through 12. The 16mm film is 17 minutes in length and can be rented for $10.00 or purchased for $100.00. The corresponding packet ($4.00) has a teacher's guide, overhead transparencies, poster, and spirit masters for duplication. The materials in the packet are designed to be presented over a total of 240 minutes, divided into 20-, 40-, or 60-minute segments. They focus on the attitudes of students and professionals about the use of safety eyewear, the various types of eyewear, and first aid measures. Members from local unions and other community resources are also encouraged to participate by serving as role models and by reinforcing the necessity of proper safety eyewear.

Additional audio-visual materials produced by the NSPB regarding eye safety in the shop or laboratory setting include the poster "See Your Future . . . Wear Safety Eyewear" ($1.00 each); the poster "Kiss Your Eyes Goodbye—If You Don't Protect Them, You Might as Well Throw Them Away" ($1.75 each); and the film *Eye and Face Protection in Chemical Laboratories* (13-1/2- or 22-minute versions, $10.00 rental fee, or $120.00 or $150.00 purchase price). Furthermore, the Southern California Society to Prevent Blindness produces the 24-page pamphlet *Eye Protection in Educational Institutions* ($1.00) which uses California's regulations and guidelines as an example.

Finally, the NSPB also coordinates the Wise Owl Club of America. For a one-time fee of $5.00, schools and laboratories can become chapters of this club. Its sole purpose is to promote the use of safety eyewear in all appropriate settings. Then, should any persons in that chapter save their vision by using safety eyewear, they become official members of the club and receive a special pin. Since everyone likes a reward, the club adds an incentive for students to wear their safety eyewear. (Some instructors provide an even stronger incentive: they immediately fail any student who was not wearing his or her safety eyewear at an appropriate time!)

Early in the school year, nurses who work in school settings should review with instructors of laboratory and shop classes safety procedures and first aid measures for those classes and the ways students will be instructed in these areas. Also review at this time the cleansing and dispensing of safety eyewear, and ensure that special faucets for washing chemicals out of eyes are easily accessible and not surrounded by laboratory or other equipment.

Sunviewing

Remind children never to look at the sun directly, even if they are wearing sunglasses or holding tinted glass or film before their eyes. Also encourage them to wear sun goggles (not sunglasses) when in the snow or near a sun lamp, although they may not be directly facing the source of ultraviolet rays (for instance, when lying prone by a sun lamp). The glare can be reflected into the eye from any angle. (Sunglasses are discussed in further detail at the end of this chapter.)

Children with Vision in Only One Eye

Parents of a child who has vision in only one eye should encourage their child to wear impact-resistant glasses during all times of play and sports. In fact, some ophthalmologists recommend that these children wear such glasses during all waking hours, and others advise their patients not to participate in contact sports. Since the purpose of the safety glasses is to protect the child's remaining vision, it does not matter whether the child has a refractive error; clear glass can be inserted into the frames for children who have normal vision without correction.

Fireworks

The handling of fireworks can be detrimental to the vision of any person, regardless of age. However, children seem even more vulnerable because of their decreased cognitive and motor skills.

Table 12-2 lists the types of fireworks currently allowed by the various states. Class C fireworks contain 50 mg or less of gunpowder and include bottle rockets

Table 12-2
Firework Control Laws

I.	**States having no fireworks laws, except at county level:**		
	Hawaii	Nevada	
II.	**States that allow Class C fireworks:**		
	Alabama*	Louisiana	South Dakota
	Alaska	Mississippi	Tennessee
	Arkansas	Missouri	
III.	**States that allow Class C fireworks as approved by enforcing authority, or as specified by law:**		
	California	Kentucky	District of Columbia
	Oklahoma	Michigan*	South Carolina
	Idaho	Nebraska	Texas
	Indiana*	Montana	Virginia*
	Kansas	New Mexico	Washington
	North Dakota	Wyoming	
IV.	**States that allow only sparklers or snakes:**		
	Colorado (sparklers)	Pennsylvania (sparklers)	
	Florida (sparklers)	Utah (sparklers)	
	Illinois (sparklers)**	Iowa (sparklers and snakes)	
	Maine (sparklers)	Oregon (sparklers and snakes)	
	Maryland (sparklers)	Wisconsin (sparklers and snakes)	
V.	**States that ban all Class C fireworks:**		
	Arizona	Minnesota	Ohio
	Connecticut	New Hampshire	Rhode Island
	Delaware	New Jersey	Vermont
	Georgia	New York	West Virginia
	Massachusetts	North Carolina	

From "Fireworks: Spectacles not Toys" by N. Acocella, page 7
 *Previously in Group IV.
**Previously in Group V.

and firecrackers. Class B fireworks contain more (sometimes much more) than 50 mg of gunpowder and include, but are not limited to, cherry bombs and M-80 fireworks. Class B fireworks can be sold on an interstate basis only for use in public displays and not for commercial or consumer use; enforcement of this federal law, however, is quite difficult. Relatively new federal regulations also require that all fireworks have a lighting-to-explosive time of 3–6 seconds.

In 1975 a bill that proposed to ban the commercial sale of fireworks in all states was before Congress. However, it did not pass. Currently, some states are actually relaxing their regulations. As a result, the NSPB is attempting to gather accurate statistical information on the number of eye injuries occurring from consumer handling of fireworks and can use input from nurses regarding this matter. Nurses should also help support more restrictive legislation regarding consumer use of fireworks and should become involved in teaching persons of all ages, but especially children, the danger of handling fireworks.

Safety Councils

Depending on your setting, you may wish to support the development of a safety coordinator or council or to participate in one that already exists. Of course, the coordinator or council would be concerned with all aspects of safety and not just those matters related to the eye. However, the enforcement of safety principles in general would obviously have an impact on decreasing eye injuries.

Increased safety could be accomplished through more accurate data collection, analysis of accident reports, and education of staff, students, patients, and their parents through in-service training, parent meetings, or school classes. Pamphlets on safety can be distributed in offices and waiting areas, and first aid measures can be reviewed.

To assist in these efforts, obtain a copy of the book *Teaching About Vision,* which was produced as a joint effort by the American School Health Association and the NSPB. It offers specific information about promoting the safety of children's vision and discusses approaches and interventions for the various age ranges. In addition, it covers classroom illumination, emergencies, shop safety, and so on. It currently is in its second edition and can be purchased from the NSPB for a cost of $2.00.

Finally, the NSPB has also produced the *Magic of Sight* for children in grades 5 and 6. This 13-minute filmstrip with corresponding audiocassette is available for $12.50 and explores vision, eye health, and safety in an interesting format.

Types of Safety Eyewear

Eyewear can be classified according to its purpose and its structure. Although the obvious purpose of all safety eyewear is to protect the eyes, this can be accomplished in a variety of ways, as discussed in the following paragraphs. The various structures for safety eyewear are spectacles, goggles, face shields, and helmets.

Spectacles are what most people refer to as *glasses* and provide little or no protection to the peripheral eye area. In essence, their main purpose is to hold lenses (clear or tinted, with or without correction), although some safety spectacles also have small brow and peripheral shields to prevent flying particles from touching the eyes. Spectacles fit the eye by ear loops. In contrast, goggles have significant brow and side shields and are held in place with a headband. In general, they are preferred when working with liquids, particles, or sparks that may fly into the eyes or for disseminating the impact from any object to the eye area (for example, in racquetball). Some goggles provide ventilation when one is working near fumes. If the face, as well as the eyes, needs protection, a face shield is used; if a very sturdy material is required to reduce impact to the eyes and face further, a helmet is recommended. Many agencies and states offer specific directions as to which type of safety eyewear is necessary for which circumstances.

Safety eyewear can protect the eyes in several ways. For example, all safety eyewear provides a physical barrier between the eye and foreign materials. The amount and type of barrier required depend on the type of substance(s) with which one is working. In addition, safety eyewear provides resistance against various levels of impact. Although current federal regulations require that the lenses of all glasses be made of plastic or tempered glass to provide some resistance against small impacts, industrial quality eyewear is the preferred choice for safety eyewear, as its lenses are made of a specified thickness and provide a much higher level of impact resistance. Since street glasses are rarely made of industrial quality, they are not advised for racquet sports or laboratory or shop settings.

Frames can also be designed to disseminate impact to the various facial bones, away from the eye, offering an additional safety feature. In the past, certain sport eye protectors were essentially a safety frame without lenses. Now, however, most eye safety authorities recommend the purchase of safety or sports glasses that have impact-resistant lenses. The new plastic polymer, polycarbonate, appears to be quite promising as the source from which both lenses and frames of industrial quality are made. The frames should fit well, which may be a problem for younger children, since few frames are made in children's sizes.

Most types of safety eyewear can be purchased for an additional fee with built-in prescriptive lenses. Persons who wear contact lenses should avoid wearing their lenses when near fumes or sprays that may become entrapped between the lens and eye, causing possible damage. In addition, contact lens wearers should be informed that their lenses provide absolutely no resistance against impact and can actually damage an eye if in place when an impact occurs (for example, the use of hard contact lenses during a game of racquetball, with no other safety eyewear in place).

Unfortunately, the maintenance of safety eyewear is often neglected, perhaps to such a degree that the safety features are severely compromised. Encourage coaches and instructors to teach students how to provide adequate maintenance and to examine their students' eyewear periodically. If eyewear is not the personal property of a student, it should be thoroughly cleansed and disinfected between use by different students.

Sunglasses

Despite nebulous advertisements, all glasses with tints are not sunglasses. For best effect, sunglasses need to thin out ultraviolet (UV) and infrared (IR) rays, while minimally affecting one's visual acuity and color perception.

Ultraviolet rays are light waves with wavelengths between 200 and 400 nanometers (nm). In contrast, infrared rays are longer and less energetic and have wavelengths between 800 and 1500 nm. In between are the visible light waves. Normally the cornea absorbs any rays less than 300 nm, and the lens absorbs those rays between 300 and 400 nm. However, when the UV rays are too intense, such as during sunbathing, sitting under a sunlamp, or skiing at high altitudes, the cornea can literally become sunburned, resulting in a diffuse keratitis. In addition, there is some evidence that exposure to intense UV rays can lead to the yellowing of the lens, or ''sunshine'' cataracts; intense infrared rays can cause a ''glassblowers'' cataract. In milder doses, infrared rays can cause eye fatigue and discomfort, and both types of rays can cause injury to the retina under selected conditions or in the presence of certain ocular problems. For example, a child who has had a cataract removed no longer has a natural lens to filter out the higher ultraviolet rays. (Spectacles and contact lenses can absorb rays only up to 320 nm.) In addition, children with retinitis pigmentosa, albinism, and other corneal, anterior chamber, or lens problems are also at risk for developing additional ocular problems secondary to sun exposure.

The many types of sunglasses on the market can be confusing, causing some people to make inappropriate selections. For example, some untreated darker lenses may actually increase the risk for potential eye damage because the pupils dilate behind the darker lenses, allowing more rays to enter the eye. Therefore, instruct your patients to read the labels attached to sunglasses. Persons with normal eyes who are buying sunglasses for outdoor use should look for lenses that allow 10–30 percent of light to enter the eyes in sunlight. The tint of the lenses should be gray, smoke, amber, green, or brown. Other tints usually do not allow for adequate UV and IR ray attenuation or acceptable color perception. In addition, the lenses should be inspected for flaws and held under a fluorescent light or in front of a distant vertical object to assure that they do not allow for significant distortion of objects. For example, the fluorescent light reflection on the lenses when they are held parallel to the light should appear straight.

In addition to tint variation, there are also lens differences. Photochromic lenses change their absorptive powers and intensity of tint, depending on the amount of light present. Polarizing and mirror lenses decrease reflected glare. NoIR and OLo glasses can reduce the amount of light entering the eye to 1, 2, 4, 8, or 10 percent and come in a wrap-around style for added protection against peripheral light. They range in price from $15.00 to $60.00, can be placed over prescriptive lenses, and can be made to fit more children. Also in a wrap-around style, Gargoyles by Pro-tec provide both light restriction and impact resistance and hence are beneficial for persons who participate in outdoor sports. In contrast, the CPF 550 by Corning Glass is designed only for patients with retinal degenerative diseases.

Because these brands of glasses are but a few of those available on the market, your patients and families with special needs should first consult their eye examiner for recommendations. Those persons who need only "regular" sunglasses may wish to read, *Sunglasses and Your Eyes—A Consumer's Guide to Sunglass Selection* (single copy free from Bausch and Lomb, Inc.) or *Sunglasses—Know What You're Getting, and What They Are Really For* (single copy free from the NSPB).

SELECTED PATIENT RESOURCES

American Academy of Ophthalmology

Eye Injuries: Prevention and First Aid: 8 pages, $5.00/100

American Optometric Association (add postage costs to price of materials)

To View or Not to View (re: TV): scf/SASE* $9.00/100

A Good Look at Sunglasses: scf/SASE* $9.00/100

Driving Takes Seeing: scf/SASE* $9.00/100

Open Your Eyes to Vision in Driving Safely: scf/SASE* $9.00/100

Seymour Safely Bag Puppets (with safety message): $9.00/100

Seymour Safely and Op-Tic (story about general safety, featuring robot from outer space): 12 pages, $1.00 each

Seymour Safely Safety stickers: $15.00 per 1000

Reflections of Bike Basics: 24 pages, $2.25 each

Happy Boo Day to You (Halloween safety tips for young children): 8 pages, $1.00 each

Bausch & Lomb, Inc.

Sunglasses and Your Eyes—A Consumer's Guide to Sunglass Selection: single copy free, 16 pages

National Society to Prevent Blindness (single copies are free, unless otherwise noted)

---

*single copy free with self addressed stamped envelope

Play It Safe . . . Your Child's Eyes Are At Stake (basic safety tips for parents): $4.00/100

First Aid for Eye Emergencies (sticker): $3.00/100

How to Jump-Start a Car Safely (sticker for car battery): 25¢ each, $10.00/100

Sunglasses . . . know what you're getting and what they're really for: $8.00/100

TV and Your Eyes: $9.00/100

Eye Safety Is No Accident: $8.00/100

20 Questions on Eye Safety (about safety eyewear): $4.00/100

The Wise Owl Club of America (brochure and application to establish chapter in your local school or agency)

Teaching about Vision: 72 pages, $2.00 per copy

The Eyes Have It—Teacher's Packet on Children's Eye Safety—K through 3 grade: $3.00/packet

The Eyes Have It! 16 mm, color film, 8 minutes: $10.00 rental fee or $100.00 purchase price

*The Magic of Sight—Multi-Media Kit on the Eye—*grades 5 and 6: $12.50, includes 13-minute filmstrip and cassette and teacher's packet

*An Option to See—Teacher's Packet on Lab and Shop Eye Safety—*grades 7 through 12: $4.00/packet

An Option To See—16mm, color film, 17 minutes $10.00 rental fee, or $100.00 purchase price

*Eye and Face Protection in Chemical Laboratories—*16mm, color film, 13-1/2- or 22-minutes: $10.00 rental fee, or $120.00 or $150.00 purchase price

*Kiss Your Eyes Goodbye—If You Don't Protect Them, You Might as Well Throw Them Away—*poster: $1.75 each

*See Your Future . . . Wear Safety Eyewear Now—*poster: $1.00 each

Give Your Eyes a Sporting Chance. Use Eyeguards (for all Racquet Sports) —poster: $1.00 each

Patient Information Library

I Care—Eye Care at Work, Home, and Play by R. J. Keefe, 16 pages: $1.00 each

SELECTED BIBLIOGRAPHY

Acocella N: Fireworks: Spectacles not toys. Sightsaving 51:2–7, 1982
Collet BI: Traumatic hyphema: A review. Ann Ophthalmol 14:52–56, 1982
Frey T: Pediatric eye trauma. Pediatr Ann 12:487–497, July 1983
Jones M, Tippett T: Assessment of the red eye. Nurse Prac 5:10–15, January–February, 1980
Oglesby R: Eye trauma in children. Pediatr Ann 7:11–47, January 1977
Paton D, Goldberg MF: *Management of Ocular Injuries*. Philadelphia: Saunders, 1976
Saclarides EE, Parrish RK, Saclarides TJ: Ocular emergencies. J Ophthalmic Nurs Tech 1:43–49, August 1982
Vinger PF: Sports eye injuries—A preventable disease. Ophthalmology 88:108–112, 1981
Weinstock FJ: Emergency treatment of eye injuries. Am J Nurs 71:1928–1931, 1971

Chapter Thirteen

The Child with a Visual Impairment

Persons with *impaired vision* (vision that cannot be corrected with regular prescriptive lenses) are classified either as being blind or having low vision. The functional difference between these two groups is that persons with low vision have varying amounts of residual vision, which can be augmented with various adaptations and special devices. In contrast, persons who are *functionally blind* have no useful residual vision: either they cannot see at all, or they can perceive only light or perhaps hand motions and must rely on nonvisual cues to assist them in their everyday functioning. The vast majority of persons with visual impairments are in the low-vision category. These functional classifications differ from the legal ones, which are based on visual acuity. For legal purposes, a person is usually considered to have *low vision* if their central visual acuity in the better eye is between 20/60 and 20/200. Persons who are defined as *legally blind* have a central visual acuity in their better eye of 20 degrees or less or vision of 20/200 or less in their better eye. This classification allows persons to qualify for various tax and insurance benefits, as well as for public assistance. However, many persons who are legally blind have a fair amount of residual vision, although the term *blindness* gives those around them the incorrect idea that they cannot see at all. Hence, the term *visually impaired* is gradually coming into use.

Although the majority of persons in the United States with some type of visual impairment are over 65 years of age, it is estimated that 2 out of every 500 school children have a visual impairment, and about 1 in every 2500 are legally blind. Approximately three-fourths of all these children had the onset of their impairment before their first birthday, and of these, more than 50 percent had a prenatal onset.

A child with a congenital or a hereditary cause of visual impairment needs a complete medical work-up in addition to ocular care to assess whether the child may also have problems in other organs or systems and to explore whether genetic counseling is necessary for the family.

Table 13-1 lists the most common causes of visual impairment in children. A noticeable omission to persons acquainted with visual impairment on a worldwide basis is *xerophthalmia,* or impairment secondary to vitamin A deficiency. This preventable condition is a result of malnutrition and is seen all too often in children in developing countries.

When interacting with children with a visual impairment, be careful to address your attention to their visual efficiency, rather than their visual acuity. That is, determine what they can do with any vision that they have. Too often persons compare children with similar visual acuities and expect them to see and behave in the same way. But one child may be capable of using vision in a different manner than another and hence be more functional in a particular activity. So remember to treat each child as an individual.

Also remember that the degree of visual impairment may be stable or change, depending upon the specific cause. In fact, some impairments, such as those from trauma or responsive to surgery, can improve over time, although many others become worse. Finally, some children may have associated photophobia, nystagmus, color deficiency, or visual field changes (central or peripheral), which may also decrease their vision.

DIAGNOSIS AND COUNSELING

When a diagnosis of a visual impairment in a child has been made, the family begins an intense mourning process. If the child is diagnosed at or shortly after birth, this mourning can interfere with the attachment process of parent and

Table 13-1

Common causes of visual impairment in American children and adolescents

Congenital	**Hereditary**
cataracts	achromatopsia
coloboma	albinism
corneal dystrophy	aniridia
functional amblyopia	cataracts
glaucoma	juvenile macular degeneration
keratoconus	Leber's optic atrophy
toxoplasmosis	Marfan's syndrome
Adventitious (acquired)	retinitis pigmentosa
brain tumor	retinoblastoma
infection	**Vascular**
trauma	diabetic retinopathy
uveitis	Coat's disease
	retrolental fibroplasia
	sickle cell retinopathy

From Stern EJ: Helping the person with low vision. Amer J Nurs 80:1789–1790, Oct 1980

NURSING GOALS, OUTCOME STANDARDS, AND DIAGNOSES

Since nurses work in such a diversity of settings and roles, we have various opportunities to affect the life of a child with a visual impairment positively and to assist the child's family, teachers, and other significant caretakers. This chapter's primary nursing goal, therefore, is that *every child with a visual impairment will perform age-appropriately in the social, self-care, motor, communication, and academic areas,* barring the presence of any other physical, sensory, or developmental problems. Further, nurses must recognize that certain "delays" in some of these areas are normal and age-appropriate for children with visual impairments.

Outcome Standard 1

All children with visual impairments have maximal use of any residual vision (minimizes *sensory deficit*).

Suggested Interventions:
- The nurse ensures that the child has received adequate medical care and follow-up for a particular eye problem by communicating either verbally or in writing with the child's primary care provider or ophthalmologist.
- If such information is unattainable, or if it is unclear whether the child has received complete and necessary medical care, the nurse refers the child to an ophthalmologist for a current ocular examination.
- Children who have a quantifiable visual acuity are referred to a local low-vision specialist.
- The nurse ensures that appropriate children have obtained any recommended low-vision equipment. When financial or psychosocial barriers prevent this, the nurse assists in whatever way possible to remove such barriers.
- The nurse assists in visual acuity screenings and in-service training whenever possible to ensure that all children with visual impairments are identified as soon as possible (see Chapters 1 and 2).

Outcome Standard 2

All children with a visual impairment receive the services of professionals specialized in the development and/or education of children with visual impairments when the impairment is identified and receive professional services as necessary throughout their lives.

Outcome Standard 3

Each child with a visual impairment is mainstreamed into numerous contacts and activities with sighted children and adults as soon as the visual impairment is identified.

Suggested Interventions:
- The nurse ensures that the family of a child with a visual impairment has

information about developmental and educational services available to the child from local, state, and national agencies (decreases *knowledge deficit*).

- The nurse, along with other professionals, assists the family in promoting the child's normal growth and development. At the time of diagnosis this process will focus on overcoming *self-care deficits* and *impaired physical mobility*. Also intertwined may be the parent's *knowledge deficit* about growth and development of children in general and the tendency of parents to limit their child's *potential for physical injury*. The nurse must help parents to recognize that carefully monitored risk taking is essential for a child with a visual impairment to reach full potential.

- The nurse assists the child with a visual impairment and the parents in incorporating the child into a wide variety of activities with sighted children (counteracts *social isolation, deficit in diversional activities, disturbance in self-esteem*, and such *alterations in parenting* as overprotection, pity, or shame).

- The nurse assists sighted peers in accepting the child with a visual impairment, and in understanding the child's limitations, and in promoting the child's strengths and capabilities (counteracts *knowledge deficit* or *anxiety* of peers and *social isolation* and resultant *disturbance in self esteem* of the child with a visual impairment).

- The nurse promotes the child's enrollment in the least restrictive environment in the school setting and assists teachers and other school personnel in becoming comfortable with a child with a visual impairment under their care (counteracts *knowledge deficit, ineffective coping* or *anxiety* by school staff, and helps school personnel reduce the child's *potential for injury* and *social isolation* in the school setting).

- The nurse assists the adolescent with a visual impairment, and the family and educators in exploring vocational interests and in ensuring that all influential persons (including potential employers) encourage such exploration and decisions regarding a career (counteracts *spiritual distress,* and *disturbance in self-concept* of the adolescent or *knowledge deficit* of the adolescent, the family, educators, or employers).

Outcome Standard 4

Older patients with a visual impairment and the parents of all children with a visual impairment verbalize the impact of the impairment on their daily lives and use supportive services as necessary.

Suggested Interventions:

- The nurse informs parents and significant others of various available supportive resources. These may include parent or youth groups, role models, literature, newsletters and other mailings, respite care, professional counseling, vocational rehabilitation, and national or local organizations and agencies. Such services help to counteract *alterations in parenting, ineffective coping, dysfunctional grief, social isolation* of the family or child, *alterations in family processes* (including in-laws and grandparents), *anxiety* and *fears, knowledge deficit,* and *spiritual distress.*

• The nurse recognizes that for varying time periods after the diagnosis of a visual impairment in a child the parents may be in such acute grief that they are not able to utilize many appropriate services. Therefore, the nurse gently encourages parents and other family members through the acute grief process, occasionally repeating what supportive services are available and pointing out that relatives and friends usually lag behind the parents in the grieving process. At a later time the nurse introduces the concept and process of chronic grief to the family (see nursing diagnoses in the above intervention).

• The nurse provides parents, other family members, friends, and older children numerous opportunities to discuss the impact of the visual impairment on their daily lives and provides support and guidance as necessary.

(See previous chapters for discussion of specific visual problems.)

---

child. Additionally, concerns regarding the presence or possibility of other handicaps may compound the situation. If the child is a few months old at the time of diagnosis, the attachment process is usually in full swing, and hence the needs of the parents will be slightly different. When a child experiences vision loss after infancy, both the child and parents need to grieve over the loss of the child's sight. (This is not to imply that congenitally blind children do not grieve about their own loss.) The younger the child, the more quickly the adaptation to the loss seems to occur, particularly when those around the child have positive and viable attitudes.

The grief process is a vital and necessary step to acceptance of the child's impairment. Nurses should be aware of its various stages and manifestations and remember that people take different amounts of time to go through each step in the process. Some of these steps are similar to those following the death of a significant other: shock, denial, anger, and depression, for example. However, the manifestations may be different. Anger may be evidenced by rejecting the child, by forcing the child to be independent too soon, or by acting out toward hospital or office staff. Depression may lead some parents to feelings of inadequacy or withdrawal, or cause some to overprotect their child. Guilt about some past behavior may lead a parent to believe that he or she is being punished, and thoughts such as, Why me? and Why my baby? may sink a parent into deeper depression.

In many cases, it is the child's pediatrician or family physician who first suspects that something is amiss with the child's vision, perhaps because of the parent's suspicions and findings. The child is referred to an ophthalmologist, who confirms or establishes the diagnosis and who is put into the position of telling the parents the findings. For many ophthalmologists, this is one of their most difficult responsibilities, and many of them frankly admit that they do not handle it well. In fact, they may feel so ill at ease at the time that they quite abruptly tell the parents their findings and quickly send them on their way.

Nurses who work in settings with pediatricians, family physicians, and ophthalmologists should encourage the practice of having both parents present when discouraging findings must be reported. Similarly, single parents should have a friend or relative with them. In this way, both will receive the same information and will be more likely to remember it correctly. The ophthalmologist should notify the referring pediatrician or family doctor, and the parents should consult the primary care provider at their earliest convenience for additional guidance and support.

It may be difficult for the ophthalmologist to quantify the amount of visual loss, however. For example, although optic nerve atrophy can be readily recognized, its effect on a child's vision may be much more difficult to determine, especially in a young infant. In addition, many children learn to use any residual vision to a greater extent as they grow older, thus later increasing their visual efficiency. Furthermore, certain problems such as cataracts or glaucoma can be treated with early surgical interventions, so that a child's vision may improve. Low-vision aids also may be helpful as the child grows. Because of these various possibilities, and because of the parents' fragile state, hope for useful vision should be given whenever possible.

Parents tend to be most concerned about the effect of the visual loss on their child's day-to-day functioning and may even be thinking about the child's marriage and career 20 years away. Contacting families who have coped with similar problems and now have a well-functioning and adjusted child may be helpful at this time, especially since most persons have no personal experience with a person with a visual impairment (although they may have considerable misinformation from television).

Besides providing early intervention for any ocular problems that can be treated, the ophthalmologist may also counsel the family about genetic transmission of a particular defect and may request examination of the parents or other family members to determine the potential for its being inherited or transmitted. Finally, an ophthalmologist can also treat many cosmetic ocular defects that can have far-reaching social implications for the child, even though there may be no associated improvement in the child's vision.

Newsletters and meetings, such as those of the National Association for Parents of the Visually Impaired (NAPVI) and the International Institute of Visually Impaired, 0-7, Inc. (IIVI) can be a great help, as can parent groups in the area. The American Foundation for the Blind offers *Parenting Preschoolers: Suggestions for Raising Young Blind and Visually Impaired Children* (1984, single copy free). Such books as *Get a Wiggle On* (AAHPERD, $5.00) and *Can't Your Child See?* (Baltimore: University Park Press, 1977 $11.00) should also be recommended.

Some parents benefit from several sessions with a professional counselor or member of the clergy, either to cope with their grief or to handle an associated problem, such as marital crises. Remember, however, that although parents may desire assistance (either supportive or informational), they may simultaneously reject such assistance as part of their denial.

In follow-up sessions with the primary care provider or team members, the parents need support, clarification, and encouragement about the child's impairment and development. Children who have been visually impaired since early infancy do not know what sight (or better sight) is and hence literally do not know what they are missing. If there is no evidence of other handicaps, the parents must be encouraged to view the child as normal and to strive for a balance between being overprotective and encouraging the child to be too independent too soon.

With the assistance of an early childhood specialist who is knowledgeable about the development of children with visual impairments, the family can begin a program to maximize the child's social, motor, intellectual, and sensory functions. Many home intervention programs cover wide geographical areas, and the Department of Education can identify those in your own state. These specialists can provide information, demonstrations, and support to families. If a specialist in visual impairment is not available in person, the Blind Children's Center in Los Angeles and the Variety Club's Blind Babies Foundation offer correspondence programs. Either way, remind parents that each child develops at a different pace, and that certain developmental milestones that normally require vision (sitting, walking, and so on) are delayed in children with visual impairments. However, the delay is secondary to lack of visual input and not caused by other inherent problems (assuming the child has no other problems) or poor parenting. In addition, parents without previous experience in rearing sighted children will need some reassurance about general principles of child development.

Additional crisis areas that may require counseling include dealing with well-intended but unwanted advice from relatives and friends, deciding to have additional children, and assisting siblings in dealing with their brother or sister's visual impairment. Younger siblings frequently fear that they, too, will become blind, and siblings of all ages may develop psychosomatic complaints in attempts to receive additional attention.

Finally, many parents find that taking one day at a time is much easier for them than dealing with potential future problems. Many young children also live in this one-day-at-a-time approach, and parents who can conceal their own anxieties about their child's future will be doing the child a big favor.

THE CHILD WITH MULTIPLE PROBLEMS

Unfortunately, some visually impaired children also have auditory, developmental, or physical problems. Families of these children need intense supportive services when such problems are identified. These services should include counseling, contact with other families who have successfully coped with a similar problem, services of educators who are specialized in the care of children with multiple problems, and, equally important, arrangements for regular respite care.

Children who are *multisensorily impaired* (deaf and blind) form a small but significant portion of those with multiple problems. (Remember that many of these children are not totally deaf or blind; they may have varying amounts of residual vision or hearing.) Like Helen Keller, these children can be taught to maximize their sense of touch and to communicate with signing or the manual alphabet. For example, during the infancy stage, a parent may tap the leg of the child while changing the diapers or manually spell *milk* before giving the child a bottle.

In the United States, the American Foundation for the Blind, the Perkins School for the Blind, and the Foundation for the Junior Blind provide special services for these children. For example, the Foundation for the Junior Blind and the Perkins School have residential educational programs. In addition, the Perkins School publishes the newsletter *Children of the Silent Night* as well as numerous other resources. In Great Britain, the National Association for Deaf-Blind Children publishes *A Parent's Guide to the Early Care of the Deaf-Blind Child* and other guides.

A number of other children with multiple problems are visually impaired and also have a developmental delay, seizure disorder, or cerebral palsy. These problems may not be identified until the child is several months old or later. As a result, parents of a child with a visual impairment may be quite anxious during their child's early months as they wait to see whether any of these problems will occur. To help decrease this anxiety, instruct parents about the expected delay in specific areas (described elsewhere) that occur in all children with serious visual impairments; these delays should not be confused with overall generalized delays in development.

Finally, parents must learn to coordinate the various specialists involved in their child's care so that they do not conflict with one another and so that each specialist is attuned to all the demands on the child and family. This in itself is a tedious job, so assist parents in setting limits and in overcoming any feelings of guilt or frustration they may develop because they cannot follow everyone's directions.

SOCIAL DEVELOPMENT

Unless a baby has an obvious eye problem at birth, many parents do not realize that their child has a visual impairment until the child is about 4 months of age. Hence, in these babies, the very early attachment process is not altered by the impairment.

Once a visual impairment has been identified, parents should be instructed about the child's great need for tactile and verbal expressions of love, since the child, for example, cannot see his parents smiling at him, or look at his relatives gloating above the crib. Suggest that parents hold, cuddle, talk, and sing to their baby at frequent intervals (but not every moment.) Carrying an infant in a modern-day papoose is also beneficial. Parents themselves may need considerable support during the early months following the diagnosis and may have decreased energy levels. In addition, a few infants will not like to be held, and parents will need additional support in teaching their baby to enjoy this important aspect of human socialization between parent and child. Furthermore, smiling may be delayed in the child with a visual impairment, and this can also decrease parental satisfaction.

In the early stages remind parents that the child's interactions with others depend to a great extent upon the interactions of others with the child. For example, a child who is pitied and kept hidden from the family and kids down the street may quickly form a self-identity as a pitiable child who is not to be with others. In contrast, a child who is accepted as a normal child who happens to have a visual impairment will most likely develop a healthy self-image. Such an approach also implies that the child will be disciplined as other children in the family are, will be given age-appropriate tasks, and will have the chance to try new things, even though the child may experience misunderstanding or even an occasional cruel remark. Children should be handled by other persons besides their parents from infancy, for, in this manner, they will become comfortable with other people at an early age.

As children grow, they may need assistance in learning how to "let off steam." Many children with visual impairments have temper tantrums instead of fighting because they hesitate to move around. Hence, children may need to learn where and when tantrums are acceptable and what other activities help to relieve energy.

Some disconcerting behaviors of many blind children include poking their fingers into their eyes, waving or flapping their hands, and rocking back and forth. These are called *blindisms* and are assumed to be ways some children stimulate themselves or release energy. For example, it is thought that poking a finger into one's eye releases phosphenes, which in turn cause a small-scale light show. Other actions, such as head banging, may be more serious. Although such behavior can alarm the family and is not socially acceptable, current specialists advocate ignoring it and engaging children in other activities or teaching them acceptable alternatives, such as rocking in a chair or on a horse. Just as with thumb sucking, children with visual impairments usually outgrow these actions at a fairly early age.

Still another aspect of different social development in children with visual impairments is that their body image and sense of self tend to be delayed. Children may talk about themselves in the third person instead of the first or name each part of their body but be unable to synthesize this knowledge and recognize that it makes up the whole of themselves.

The areas of communication and self-help skills discussed elsewhere also have important social implications. Even teaching children to "look" at someone who is talking to them can make a big difference in the way people interact with them.

Encourage parents to involve their child in as many social activities as possible, starting at the infancy stage. They can take their child to the grocery store, Little League games, the zoo, overnight trips, and so on. The more exposure children receive to various activities, the faster they will learn how to interact in them. They should also begin playing with sighted children as soon as possible.

No doubt the hardest years for children with visual impairments (as well as for most children) are the adolescent years. Adequate support will be necessary for both adolescents and parents, especially if there have been no older sighted children in the home, or if the visual impairment has had a recent onset. Adolescents and parents may have difficulty separating problems that are secondary to adolescence from those that result from the impairment. Sexual identity, formed since early childhood, will also be at a crucial stage of development, and parents may need help in recognizing and dealing with this aspect of their growing child. Parents should also encourage activities that promote independent living, such as household chores and handling finances, as well as participation in such recreational activities as sports and youth groups.

COMMUNICATION

A baby is introduced to extrinsic communication on the day of birth. At this time, the family communicates their love and affection through holding and talking to the child. However, because the baby with a visual impairment does not see the pleasure or concern on the parents' faces, the parents must express many of these feelings and thoughts verbally.

As they grow older, children with visual impairments learn to discriminate not only words, but intonations. Yet they are still not privy to many nonverbal cues, such as frowns or puzzled looks. Hence, a simple touch or hug can often reassure a child.

To help increase a child's auditory skills, the family should present a multitude and variety of sounds from early on. Toys that have sound characteristics are good for this purpose, since they help the young child identify a cause-and-relationship effect between sounds and objects. In addition, parents can move the child about the environment at frequent intervals each day so that the child can be exposed to a changing repertoire. Through their frequent verbalizations from near or far, parents can explain how the blender makes this sound, the electric shaver that one, wind chimes this one, and so on. However, warn parents not to use the television or radio indiscriminately, as babies quickly learn to ignore most or all other sounds because the TV or radio sounds they hear so frequently have become nonpurposeful.

Once a diagnosis of a visual impairment has been made, family members almost automatically begin to describe the environment in detail to help compensate for the child's lack of visual input. However, some families may need assistance in describing things concretely and explicitly. Remind parents to use consistent terms for persons and objects and that it is helpful to build a child's vocabulary in the early stages with words of familiar persons and objects, such as body parts, furniture, types of food, and names of toys. Nevertheless, parents should not be uncomfortable in using such phrases as "The grass is so green," or "You have pretty blue eyes," or "Look at that big truck," even though the child may not be able to perceive color or to see the truck.

Storybook records or cassettes and albums of children's songs and music are also quite helpful in expanding a child's language skills. These are available commercially or through the free Library of Congress Talking Book Program.

In general, children who are visually impaired but have no other disabilities develop language skills at the same pace as sighted children but may fall behind in their vocabulary at 2 years or so. Some tend to verbalize less in their infancy and to spend more time in the *echolalic,* or repetitive, phase.

Children should be encouraged to face each person with whom they are talking directly and appreciate being told when people enter or leave a room and who is present or speaking. In addition, since they cannot see nonverbal cues, others can help by explaining significant cues of this sort, such as laughter at a sibling who is acting funny. Finally, occasionally other persons must be reminded that a person with a visual impairment is not deaf or delayed and appreciates being spoken to, rather than spoken about, in a normal tone of voice.

LOW-VISION AIDS

Although the vast majority of persons with visual impairments have some functional residual vision, the use of low-vision aids did not become generally accepted until about 1950. At that time, researchers recognized that the use of one's remaining vision would not result in any additional loss but would only lead to occasional eye fatigue.

Today's low-vision devices are all intended to increase visual efficiency and are based on either object or image classification. *Object magnification* is the enlargement of an object (for example, large print) so that it occupies more space on the retina for processing. In *image magnification,* the object is not altered, but its appearance on the retina is enlarged. Magnifiers, telescopes, and the *approach method* (moving an object closer) are examples of image magnification.

Additional factors affecting low-vision devices include proper lighting with minimal glare (increased lighting does not necessarily benefit all patients) and contrast (increased contrast provides better visibility).

Low-vision aids can be divided into three main categories. The category and type of aid that provide the best vision and function vary from patient to patient. In general, the less conspicuous and the less expensive an aid, the more likely it will be used. Additional compliance factors include whether patients have accepted their low vision and whether they want to improve it with a low-vision aid.

The first low-vision aid category includes the nonoptical aids, such as the approach method and large-print books. Children with low vision should use the approach system whenever possible, that is, hold their books or toys at whatever distance they find most functional. Large-print books are normally printed in type twice the size of regular newspaper print and therefore usually benefit children with mild visual losses. The books are specifically produced to increase contrast and to decrease glare. (Magnification by photocopying does not normally offer these features.) The negative aspects of large-print books include the difficulty in obtaining them, their cost to print, and their bulkiness.

These books begin to benefit many appropriate children around third or fourth grade, since the print in school books tends to decrease in size around that time. In addition, many children with low vision are identified at that age when their reading skills decrease suddenly as the result of the change in text print size.

Large-print books can be obtained from a number of agencies, including the American Printing House for the Blind and the National Association for the Visually Handicapped. Students in elementary and secondary schools should also contact the Superintendent of Special Education in their school district or state to obtain appropriate texts. The R. R. Bowker Company is the largest commercial producer of large-print books.

Large-print calendars, phone dials, dictionaries, playing cards, watches, and calculators are some of the other everyday nonoptical items that can be found in large department stores. In addition, retail store catalogs offer lamps to decrease glare, and these are especially helpful for children with photophobia. Felt-tipped pens can also provide increased visibility, and various pinhole or slit devices can likewise decrease glare and increase visibility. Finally, although tape recorders, canes, and seeing-eye dogs are assists for those persons who are blind rather than those with low vision, they, too, are nonoptical aids.

The second major category of low-vision aids includes the optical ones, such as magnifiers and telescopes. Magnifiers can be hand-held or head-bound to allow for variability in focusing; they are also available on stands or paperweights for fixed focusing. The stronger the magnification provided, the smaller the field that can be viewed at any one time.

Although many magnifiers are available from commercial stores and are initially less expensive, it is often more cost-effective and beneficial in the long run for patients to consult a low-vision specialist for recommendations. The National Association for the Visually Handicapped offers a free listing of low-vision specialists in one's local area or state as part of their low-vision packet, and these specialists can advise a patient about all types of low-vision equipment. In addition, Lighthouse Industries of the New York Association for the Blind provides a comprehensive catalog of magnifiers and other low-vision equipment.

Nightscopes have wide-angle features in addition to their increased lighting mechanisms, to assist the patient who has limited dim light and peripheral vision. Patients with retinitis pigmentosa are one group of patients who benefit from this type of aid.

Telescopes are the only currently available means of allowing persons with low vision to improve their distant vision. They can also be hand-held or mounted on spectacles or a headband and may be monocular or binocular. Normally, the field viewed through a telescope is quite small. The classic one developed by Galileo is still the most commonly used today and costs $200.00 to $1200.00, depending upon variations. Younger children often prefer the hand-held telescopes, as they can magnify six to eight times and are less threatening to a child's self-image than those mounted on spectacles.

Many low-vision specialists feel that the earlier a child receives a low-vision aid, the greater is the likelihood of the child's using it. To provide role modeling, the National Association for the Visually Handicapped has produced four small books about children in the elementary school years who use low-vision aids. *Monocular Mac* focuses on a boy who uses a monocular telescope both at home and at school to help him see better. *Cathy* is about a young girl who has low vision secondary to cataracts; *Larry* is about a boy who has low vision secondary to albinism; *Susan* is the story of a sighted girl who is new in school and doesn't want to be friends with a popular classmate who has low vision. Each book costs about $1.00, and all discuss sensitive issues about children with low vision and the responses of their sighted peers and families in a pleasant and entertaining manner.

The third category of low-vision aids includes the closed-circuit machines. For example, the Voyager by Visualtek of Santa Monica, California, has a portable TV screen and a camera with a zoom lens. It can magnify normal print up to 45 times and can also assist a student in writing. Although aids in this category are quite expensive ($1000.00–$3000.00), patients with significant visual losses can often utilize normal reading materials with their use.

BRAILLE

Braille is a tactile method of transcribing letters, punctuation, abbreviations, numbers, and musical and scientific notations. It was developed in the nineteenth century by Louis Braille, who was blinded at an early age, as a response to his desire to read.

Each notation (letter, number, and so on) is a variation of six raised dots, based upon a "cell" two columns wide (⁞⁞) For example, the following dots, if they were raised, would spell the word *nurse*.

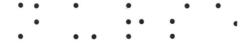

Braille is now only taught to persons who have no useful vision. It takes about 1–2 years to become proficient in reading it, and elementary school students are placed in various levels of braille classes, depending upon their proficiency. They also learn to use a special typewriter to type it, and a slate and stylus are available for manual note taking.

Books printed in braille are quite large and bulky. In addition, braille reading can be laborious, and it takes even the most proficient reader twice as long to read a given passage as a sighted person who is reading the same passage from print. Furthermore, many materials are not available in braille. (Hence, the Library of Congress, through its Talking Book Programs, provides free rental of cassettes or records.) The parents of a child who is learning braille should themselves learn to visually read it, so that they can help the child with vocabulary and assignments. And children who type in braille should also learn to use a regular typewriter so that teachers and others can read their notes.

The American Printing House for the Blind and the Howe Press of the Perkins School for the Blind carry a wide variety of equipment needed by persons who write or read in braille. (When finances are a problem, the Lions Clubs can often assist with the purchase of such equipment.) In addition, the Howe Press sells a number of illustrated children's printed books with braille overtype, so that both sighted persons and those with visual impairments can enjoy reading them together. The American Brotherhood for the Blind also carries such "twin books" for persons of all ages, and the American Printing House for the Blind and the National Braille Association carry a large assortment of books printed in braille only, including textbooks. Finally, the American Foundation for the Blind has a large assortment of household items (clocks, watches, phone dials, oven dials, and so on) with braille imprints.

GROSS MOTOR DEVELOPMENT

The gross motor development of children with serious visual impairments has given developmental specialists some of the most interesting data to date on the gross motor development of all children. It has now been well established that children with visual impairments are delayed in some, but not all, gross motor tasks; therefore, those they are delayed in must normally benefit from visual input.[1]

For example, infants with visual impairments develop head control when placed in a position that necessitates it, such as lying over their parent's shoulder or sitting in someone's lap. However, they do not use this head control or develop associated trunk and arm control when placed in a prone position until about the age of 10 months, when ear–object association begins to develop. In contrast, sighted children develop these skills at a quite early age, because of the visual benefits of looking around. Some specialists postulate that children with visual impairments do not care for the prone position at all but should be taught to tolerate it.[2]

Children with visual impairments roll over at the same age that sighted children do. They also sit and bridge (that is, get up on their hands and knees) at the same ages. Nevertheless, parents should encourage the development of these skills by frequently propping the child in a sitting position, sitting the child on their lap, and frequently changing the child's position during the day.

In contrast, children with visual impairments do not go from lying to sitting or sitting to standing until several months later than sighted children. Again, they are more likely to accomplish these tasks once they learn to discriminate auditory cues.

Many children with visual impairments have a very short crawling period (or no crawling period at all) but a longer *cruising* (standing while holding onto furniture) period. Their average age for walking independently is 18–24 months, versus 12–16 for sighted children. In addition, children with visual impairments may have an abnormal gait caused by their instability in walking, and many have an inherent hesitancy to walk. You may also note that some hold their head in a forward position, about 30 degrees, to provide maximal input into the vestibular canals.

Parents need much encouragement as their child develops mobility skills, so that they do not become overly protective. For example, the parents must learn to refrain from anxious comments when the child bumps into furniture or falls over items. And although the family should keep doors closed and furniture and toys in a consistent location, they should not clear out rooms to provide the child a "bump-free" environment. If parents have older children, they should recall the times that these children were learning to walk and provide the child with a visual impairment the same opportunities for exploration. (As children with visual impairments improve in their walking skills, they will often "trail" a wall with their hand as they walk along it.) To assist toddlers in developing balance and spatial awareness, encourage families to let the child use swings, rocking horses, tricycles, wagons, wheelbarrows, pools, and other general playground equipment as often as possible.

Orientation and *mobility training* are the terms used to describe the teaching of older children with visual impairments how to get around in unfamiliar locations. If a child has some residual vision, a low-vision device such as a monocular telescope may be useful. Older children with no useful vision may benefit from cane training, a dog (not for persons under 16 years of age), or the more recently developed ultrasonic devices that provide feedback about the distance between the child and nearby objects. (Some persons can actually determine this information themselves, without any assistive devices.)

If you work with children who have recently become seriously visually impaired or who are temporarily impaired secondary to double patching, keep the following points in mind. When walking with them, have them take hold of your arm and walk slightly behind you. Go through doors before them in the same manner. If you need to turn around in a limited space, such as in an elevator, come to a stop, drop arms, then turn toward each other, rather than trying to swing the child around. Going up stairs is much easier for persons with visual impairments than descending them, and they may feel more comfortable if someone walks in front of them while going down. In addition, teach children to swing an arm in an arc in front of them when walking along or before they bend over.

FINE MOTOR DEVELOPMENT

Although many persons believe that children with visual impairments have a natural tendency for increased tactile skills and use of their hands, such skills are really learned responses. Therefore, once a diagnosis of a visual impairment is made, parents should encourage their child to develop their tactile skills.

For small infants, this implies providing the child with a wide variety of sensations: stuffed animals, crumbs, water, plastics, grass, leaves, foods, clothes, and so forth. Some children are initially fearful of new tactile sensations, even of the warmest, fuzziest stuffed animal available. Therefore, the more sensations presented early on, the better exposure children will have and the faster they will develop their ability to discriminate.

Once the babies begin reaching with their hands, parents should place small items slightly out of reach to encourage them to move and explore and to develop awareness of *object permanence*. That is, they will learn to realize that just because something is out of touch does not imply that it no longer exists. (Children with visual impairments develop the concept of object permanence after sighted children.)

Infants with a visual impairment also go through the mouthing stage, exploring most items with their mouths as well as their hands. Parents may marvel at the detailed inspection that each item receives and should, of course, select items that are safe for the child's age and skills. And don't let parents forget that the feet are another excellent area for tactile stimulation. Hence, children should go barefoot whenever safe, on carpets, grass, sand, and dirt.

Two main disadvantages for children with severe visual impairments in developing touch and fine motor skills are that they cannot learn by imitation (a pincer grasp, for example) and that they get little, if any visual feedback. For example, they cannot see their parents hit their hands together in "patty-cake," nor can they see themselves bringing their hands together correctly or missing them in mid-air. As they get older, they will receive some feedback from sounds, but even this does not occur until about 8–10 months of age.

FEEDING

The principles for promoting satisfactory feeding skills in a child with a visual impairment are essentially the same as for children without any such impairment. That is, each skill is divided into parts, and one part is pursued at a time. However, parents of children with visual impairments must be more diligent in their efforts, to compensate for those skills that are normally visually reinforced and to overcome the hesitancy and passivity toward eating that have been noted in some children with visual impairments.[3]

Feeding should be associated with human contact as much as possible so that it not only has the additional component of touch but is also recognized at an early age as a social activity. Parents should be advised not to prop bottles or to feed the baby while the child lies in bed (unless the parents are in bed, too—quite possible at 3:00 A.M.!)

Around 2 months of age, bottle-fed babies should have their hands placed on the bottle and gradually be taught how to hold it themselves. Once a baby has learned to sit fairly well around 5–7 months of age, both a cup and finger foods can be introduced. The baby should learn to hold the cup first without any liquid for exploration and then with a small amount of liquid for drinking purposes. Finger foods, crackers and thin potato chips are good starters.

Children with visual impairments tend to be skeptical about new foods, so they should be introduced one at a time at an early age. Parents can also leave foods near children and around the house so that the children will try them when they are exploring. Foods of different substances should also be encouraged and repeatedly given (one at a time) until the child accepts them. Remarks about foods should be on the positive side and the names of each food should be stated at each meal. Foods that require chewing may require even more persistence, and a number of blind children have been known to take only pureed foods at the age of 3 years because the parents were unaware of this point. (Chewing is partly a visually learned skill.) Although it may seem harsh, young children should not be fed between their normally scheduled meals when new foods have been introduced and quickly rejected. The parent must remember that the child is probably not rejecting the new food because of taste but precisely because it is new. (Parents of children who have normal vision go through similar games, to a lesser degree.)

The use of a spoon should be introduced also at an early age. Once the child has developed a good grasp, the parents can place the child's dominant hand on the spoon and, while behind or next to the infant, guide the spoon into the child's mouth. Children with severe visual impairment become independent in the use of a spoon at about 2 years of age, versus sighted children, who learn to use a spoon independently around 16–18 months of age. Using plates with straight sides and allowing the child to use fingers to help push or place the food on the utensil is also helpful.

Needless to say, expect a mess when children (with or without a visual impairment) are learning to feed themselves. Parents should plan for this by placing plastic (or a dog!) under the high chair or occasionally feeding their child outside on days with nice weather. Also remind parents to be patient. Support groups or a parent tree can prove helpful at these times, as can the services of a nurse or educator who specializes in the early childhood development of children with visual impairments.

As children get older and polish these early skills, they will learn to use bread instead of fingers to help push food onto their utensils and to approach their plate by moving their hands first onto the table and then forward to the plate. Those of us who have seen *The Miracle Worker*, the movie about Helen Keller, have dramatically seen the difference that good feeding skills can make in a child's life, and we should encourage all children to develop these skills.

GROOMING

The attainment of a child's independence in grooming skills marks an exciting milestone for both the child and parents. Yet it takes time and patience for any child, whether visually impaired or sighted, to acquire adequate skills in dressing, washing, dental care, hair care, and toileting. Remind parents, therefore, not to try to teach their child any of these skills in a short span of time.

As in teaching feeding skills, a main point in teaching grooming skills is to divide each skill into numerous steps and to teach the simpler ones first. For example, it is easier for a child to undress than dress or to remove socks than pants. This breakdown process may seem complicated at first for the parents, but by verbalizing each step to the child as it is done, they will find the entire skill already broken into steps, and the child will be gradually learning them at the same time.

Successful dressing skills require that a child be able to identify different types of clothing, different fabrics, outside from inside, top from bottom, and color (a social necessity) by various means. A child with a severe visual impairment may complain about wearing hats with ear covers, which can decrease the amount of auditory and vestibular information that the child receives.

The teaching of other skills can also be intertwined with the teaching of self-care skills. For example, children can learn responsibility by putting clothes away on hooks that have been placed within reach. They can learn decision making by choosing what they like to wear. Dressing is also a good time to increase their body awareness and to learn opposites such as left and right and in and out.

Teaching toileting skills to children with serious visual impairments may initially be somewhat tricky, as children must not only be physiologically capable but must also be able to understand what they are supposed to accomplish. Having a footrest so that feet do not dangle and having support for their hands and trunk (for example, by placing the potty in a corner) can also be helpful. Most children with visual impairments become toilet-trained between 2 and 3 years of age. During the training period parents may enjoy reading the pamphlet

Toilet Habits: Suggestions for Training a Child Who is Blind (1980 reprint), produced by the American Foundation for the Blind.

SLEEP

Some children develop a sleep reversal, either shortly after birth or around the age of 2 years. Having a child wide awake at 2:00 A.M. and sound asleep at noon can indeed be difficult for any parent. The successful normalizing of a child's sleeping pattern focuses on the parent creating an environment that is as quiet and dark as possible at night (because many children have light perception) and bright, noisy, and active in the day. Parents should give minimal attention to the child at night when they are assured that the child is safe, adequately fed, and changed. However, some excess attention can be given during the daytime periods while the sleep pattern is reversing toward normal. Some authorities feel that children with a visual impairment also tend to have less need for naps and night sleep. Others, however, dispute this idea.

SCHOOL

As stated earlier, as soon as a visual impairment is identified, parents should receive information about early childhood specialists who are trained in the development of children with visual impairments. These specialists may come to the child's home, or the child may be brought to the specialist at a school or agency. In areas without access to a specialist the parents can contact the Blind Children's Center or the Variety Club Blind Babies Foundation for a correspondence program. In addition, all parents can enroll their child in a nursery or preschool with sighted children at their earliest convenience.

As for elementary and high school, up until the mid-twentieth century children with severe visual impairments were often placed in residential schools. They had no interactions with sighted children and only saw their families on holidays and vacations. But nowadays the situation is much different, especially with the advent of Public Law 94-142 (1977). Basically, this law states that all children are entitled to an appropriate, free public education in the least restrictive environment. Hence, many children with disabilities have now been ''mainstreamed'' into regular school settings. For children with visual impairments, the least restrictive alternative may be a regular school setting with an itinerant teacher who visits the school at regular intervals to assist both the student and the classroom teacher. Or, depending upon the number of visually impaired students in the school, a resource room or special class may be available in a regular school setting to teach the students braille, typing, and spatial orientation or to assist them in other ways to carry out their regular classroom assignments. A more restrictive setting is to have the child attend a special school. (Residential schools now usually specialize in teaching children with multiple handicaps.) In some school districts, these services are available for children when they are 3 years old.

Parents should begin to contact their public school district about 3–9 months before the date of their child's expected enrollment because it will take time to gather appropriate medical records and to determine the child's level of visual and developmental functioning. This is especially true if the school or district has had limited experience with a child who has a visual impairment.

A meeting to formulate the individual education plan (IEP) or program plan (IPP) will be arranged, with specialists in the area of visual impairment, classroom teachers, a psychologist, school nurse, administrators, and the child's parents invited. These meetings must be rescheduled at least annually, so that new goals and objectives can be formulated on the basis of the child's progress and development. If parents do not agree with the selected school setting or plan, they can request a due process hearing.

One significant factor influencing the decision about where to place a child will be the attitude of the anticipated classroom teacher. If they feel overwhelmed or feel that supportive resources will be limited (for example, there is currently a shortage of itinerant teachers credentialed to work with students who are visually impaired) teachers may be disinclined to accept the student, despite what the law mandates. Parents should feel free to provide supportive services in whatever way they can and mention this at the time of the IEP. For example, it is helpful if they can read homework assignments to the child. To assist teachers and other school staff in becoming comfortable with a child with a visual impairment in their class or school, the American Foundation for the Blind offers *Good Start—A Multi-Media Approach to Meeting the Needs of Visually Handicapped Students* ($350.00 purchase price from Phoenix Films, Inc.), and *A Different Way of Seeing* (1983), a pamphlet in letter form to classmates of a child with a visual impairment (single copy free). In addition, the Foundation has made available *When You Have a Visually Handicapped Child in Your Classroom: Suggestions for Teachers* (single copy free), and other materials.

At the IEP, necessary educational aids for the student are recommended. Equipment for children with low vision is described elsewhere in this chapter. Besides braille materials for children with no useful vision, equipment may include tape recorders or cassettes, an Optacon (a fairly new and expensive device from Telesensory Systems Inc. that can make print raised, so that it can be tactually felt by the student), or the free services of Recording for the Blind. The determination of whether the child can read print or has no useful vision is another important factor in deciding which school setting is most appropriate.

Nurses who work in school settings have various opportunities to assist the child with a visual impairment. They may help obtain and interpret medical reports and assess whether the student needs additional medical follow-up (for example, for students with glaucoma or retinal disorders). They may attend IEP meetings, an excellent time to integrate the student's normal development into the plan (for example, by promoting participation in physical education classes). There may also be opportunities for educating or sensitizing sighted peers about the student's visual impairment or for counseling the student in peer relationships and development.

VOCATIONAL ASPECTS

During junior high school, children will need assistance in considering their vocational interests. Students should be encouraged to begin exploring their interests through various classes, work-study experiences, and extracurricular activities.

Usually students with visual impairments are quite realistic about their vocational selections, although some may be negatively influenced by well-meaning but erroneous adults who discourage them from pursuing certain vocational interests because "they are inappropriate for someone who is blind." Persons with serious visual impairments have blazed many trails in vocations previously felt to be inappropriate, and work in such areas as teaching, linguistics, law, physical education, social work, and electrical engineering. Therefore, it is recommended that students explore interests through various means and decide for themselves what is realistic and what is not, in view of their own capabilities and limitations. The popular book *If You Could See What I Hear* by Tom Sullivan is a good overview, written in an autobiographical style, which gives the reader the breadth and depth of a particular blind person's capabilities. Students should also contact their local department of vocational rehabilitation.

REFERENCES

1. Frailberg S: Parallel and divergent patterns in blind and sighted infants. Psychoanalytic Study of the Child 23:264–300, 1968
2. Adelson E, Frailberg S: Gross motor development in infants blind from birth. Child Development 45:114–126, 1974
3. Frailberg S: *Insights From the Blind*. Ann Arbor: Univ. of Michigan Press, 1977

SELECTED BIBLIOGRAPHY

Brown MS: The Gordons needed all the help they could get. Nursing 77 7:40–43, October 1977 (An account of a family with a deaf-blind child)

Ende ML: Three congenitally blind infants and their mothers. Matern Child Nurs J 1:55–65, Spring 1972

Frailberg S: *Insights From the Blind*. Ann Arbor: Univ of Michigan Press, 1977 (About congenitally blind children)

Jan JE, Freeman RD, Scott EP: *Visual Impairment in Children and Adolescents*. New York: Grune & Stratton, 1977

National Association for Visually Handicapped: *Growth and Development of the Partially Seeing Child: Professional Guide*. New York, 1975

National Association for Visually Handicapped: *Low Vision Packet*. New York, 1984

O'Brien R: Education of the child with impaired vision. Pediatr Ann 9:434–440, 1980

Pagon RA: The role of genetic counseling in the prevention of blindness. Sight Sav Rev 49:157–165, winter 1979-1980

Raynor S, Drouillard R: *Get a Wiggle On: A Guide for Helping Visually Impaired Children Grow*. Reston, Virginia: AAHPERD, 1978 (Sequel: *Move It!!!*)

Scheiner AP, Moomaw M: Care of the visually handicapped child. Pediatr Rev 4:74–81, September 1982

Scott EP, Jan JE, Freeman RD: *Can't Your Child See?* Baltimore: University Park Press, 1977

Swallow RM: Fifty assessment instruments commonly used with blind and partially seeing individuals. J Vis Impairment and Blindness 75:65–72, February 1981

Variety Club Blind Babies Foundation: *Information Packet: A Compilation of Materials Addressing the Unique Perspective of Blind and Severely Visually Impaired Young Children*. San Francisco, 1984 (About $10.00)

Wiley L (ed): Traumatic blindness: a flexible approach for helping a blind adolescent. Nursing 79 9:37–41, January 1979

Chapter Fourteen

Dyslexia

T he term *dyslexia* literally means "bad reading." In earlier decades it usually referred to the neurologic sequelae of a stroke or accident in which a patient developed difficulty in reading because of alterations in visual perception. Now dyslexia is also recognized as a learning disability, and this type is often called *developmental* or *primary dyslexia*.

Yet a widely used definition of learning disabilities formulated by the National Advisory Committee on Handicapped Children in the late 1960s clearly states that dyslexia, or any other learning disorder, is *not* "due primarily to visual, hearing or motor handicaps, to mental retardation, emotional disturbance or to environmental disadvantage." Instead, it is assumed that the learning disability is secondary to altered or nonconventional processing of visual or other types of sensory input, or any corresponding motor output. Many authors believe that the altered processing is due to a prenatal, perinatal, or postnatal insult, which often remains unidentified. In addition, because dyslexia and other learning disabilities frequently appear in several generations of the same family, a hereditary tendency is being sought.

Estimates of the incidence of learning disabilities range from 2-20 percent of the general population, and persons with some type of dyslexia are estimated to comprise 2-5 percent of the general population.[1,2] Children with dyslexia may also have other learning disabilities, such as problems with speech, numbers, time, space, laterality, hyperactivity, coordination, balance, attention span, dominance, memory, auditory discrimination, or emotional lability. Although most children have problems in a few of these areas, children with a learning disability tend to have more of these problems, which they do not outgrow.

The incidence of dyslexia is about four times greater in boys than in girls. Such famous persons as Nelson Rockefeller, Leonardo da Vinci, Hans Christian Anderson, Woodrow Wilson, Albert Einstein, and Thomas Edison all had some degree of dyslexia; therefore, the identification of dyslexia in a child does not imply a limited or bleak future.

Yet children with dyslexia who are not identified early may develop numerous psychosocial stresses because of their own or other people's misconception that they are stupid, lazy, or uninterested. Unfortunately, many children who have never been properly identified with dyslexia eventually drop out of school and take low-paying jobs; their continued array of failures despite early efforts to try hard and to please may well have contributed to their later underachievement. Children known to have dyslexia may also be shy, withdrawn, serious, easily frustrated, or silly. Some may have increased complaints of head or stomach aches, and many have altered self-concepts. Their families may place the child in an overprotective or strict environment, may resent the child, or may not fully understand the learning disability. For these reasons, many professionals don't use the label *dyslexia* but instead refer to any processing alterations in descriptive terms, with no overall label.

Diagnosis

Most commonly a child with dyslexia is first noticed because of poor school performance or difficulty in reading. Usually a 1-year discrepancy in reading in children in the first grade or a 2-year discrepancy in older children indicates dyslexia. This operational definition implies an approximate 50 percent minimal difference between the child with dyslexia and the "normal" child for that grade, indicating a vast difference between the performance levels of these two groups and a vast difference between the dyslexic child's potential and achievement levels. (Remember that children with dyslexia usually have average or above-average intelligence.) The classic symptom of letter or word reversal, such as reading or writing *b* for *d*, or *was* for *saw*, is normal in up to one-fourth of first graders. Hence, it is not an exclusive diagnostic clue to the early identification of the child with dyslexia.

Therefore, when a child is suspected of having dyslexia or another learning disability, vision, hearing, and other physical problems must first be ruled out. The medical evaluation should also include a thorough birth, developmental, social, and family history (for example, whether anyone else in the family has a learning disability), as well as a general physical examination and general neurologic assessment. A number of children with learning disabilities have some evidence of "soft signs" in the neurologic assessment. Although this term is ambiguous, it often indicates that no firm neurological abnormality is associated with the finding, and that the finding is often found in many younger children (for example, abnormal pencil grip). A specific assessment by a neurologist is rarely necessary, however. (For further discussion of such signs the reader may wish to refer to the Bibliography for works by Levine, Desmond et al, or Grossman.) Also necessary are psychologic or behavioral, speech, and nutritional assessments. All of these help exclude an obvious physical or environmental explanation for the child's decreased performance and may occasionally provide a clue to the cause of the learning disability. However, minimal effort should be devoted to identifying a cause, since one frequently cannot be determined, and its identification rarely serves any useful purpose.

After these assessments the child receives a Wechsler Intelligence Scale for Children—Revised (WISC—R) or other intelligence test to determine academic potential, followed by reading and math achievement tests. Some of these tests should be given on an individual basis, by a school or other licensed psychologist. In addition, some process tests, such as the Frostig Test of Visual Perception, may also help to identify how a particular child "processes" sensory input.

From this discussion one can see that the identification of dyslexia in a child is a complex process requiring an interdisciplinary approach. During the diagnostic phase nurses frequently perform the developmental, family, social, and nutritional assessments. In addition, nurse practitioners may provide the physical and neurologic assessments. The school nurse often collects the information from other team members and presents it at the individual educational planning meeting.

Treatment

Once a child with dyslexia is identified, an individual educational plan is arranged. (Unfortunately, P.L. 94-142 allows for the remedial education of only 2 percent of the population.) A curriculum is planned around a child's educational strengths and particular patterns of learning and to assist the child in overcoming or dealing with significant weaknesses. This approach requires special teachers who are well-versed in a variety of techniques, for merely giving a child more of the same conventional techniques that have not worked in the past is of no help. Such techniques may include having the child orally repeat selected information many times, trace words with a finger or pen, or use a tape recorder. Adults with dyslexia who are in the position to do so hire a secretary to free themselves from their learning disability. (Remember, many children do not outgrow their dyslexia but merely learn to work around it.)

Often a child with dyslexia will be placed full- or part-time in special classes for the educationally handicapped. However, a common drawback of these classes is that children with emotional problems and developmental disabilities are often placed in the same classes with children with learning disabilities, leading to an altered self-concept for the child with the learning disability and decreased time available with the teacher. Yet when properly done, a 1-year special teaching program can result in a 3-year increase in the child's reading skills. Other sources of educational programs include private or university learning centers and clinics, resource rooms, private schools, and special tutors. (Adolescents with dyslexia can make advance arrangements with the College Entrance Examination Board to have college board tests read to them.)

Another source of treatment is that provided by optometrists in their visual training programs. These methods continue to be a source of great controversy, however. For example, do children have dyslexia because of poor eye teaming, or do they have poor eye teaming because of dyslexia? Is a child responding to a particular treatment modality, or because of the one-to-one method in which it is being taught? In 1972 the American Academy of Pediatrics, along with the American Association of Ophthalmology and several other organizations, produced a statement on the eye and learning disabilities, parts of which read: "Eye care should never be instituted in isolation when a patient has a reading problem" and "studies have shown that there is no peripheral eye defect which produces dyslexia and associated learning disabilities."[3] A more recent statement by these organizations continues to support this, reemphasizing that "no known scientific evidence supports claims for improving the academic abilities of dyslexic or learning-disabled children with treatment on (a) visual training . . . or (b) neurological organizational training . . ."[4] However, to help clarify the role of optometrists in regard to children with learning disabilities, the December 1981 issue of the *Journal of Learning Disabilities* featured "Focus on Optometry."[5]

Finally, a child with a significant learning disability may require the services of a counselor, especially during any crisis periods. Family counseling may also be appropriate for selected cases, and the nurse can often assist with these referrals.

Additional Nursing Interventions

In addition to collecting and coordinating assessments during the diagnostic phase and making referrals to mental health services as needed, the nurse has several other opportunities to assist a child with a learning disability. For example, the nurse can provide information on relevant national organizations, such as the Association for Children with Learning Disabilities (which has numerous local chapters), the Orton Dyslexia Society, and the Learning Disabilities Program of the Bureau of Education for the Handicapped. In addition, the Council for Exceptional Children provides numerous materials on learning disabilities for teachers and other school personnel.

Nurses who work with a number of children with learning disabilities may wish to attend continuing education courses on physical and neurological assessment. Similarly, any nurse who is knowledgeable about children with learning disabilities should share such knowledge through appropriate in-service sessions, particularly for colleagues in school and ambulatory settings.

Another important role for all nurses is to promote the normal growth and development of children with learning disabilities. This includes encouraging these children to develop hobbies and peer activities in which they can experience success and self-confidence. In addition, nurses may need to remind parents to refrain from comparing one child to another and to reinforce each child's strengths while downplaying weaknesses.

Finally, a number of nurses become significant advocates for children with learning disabilities. They can ensure that children's learning disabilities are properly identified and promote the most optimal and least restrictive school settings and resources.

REFERENCES

1. Association for Children with Learning Disabilities. Taking the first step . . . to solving learning problems. Pittsburgh (no date)
2. American Association of Ophthalmology (now consolidated with American Academy of Ophthalmology) Dyslexia. Washington D.C. (now San Francisco), 1979.
3. American Academy of Pediatrics Joint Organizational Statement. The eye and learning disabilities. Pediatrics 49:454–455, 1972
4. Committee on Children with Disabilities of the AAP and Ad Hoc Working Group of the American Association for Pediatric Ophthalmology and Strabismus and American Academy of Ophthalmology: Learning disabilities, dyslexia, and vision. Pediatr 74:150–151, 1984
5. Seiderman AS (ed). Focus on Optometry. J Learning Disabilities 14:564–590, 1981

SELECTED BIBLIOGRAPHY

Desmond MM, Vorderman AL, Fisher ES: Assessment of learning competence during the pediatric examination. Curr Prob Pediatr 8:1–64, June 1978

Forness SR: Diagnosing dyslexia. Am J Dis Child 136:794–799, 1982

Goldberg HK, Schiffman GB, Bender M. *Dyslexia—Interdisciplinary Approaches to Reading Disabilities*. New York: Grune & Stratton, 1983

Grossman HJ: Neurologic assessment and management of learning disorders. Pediatr Ann 7:326–329, May 1978

Heinlein D: The nurse's role in helping to assess learning disabilities in the school setting. J Sch Health 50:15–17, January 1980

Levine MD, Brooks R, Shonkoff JP: *A Pediatric Approach to Learning Disorders*. New York: Wiley, 1980

Levine MD, Meltzer LJ, Busch B, et al: The pediatric early elementary examination: Studies of a neurodevelopmental examination for 7- to 9-year-old children. Pediatrics 71:894–903, 1983

Metzgar RL, Werner DB: Use of visual training for reading disabilities: a review. Pediatr 73: 824-829, 1984

Appendix A

Interpreting Results from Professional Eye Examiners

Perhaps the biggest complaint about professional eye examiners is that they write their notes in a secret code. Many nurses and primary care providers have tried to decipher these notes, only to throw their hands up in despair and call the eye examiner for a verbal explanation. However, if you have become familiar with much of the information in this book (and with the help of Appendix B), you should be able to interpret most notes from professional eye examiners intelligently.

For example, the following is a note made by an ophthalmologist subsequent to an eye examination of a 7-year-old-girl. How do you interpret it?

A $V_{A\overline{sc}} <^{20/25}_{20/20^{-2}}$

B Pupils 5 2+ RL neg MG
        5 2+

C EOMs
      D & N s̄c straight
      D & V full

D Stereo–40 arc sec

E Color–nl

F SLE: L/L WNL
           conj–quiet
           cornea–clear ou
           AC–D & C
           iris WNL

G T_{AP} 16
         14 @1500

H	Dil	1% cyclo ou
I	ret	+ 0.50 sph
		+ 1.00 sph
J	lens/vitr clear	
	DMV WNL, C/D 0.5 ou	

This represents a normal eye examination. Section A states that her distance visual acuity (V_A) without glasses or contact lenses is 20/25 in the right eye and 20/20 in the left eye; the patient misses two figures on the 20/20 line, however, with the left eye. Since no mention of the type of visual acuity test is made, it is assumed (often incorrectly) that letters were used. (Review Chapter 1 if you are unclear about these findings.) No mention of near vision testing is made, and pinhole testing was not necessary since the patient had normal visual acuity for her age.

Section B indicates that both pupils were 5 mm in size, and that on a scale of 0 to 4, they both reacted to light at a 2+ level. In addition, there is no Marcus-Gunn (afferent pupillary defect) present (Chapter 8).

As for the extraocular muscle movements described in Section C, the child's eyes remained straight when she looked at distant stimuli as well as near ones, without the use of any glasses or special lenses. Furthermore, she had full or complete eye muscle movements when her ductions and versions were tested (Chapter 5).

During stereotesting (Chapter 4), the child passed up to and including those stereograms representing 40 seconds of arc. Furthermore, her color vision (Section E) was normal (Chapter 6).

The slit-lamp examination discussed in Section F tells us that the lids, lashes, and the iris were within normal limits. The cornea was clear in both eyes; the anterior chambers also were deep and clear (Chapter 11). The child's intraocular pressure, shown in Section G, was measured with an applanation tonometer and shows that the right eye had 16 mm of pressure and that the left had 14 mm. This test was taken at 3 o'clock in the afternoon (Chapter 7).

The child's eyes were then dilated with 1 percent Cyclogyl (Alcon Laboratories), and after an appropriate waiting time retinoscopy was performed (Sections H and I). The refraction showed the child to be mildly hyperopic in both eyes, with the left eye more hyperopic than the right. These refractive errors were equal in all directions ("spherical"), and hence, no astigmatism was seen (Chapter 3).

Finally, Section J shows that the lens and vitreous are clear, and that the optic disc, macula, and retinal vessels appear within normal limits during the examination of the fundus. In addition, the cup of the optic disc is half the size of the optic disc itself, which can imply glaucoma. However, in view of the child's normal ocular tension, this is considered normal (Chapter 7).

Now look at the following example and try to interpret the findings.

History: 8 yo boy, complaining of ocular redness when reads or watches TV; also complaining of pain at these times; no significant medical or surgical history; no known allergies

A $V_{A\overline{s}c}$ ⟨ $\begin{array}{l}$-20/50$\\$-20/40$\end{array}$ ph 20/30
                              ph 20/25

B   EOMs–appears straight
         full D & V

C   pupils–5 RL $\begin{array}{l}3+\\3+\end{array}$ no MG
            5

D   stereo 5/9 circles + fly

E   SLE: lids–no blepharitis
              conj–no papillae or follicles
              cornea–clear
              A/C–deep, clear
              iris–WNL

F T_A $\begin{array}{l}12\\12\end{array}$

G   Cyclopleged with Neo 2-1/2% and Cyclo 1% × 3
         +1.50 +2.25 ×90 ⟶ 20/25
         +2.00 +1.50 ×90 ⟶ 20/25

H   RTC in 1–2 wks for postcycloplegic refraction

Section A's data base indicates that the child does not have normal visual acuity, with his left eye seeing slightly better than his right. (Remember that the results of the right eye are always written first.) However, when a pinhole occluder is used, the child's acuity is improved, implying that he has a refractive error.

Sections B, C, E, and F are similar to the first case history and are normal findings. The results in Section D refer to the older Titmus stereotests and state that the child correctly selected five of the nine circles on one part of the test, and correctly responded to the Fly Test. These are acceptable responses (refer to Chapter 4).

In Section G we see that the child was given eyedrops to eliminate his ability to accommodate; his eye muscles were paralyzed so that they could not carry out one of their normal functions of helping to refract light rays as they enter the eye. When the paralysis was complete, a refraction examination was performed. The numbers in the left column indicate that the child has hyperopia, as they are preceded by a plus sign. (Results indicating myopia are preceded by a minus sign.) In addition, the figures in columns 2 and 3 indicate that the child has astigmatism. (If the child had hyperopia only, the numbers in columns 2 and 3 would be replaced by the abbreviation "sph.")

Finally, Section H tells us that before the examiner gives a prescription for glasses to the patient, the examiner wishes the child to return and have his refraction checked when the child's accommodative powers are at their maximum and not affected by any eye medications. In this way, the examiner can prescribe the best lenses for the child, allowing for a balance between the new prescriptive lenses and the child's own accommodative powers.

The third example involves a 9-month baby with a history of his eye turning in since the age of 7 months. Other significant past history includes episodes of hypoglycemia at birth secondary to maternal diabetes. The following are significant findings from the baby's first complete eye examination (other findings were noncontributory and are not listed here.)

A	V_A	F & F Fixes	prefers OD, briefly holds with OS, objects to having OD covered
B		EOMs:	ET, variable 20Δ
C		L/L:	broad epicanthus
D		lens:	OD clear OS lamellar opacity with some cortical component

Section A tells us that the baby's right eye sees well, but that the left eye is fixing but not following. This implication of laziness makes one think about amblyopia ("lazy eye") and is further supported by the child's aversion to having his right eye covered (Chapter 4).

Section B tells us that the child has an esotropia, or eye wandering in, of about 20 prism diopters (Chapter 5). Section C contains a note that the child has a broad epicanthus, which is known to cause the appearance of esotropia (see pseudostrabismus in Chapter 5). However, since the examiner specifically notes the broad epicanthus, it can be assumed that the presence of a true esotropia was verified in a more reliable fashion than mere observation.

Finally, we see in section D that the child has a cataract in his left eye, which, together with the esotropia may have contributed to the amblyopia of the left eye. Hence, the initial treatment plan focused on patching the right eye for 8 hours a day to force the left eye to see better (Chapter 10).

Appendix B

A List of Abbreviations Commonly Used in Ophthalmology

A	applanation; also, in the SOAP charting system, assessment
A/C; AC	anterior chamber
Acc	accommodation
AC/A	accommodative convergence–accommodation ratio
AgNO$_3$	silver nitrate
ANA	antinuclear antibody
AO-HRR	American Optical Hardy, Rand & Rittler Color Test
Ap	ocular tension measured by the applanation method
APD	afferent pupillary defect
Appl	ocular tension measured by the applanation method
ARC	abnormal or anomalous retinal correspondence
b.c.	base curve, a measurement of contact lenses
b.i.d.	twice a day
BLL	brows, lids, lashes
B.O.	base-out (referring to a prism)
B.U.	base-up (also referring to a prism)
BW	birth weight

For many abbreviations, upper- or lowercase letters may be used. In addition, the use of periods after each initial varies.

CAB	cellulose acetate butyrate; a polymer from which gas-permeable lenses are made
Cat	cataract
cc	cubic centimeter
c̄c	with correction
C.C.	chief complaint
C/D	cup disc ratio of optic nerve
C.F.	counts fingers
CL	contact lens
CN	cranial nerve
CNS	central nervous system; also, clinical nurse specialist
C.O.	certified orthoptist
COA	certified ophthalmic assistant
c/o	complains of
COMT	certified ophthalmic medical technologist
conj	conjunctiva
C.O.T.	certified ophthalmic technician
D	diopter; also, distance vision; less often, optic disc
D.A.	dark adaptation
D& C	deep and clear (referring to anterior chamber)
D & V	ductions and versions
dc	discontinue; also, discharge
DCR	dacryocystorhinostomy
DD (dd)	disc diameter; also, developmental disability
DDST	Denver Developmental Screening Test
DEST	Denver Eye Screening Test
Dil	dilate
D.M.	diabetes mellitus
DMV	disc, macula, vessels
E	esophoria
E'	esophoria at near

ECCE	extracapsular cataract extraction
EENT	eye, ear, nose, and throat
EKC	epidemic keratoconjunctivitis
ENT	ear, nose, and throat
EOG	electrooculogram
EOMs	extraocular muscles
ERG	electroretinogram
ET	esotropia
ET′	esotropia at near
E(T)	intermittent esotropia
E(T′)	intermittent esotropia at near
EUA	examination under anesthesia
Ext	external
FA	fluorescein angiogram
F.B.	foreign body
F & F	fixes and follows
FH	family history
FM–100	Farnsworth–Munsell 100-Hue Color Vision Test
FTC	full to confrontation; ft-c for foot candle
F₃T	Trifluridine (antiviral ophthalmic ointment)
FTO	full time occlusion
GC	*Neisseria gonorrhoeae*
GCM	good, central, maintained
G.F.	Goldmann visual fields
gtts	drops
$\mathbf{H}\,{}^{-1}_{+4}$	indicates underacting (–) or overacting (+) extraocular muscles of each eye and their location (Fig. 5-2)
HCL	hard contact lens
HEMA	hydroxyethylmethacrylate, a polymer from which soft contact lenses are made
H.M.	hand motions or movements
HOTV	method of screening preschool children for distance vision

HPI	history of present illness
HSV	*Herpes simplex* virus
HT	hypertropia
HW	holds well (regarding the fix and follow test)
ICP	intracranial pressure
IDU	idoxuridine (antiviral ophthalmic ointment)
IEP	individual educational plan
I & D	incision and drainage
IO	inferior oblique muscle
IOL	intraocular lens
IOP	intraocular pressure
IPD	interpupillary distance
IPP	individual program plan
IR	inferior rectus muscle
J	Jaeger near vision test
JRA	juvenile rheumatoid arthritis
K	Krimsky test for strabismus; also, keratometry (corneal) measurements (readings)
L	left, as in LIO, or left inferior oblique muscle
L/D	light/dark ratio
LE	left eye
LL	lower lid; also, lids and lashes
LP	light perception
LR	lateral rectus muscle
M	macula; also, manifest refraction
M.G.	Marcus Gunn (afferent pupillary defect)
mm	millimeter
MR	medial rectus muscle
N	near visual acuity; also, near point vision system
Neo	Neosynephrine
NI	no improvement
NKA	no known allergies

NLD	nasolacrimal duct
NLP	no light perception
nm	nanometer, a measure of light wave frequency
NPC	near point of convergence
NPL	no perception of light
NRC	normal retinal correspondence
NS	Neosynephrine; also, normal saline
NSPB	National Society to Prevent Blindness
O	in the SOAP charting system, objective
OA	overacting extraocular muscle
OD	right eye; also, doctor of optometry
OKN	optokinetic nystagmus
O.N.	optic nerve
ortho	straight
O.S.	left eye
O.T.	ocular tension
OU	both eyes
P	pupil; also pilocarpine; in SOAP charting system, plan
P$_x$	strength of Pilocarpine
P.D.	pupillary distance; also, prism diopter
PE	physical examination; also, physical education
PERRLA	pupils equal, round, and react to light and accommodation
PF	Pred-forte (steroid eyedrops)
PH	pin-hole
PHPV	persistent hyperplastic primary vitreous
PI	phosphate iodine
pl	plano (''plain'' lens containing no correction)
PL	perceives light
PLL	perceives and localizes light
PMMA	polymethylmethacrylate; a polymer from which some hard contact lenses are made
PNERLA	pupils normal (in size and shape), equal and react to light and accommodation

P.P.	nearest point (punctum proximum) at which a person can see clearly; implies total accommodation
P.R.	far point (punctum remotum); that point at which accommodation ceases
PT, PTT	prothrombin time; partial thromboplastin time
q.d.	every day
q.h.	every hour
q.i.d.	four times a day
q.o.d.	every other day
R	right, as in RIO, or right inferior oblique muscle
RA	react to accommodation (referring to pupils)
RB	retinoblastoma
RC	retinal correspondence
RD	retinal detachment
RDE	Random Dot E stereogram
RE	right eye
Ref	refraction
Ret	retinoscopy
RL	react to light (referring to pupils)
RLF	retrolental fibroplasia
r/o	rule out
ROP	retinopathy of prematurity
RP	retinitis pigmentosa
R/R	resect/recess (strabismus surgery)
RTC	return to clinic (refers to follow-up appointment)
Rx	prescription
S	in the SOAP charting system, subjective data base
s̄c	without correction
SCL	soft contact lens
sl	slightly
SLE	slit lamp exam; also, systemic lupus erythematosus
SO	superior oblique muscle

s/p	status post
sph	sphere; indicates no astigmatism
SR	superior rectus muscle
ST	esotropia (rarely used nowadays)
STORCHES	variation of the abbreviation TORCH
STYCAR	Screening Test for Young Children and Retardates, a distance vision screening tool for preschool children
T	tension (intraocular pressure); also, Timolol
T_A or T_{AP}	intraocular pressure measured by the applanation method
TCU	The City University Color Vision Test
T_S	intraocular pressure measured by the Schiotz method
Tx, T_X	treatment; also, the strength of Timolol
t.i.d.	three times a day
TNO	the name of a specific stereo test
TORCH	acronym for a number of organisms that can cross the placenta: toxoplasmosis, rubella, cytomegalovirus, herpes
TRIC	trachoma inclusion conjunctivitis
UA	underacting muscle; less often in ophthalmology, urinalysis
UL	upper lid
URI	upper respiratory infection
V, VA	visual acuity; VA_{cc} indicates the use of corrective lenses; VA_{sc} indicates that no corrective lenses were used during the visual acuity screening
V	vitreous or vessels, depending on context
VEP	visually evoked potential
VER	visually evoked response
VF	visual fields
W	wearing
W4D	Worth four-dot test for suppression
WNL	within normal limits
X	exophoria
X′	exophoria at near

XT	exotropia
X(T)	intermittent exotropia
Δ	prism diopter
+	indicates hyperopia or overacting extraocular muscles
–	indicates myopia or underacting extraocular muscles

Appendix C

List of Agency and Company Addresses

AAHPERD - American Alliance for
Health, Physical Education,
Recreation and Dance
1900 Association Drive
Reston, Virginia 22091

American Academy of Pediatrics
P. O. Box 1034
1801 Hinman Avenue
Evanston, Illinois 60204

American Academy of Ophthalmology
P. O. Box 7424
San Francisco, California 94120-7424

American Brotherhood for the Blind
18440 Oxnard Street
Tarzana, California 91356

American Foundation for the Blind,
Inc.
15 West Sixteenth Street
New York, New York 10011

American Optical Corporation
(now Reichert Scientific Instruments)
Box 123
Buffalo, New York 14240

American Optometric Association
243 North Lindbergh Blvd.
Saint Louis, Missouri 63141

American Printing House for the
Blind, Inc.
1839 Frankfort Avenue
Louisville, Kentucky 40206-0085

American School Health Association
P. O. Box 708
1521 So. Water Street
Kent, Ohio 44240

Arizona Department of Health
Services
Vision Consultant, MCH Bureau
Arizona Children's Hospital
200 North Curry Road
Tempe, Arizona 85281

Association for Children with
Learning Disabilities
4156 Library Road
Pittsburgh, PA 15234

Association for the Education of the
Visually Handicapped (The
Alliance)
206 No. Washington Street
Alexandria, Virginia 22314

Bausch & Lomb, Inc.
P. O. Box 450
Rochester, New York 14602

Agencies may charge extra for the costs of postage and handling.

Beiersdorf, Inc.
P. O. Box 5529
South Norwalk, Connecticut 06856

Blackbird Vision Screening System
P. O. Box 7424
Sacramento, California 95826

Blind Children's Center
4120 Marathon Street
Los Angeles, California 90029

Burroughs Wellcome Co.
3030 Cornwallis Road
Research Triangle Park, North
   Carolina 27709

CooperVision Pharmaceuticals, Inc.
P. O. Box 367, San Germaine
Puerto Rico, 00753, USA

CooperVision Surgical/Systems
   Division
17701 Cowan Avenue
Irvine, California 92713

Corning Medical Optics
MP 21-2
Corning Glass Works
Corning, New York 14831

Council for Exceptional Children
1920 Association Drive
Reston, Virginia 22091-1589

Da-Laur Incorporated
140 Crescent Road
Needham Heights, Massachusetts
   02194

Eye Bank Association of America
6560 Fannin—Level 8
Houston, Texas 77030

Foundation for the Junior Blind
5300 Angeles Vista Boulevard
Los Angeles, California 90043

Good-Lite Company
1540 Hannah Avenue

P. O. Box 26
Forest Park, Illinois 60130

Howe Press
Perkins School for the Blind
175 No. Beacon Street
Watertown, Massachusetts 02172-9982

Infant Stimulation Educ. Association
c/o Dr. Ludington-Hoe
UCLA Center for the Health Services
Factor 5-942
Los Angeles, California 90024

International Institute for Visually
   Impaired, 0-7, Inc.
1975 Rutgers Circle
East Lansing, Michigan 48823

IOLAB Corporation
861 South Village Oaks Drive
Covina, California 91724

Keeler Optical Products, Inc.
456 Parkway
Broomall, Pennsylvania 19008

LADOCA Publishing Foundation
East 51st Avenue and Lincoln Street
Denver, Colorado 80216

Learning Disabilities Program
Bureau of Education for the
   Handicapped
7th and D Streets, SW
Washington, D.C. 20202

Library of Congress
Division for the Blind and Visually
   Handicapped
1291 Taylor Street N.W.
Washington, D.C. 20542

Lighthouse Industries/The New York
   Association for the Blind
36-02 Northern Boulevard
Long Island City, New York 11101

Maryland Society for the Prevention
   of Blindness

1313 West Old Cold Spring Lane
Baltimore, Maryland 21209

Mead Johnson and Company
Evansville, Indiana 47721

Munsell Color of MacBeth
2441 No. Calvert Street
Baltimore, Maryland 21218

National Association for Parents of
the Visually Impaired (NAPVI)
P. O. Box 180806
Austin, Texas 78718

National Association for Deaf-Blind
and Rubella Children
164 Cromwell Lane
Coventry CV4 8AP England

National Association for the Visually
Impaired
305 East 24th Street
New York, New York 10010

or

3201 Balboa Street
San Francisco, California 94121

National Braille Association
422 South Clinton Avenue
Rochester, New York 14620

National Federation of the Blind
1800 Johnson Street
Baltimore, Maryland 21230

National Foundation for Educational
Research
NFER-Nelson Publishing Company
Ltd.
Darville House, 2 Oxford Road East
Windsor, Berkshire SL4 1DF,
England

National Retinitis Pigmentosa
Foundation
8331 Mindale Circle
Baltimore, Maryland 21207

National Society to Prevent Blindness
79 Madison Avenue
New York, New York 10016

NoIR/Recreational Innovations
Company
P. O. Box 159
6155 Pontiac Trail
South Lyon, Michigan 48178

OLo Products, Inc.
P. O. Box 613
Manhasset, New York 11030

Ophthalmix
P. O. Box 92
La Grange, Illinois 60525

The Orton Dyslexia Society
724 York Road
Baltimore, Maryland 21204

Patient Information Library (minimum
order $25.00)
Krames Communications
312 90th Street
Daly City, California 94015-2621

Perkins School for the Blind
(See Howe Press)

Phoenix Films, Inc.
468 Park Avenue South
New York, New York 10016

Pro-tec, Inc.
11108 Northrup Way
P. O. Box 4189
Bellevue, Washington 98004

Psychological Corporation
7500 Old Oak Boulevard
Cleveland, Ohio 44130

Recording for the Blind, Inc.
20 Roszel Road
Princeton, New Jersey 08540

Reichert Scientific Instruments
Box 123
Buffalo, New York 14240

Richmond Products ($20.00 minimum order)
4089 South Rogers Circle, Suite 6
Boca Raton, Florida 33431

R. R. Bowker & Co.
1180 Avenue of the Americas
New York, New York 10036

Stereo Optical Company
3539 North Kenton
Chicago, Illinois 60641

Southern California Society to Prevent Blindness
249 E. Emerson Avenue, F
Orange, California 92665

Telesensory Systems Inc.
455 North Bernardo
P. O. Box 7455
Mountain View, California 94039-7455

Texas Association for Retinitis Pigmentosa
P. O. Box 8388
Corpus Christi, Texas 78412-0388

3M Center—Personal Care Products Division
St. Paul, Minnesota 55144

Titmus
P. O. Box 191
Petersburg, Virginia 23803

Variety Club
Blind Babies Foundation
544 Golden Gate Avenue
San Francisco, California 94102

Visualtek
1620 26th Street
Santa Monica, California 90404

WCO Ophthalmic Instrument Division ($50.00 minimum order)
925 26th Avenue, East
Bradenton, Florida 33508

Wisconsin Optometric Association
5721 Odana Road
Madison, Wisconsin 53719

Appendix D

General Ophthalmological References

Crawford JS, Morin JD (eds): *The Eye In Childhood*. New York, Grune and Stratton, 1983

Duane TD (ed): *Clinical Ophthalmology*, vols 1–6 (rev ed). New York, Harper & Row, 1982

Harley RD: *Pediatric Ophthalmology*, vols 1–2 (ed 2). Philadelphia, Saunders, 1983

Havener WH: *Ocular Pharmacology* (ed 4). St. Louis, Mosby, 1978

National Society to Prevent Blindness: *Understanding Eye Language*, New York, 1977 (40¢ each)

Nelson LB: *Major Problems in Clinical Pediatrics* (Vol. 25). Pediatric Ophthalmology. Philadelphia, Saunders, 1984

Physicians' Desk Reference for Ophthalmologists (ed 12). Oradell, N.J., Medical Economics, 1984

Robb RM: *Ophthalmology for the Pediatric Practitioner*. Boston, Little, Brown, 1981

Rooke FCE, Rothwell PJ, Woodhouse DF: *Ophthalmic Nursing—Its Practice and Management*. New York, Churchill Livingstone, 1980

Saunders WH, Havener WH, Keith CF, et al: *Nursing Care in Eye, Ear, Nose, and Throat Disorders* (ed 4). St. Louis, Mosby, 1979

Smith JF, Nachazel DP: *Ophthalmologic Nursing*. Boston, Little, Brown, 1980

Stein HA, Slatt BJ: *The Ophthalmic Assistant* (ed 4). St. Louis, Mosby, 1982

Index

Page numbers in *italics* indicate illustrations.
Page numbers followed by *t* indicate tables.

TNO stereotest, *85,* 86, 94
Tonic pupil, 169
Tonographs, 189, 223
Tonometry, 187–189
Topical anesthetics, 56–57
Torticollis, 171, 172
Toxocariasis, 155
Toxoplasmosis, 155
Trabecular angle, *183,* 185
Trabecular meshwork, 182, *183*
Trabeculectomy, 192
Trachoma, 236
Transillumination of iris, 245
Trephining, 192
Trial lens/frame, 53
TRIC agent, 235
Trichromatic color vision, 118, 119, 129
Trifluridine, 240
Trisomy, 13, 199
Tritanopia, 120, 128
Tropia, 101, 107. *See also* Esotropia, Exotropia
Tropicamide, 54, 56, 147
Tucking, 112
Tumors, 105, 149–152, 169, 180
Tunnel vision, 153, 185
Type I, II, and III color deficits, 117–118*t,* 121
Tyrosinase, 245

Ulcers, corneal, 241
Ultrasonic devices for the visually impaired, 286
Ultrasound, 142–143, 149
Ultraviolet burns, 252–253
Ultraviolet rays, 268
Urea, 191
Usher's syndrome, 153
Uveal tract, 155, 243
Uveitis, 155, 244

Vagus nerve, 111
Varicella, 235, 241, 244
Variety Club's Blind Babies Foundation, 278, 290, 293
Vasoproliferation, 144, 156
Vergence, 48–49, 101
Vernal conjunctivitis, 236–237
Versions, 97, 107–*108,* 299–301
Vessels retinal, *138,* 139, 144, 156
Vidarabine, (VIRA-A) 240
Visceral larva migrans, 155
Visual acuity
   amblyopia, 79*t,* 83–84
   cataracts, 197, 200, 201
   color vision deficits and, 120, 121
   definition of, 2

external eye problems and, 210, 214*t*
first aid and, 250–251
formal determination of, 2
glaucoma and, 186
of infants, 22
in neuroophthalmology, 167
of preschool and school-aged children, 18
in retinal disorders, 140
and strabismus, 97
versus visual efficiency, 273
Visual acuity screening, 1–41
   appropriate tests for various groups of children, 8*t*–9*t*
   borderline results, 36
   criteria for passing, 18
   equipment, suggested, 11–13*t*
   example of notation, 16, 299–302
   failure in, 18–21
   follow-up, 21
   glasses, children with, 6, 16–17
   guidelines, 6–21
   in home, 10
   implications, 1–2
   of infants and toddlers, 8*t*–9*t*, 22–30, 181
   machines for, 13*t,* 37
   preparing the child for, 10*t,* 12
   of preschool and school-aged children, 8*t*–9*t*, 30–37
   recording findings, 16–17
   referrals, 18–21
   reliability of tests, 10
   results, 15, 17
   value of, 2
   volunteers for, 5
   who to screen, 6
   See also Allen cards, Blackbird Vision Screening System, Denver Eye Screening Test, E Test, Fixation Test, STYCAR, Sjögren's Hand, Landolt Rings, Letter charts, H:O:T:V Test, Near tests
Visual angle, 2, 17
Visual axis, 2, 95
Visual cortex, 2
Visual efficiency, versus visual acuity, 273
Visual evoked potential/response, 180–181, 201
Visual exercises, 103, 110, 296–297
Visual fields, 2, 168*t, 173,* 177–180
   and color vision, 121
   and glaucoma, 185, 186
   and optic nerve disorders, 173–174
   and retinal disorders, 143
Visual impairment, 272–292
   attachment between parent and child, 273, 276–278, 279